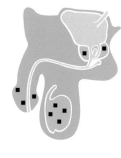

ATLAS OF SURGICAL PATHOLOGY OF THE MALE REPRODUCTIVE TRACT

ATLASES IN
DIAGNOSTIC SURGICAL PATHOLOGY

Consulting Editor

Gerald M. Bordin, M.D.
Department of Pathology
Scripps Clinic and Research Foundation

Published:

Wold, McLeod, Sim, and Unni:
ATLAS OF ORTHOPEDIC PATHOLOGY

Colby, Lombard, Yousem, and Kitaichi:
ATLAS OF PULMONARY SURGICAL PATHOLOGY

Kanel and Korula:
ATLAS OF LIVER PATHOLOGY

Owen and Kelly:
ATLAS OF GASTROINTESTINAL PATHOLOGY

Virmani:
ATLAS OF CARDIOVASCULAR PATHOLOGY

Wenig:
ATLAS OF HEAD AND NECK PATHOLOGY

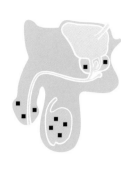

ATLAS OF SURGICAL PATHOLOGY OF THE MALE REPRODUCTIVE TRACT

Jae Y. Ro, M.D., Ph.D.
Professor of Pathology
The University of Texas
    M.D. Anderson Cancer
    Center
Houston, Texas

Mahul B. Amin, M.D.
Senior Staff
Department of Pathology and
    The Bone and Joint Center
Henry Ford Hospital
Detroit, Michigan
Assistant Professor of Pathology
Case Western Reserve University
    School of Medicine
Cleveland, Ohio

David J. Grignon, M.D.
Associate Professor
Department of Pathology
Wayne State University
Harper Hospital
Detroit, Michigan

Alberto Ayala, M.D.
Professor of Pathology
The University of Texas
    M.D. Anderson Cancer Center
Houston, Texas

W.B. SAUNDERS COMPANY
A Division of Harcourt Brace & Company
Philadelphia ■ London ■ Toronto ■ Montreal ■ Sydney ■ Tokyo

W.B. SAUNDERS COMPANY

A Division of Harcourt Brace & Company

The Curtis Center
Independence Square West
Philadelphia, Pennsylvania 19106

Library of Congress Cataloging-in-Publication Data

Atlas of surgical pathology of the male reproductive tract / Jae Y. Ro . . . [et al.]. —
1st ed.

p.   cm.

ISBN 0–7216–5284–0

1.   Generative organs, Male—Histopathology—Atlases.   2. Pathology, Surgical—
Atlases. 3. Generative organs, Male—Surgery—Atlases.   I. Ro, Jae Y.
[DNLM: 1. Genitalia, Male—pathology—atlases. 2. Genitalia, Male—
surgery—atlases. 3. Genital Diseases, Male—surgery—atlases. 4. Genital
Diseases, Male—pathology—atlases.
WJ 17   A88173 1997]

RD586.A85   1997   616.6′507—dc20

DNLM/DLC   96–6969

ATLAS OF SURGICAL PATHOLOGY OF
THE MALE REPRODUCTIVE TRACT   ISBN 0–7216–5284–0

Printed in the United States of America

Last digit is the print number: 9   8   7   6   5   4   3   2   1

To our families—

For my wife, Jungsil, and son, Bobby

JAE Y. RO

For my wife, Laurie, and sons, Robert and Mark

DAVID J. GRIGNON

For my wife Ushma, children, Anmol and Aneri, and father, Dr. B.N. Amin

MAHUL B. AMIN

For my wife, Mary, and children, Tom, Al Jr., and Maria

ALBERTO AYALA

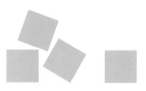

PREFACE

The last one or two decades have witnessed dramatic changes in the understanding and management of neoplasia of the organs of the male reproductive system, notably the prostate and the testis. Prostate carcinoma is now the most common noncutaneous malignancy and is second only to lung cancer in mortality among all cancers. The advent of serum prostate specific antigen (PSA) as a screening technique and the development of transrectal ultrasonography, which not only permits visualization of the prostate but also accurately allows for placement of the needle in areas of suspected lesions or in different zones of the prostate, has contributed to detection of increased numbers of localized cancer lesions, often among younger men. Breathtaking events have also taken place at the forefront of treatment for testicular neoplasia, which inexplicably is on the increase and affects men in their prime. Development of successful chemotherapy protocols aided by the availability of serum biomarkers to monitor this disease has led to the possibility of cure for more than 90% of these patients, particularly those with early-stage disease.

Advances on the clinical front have a direct impact on pathology practice. With regard to the prostate, surgical pathologists are faced with increased numbers of needle biopsies; this is attributable to PSA screening and to the automatic spring-driven 18-gauge needle core biopsy gun, which permits relatively easier sampling of greater portions of the prostate gland with minimal complications. The pathologist also plays an important role in evaluating and staging prostate cancer in prostatectomy specimens. Finally, alternative modalities to therapy, for prostate cancer with or without adjuvant surgery, including androgen-deprivation therapy, laser surgery, and cryosurgery have and will further change the nature of surgical pathology material, posing further challenges for pathologists. Regarding testicular neoplasia, pathologists play a vital role in triaging further therapy based on the classification of germ cell neoplasms into seminomatous or non-seminomatous germ cell tumors. Keeping abreast of events and developments continues to influence our practice and to require us to constantly update our diagnostic base.

The *Atlas of Surgical Pathology of the Male Reproductive Tract* is intended to serve two important roles: (1) to be a user-friendly and handy resource for easy reference for practitioners of routine surgical pathology, and (2) to provide a fundamental yet relatively comprehensive overview of the subject using numerous illustrations and abbreviated, yet succinct, text. We hope the latter function serves and complements the training of pathology and urology residents. We have also placed emphasis on the gross dissection and sampling technique in the prostate and the testis sections, as this is critical for optimal pathologic evaluation. The penis and scrotum section is the shortest among the three sections of the atlas. In this section we concentrate on lesions that are more commonly encountered in daily surgical pathology. Sexually transmitted diseases are included, but only seminal features are highlighted. Because tumors and tumorous conditions form the overwhelming majority of cases encountered routinely in testicular pathology, our focus of presentation in the testis section is restricted to the tumors and tumorous conditions of the testis and paratestis. Testicular biopsies for infertility are performed fairly infrequently, chiefly in specialized centers. Their interpretation requires excellent correlation with the clinical and laboratory findings; therefore, coverage of this topic is beyond the scope of this atlas. Finally, in the prostate section we have assigned a Gleason's grade (when applicable) to illustrations of adenocarcinoma. Grading is a powerful tool, but an exercise that, unfortunately, has been inaccurately performed. We hope to aid and enhance diagnostic skills by illustrating many of the myriad of patterns of prostate cancer.

In conclusion, we are delighted to offer this *Atlas of Surgical Pathology of the Male Reproductive Tract* and sincerely hope that it is not only a valuable source of information and visual impressions, but also an easy and reliable reference on urologic pathology.

Jae Y. Ro
David J. Grignon
Mahul B. Amin
Alberto Ayala

CONTENTS

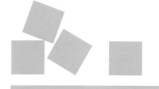

THE PROSTATE

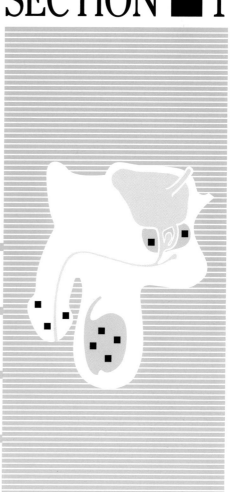

CHAPTER 1

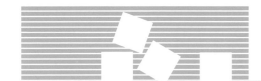

Normal Anatomy and Histology of the Prostate and Handling of Surgical Specimens

■ Anatomy

- Retroperitoneal organ located between the urinary bladder and the pelvic diaphragm.
- Rectum is posterior.
- Pubic bone is anterior.
- Urethra passes through the gland; it is divided into two halves: the proximal and distal.
- Sharp 35-degree anterior angle at midpoint (base of verumontanum).
- Verumontanum is a bulge along the posterior aspect of the urethra in the proximal one half of the distal urethra.
- Ejaculatory ducts, central and transition zone prostatic ducts empty into the urethra around the verumontanum.
- Peripheral zone ducts empty bilaterally and posteriorly on the distal one half of the urethra.
- Historically, divided into lateral, posterior, and median lobes.
- Currently the prostate gland is thought of as consisting of three zones: peripheral, central, and transition.
- Peripheral zone makes up 70% of normal prostate; consists of the apex and extends posteriorly to the base along the ejaculatory ducts, enveloping the transition and central zones.
- About 80% of prostate cancers originate in the peripheral zone.
- Transition zone makes up 5% of normal prostate; consists of two pear-shaped lobes located lateral to the proximal one half of the urethra, extending to the bladder base.
- Nodular (benign) prostatic hyperplasia (BPH) arises in the transition zone. When this process occurs, the transition zone may make up the bulk of the gland.
- Approximately 10% to 20% of prostate cancers arise in the transition zone.
- Central zone makes up 25% of normal prostate; is cone-shaped beginning around the angle of the urethra and extending along the ejaculatory ducts to the bladder base;

approximately 5% of prostate cancers arise in the central zone.
- The so-called prostatic capsule is an incomplete structure best defined along the posterior surface and the posterior one half of the lateral borders.
- Along the lateral sides of the gland, fibrous septa traverse the periprostatic fat and merge with the fibromuscular stroma of the prostate gland.
- Anteriorly, the stroma of the prostate merges imperceptibly with the fibromuscular tissue of the pelvic musculature forming the anterior fibromuscular stroma of the gland.
- Normal prostatic glands can be found within skeletal muscle at the apex, anteriorly, and in the distal posterolateral region.
- The nerve and blood supplies of the prostate originate in the neurovascular bundles which extend along the posterolateral aspect of the gland in the periprostatic adipose tissue.
- The major nerves and blood vessels enter near the bladder base and extend downward within the prostate substance.

■ Histology

- Prostate is composed of tubuloalveolar glands embedded in a fibromuscular stroma.
- Ducts and acini are lined by a double cell layer: a basal and a secretory cell layer.
- Tall columnar secretory cells line the luminal space. These cells produce prostate-specific antigen (PSA) and prostatic acid phosphatase (PAP).
- Lipofuscin pigment can be found in normal prostatic epithelium.
- Flattened basal cells, oriented parallel to the basement membrane, sit between the secretory cells and the basal lamina. They do not produce PSA or PAP.
- Basal cells in the normal prostate are not myoepithelial

cells and have been proposed by some to represent reserve cells.
- Neuroendocrine cells, which communicate with the lumen and have long dendritic processes, are present and scattered in normal epithelium.
- The proximal 1 to 2 mm of the ducts is lined by transitional epithelium.
- Ducts and acini of the peripheral and transition zones are similar in makeup and are simple, small, and rounded.
- Central zone ducts and acini are larger and more irregular in contour. The glands are complex with intraluminal ridges and papillary infoldings.
- The peripheral zone has a loose fibromuscular stroma.
- The transition zone has more compact fascicles of smooth muscle.
- In the central zone the stroma is dense, compact, smooth muscle.
- Paraganglia, appearing as small clusters or nests of cells with clear or eosinophilic cytoplasm arranged in "zell-ballen," can be found within the prostatic stroma or, more frequently, in the periprostatic soft tissues.
- The ejaculatory ducts are lined by a double or pseudostratified cell layer; large, hyperchromatic nuclei may be present. The presence of golden-brown pigment (lipofuscin) aids in its identification.

- Seminal vesicle epithelium also is double-layered, and large, bizarre (monstrous) nuclei can be seen; intranuclear inclusions may be seen; lipofuscin pigment is characteristically present.

References

Ayala AG, Ro JY, Babaian R, et al. The prostatic capsule: Does it exist? Its importance in the staging and treatment of prostatic carcinoma. Am J Surg Pathol 13:21–27, 1989.

Brennick JB, O'Connell JX, Dickersin GR, et al. Lipofuscin pigmentation (so-called "melanosis") of the prostate. Am J Surg Pathol 18:446–454, 1994.

Carstens PHB. Perineural glands in normal and hyperplastic prostates. J Urol 123:686–688, 1980.

Kuo T, Gomez LG. Monstrous epithelial cells in human epididymis and seminal vesicles: A pseudomalignant change. Am J Surg Pathol 5:483–490, 1981.

McNeal JE, Stamey TA, Hodge KK. The prostate gland: Morphology, pathology, ultrasound anatomy. Monogr Urol 9:36–54, 1988.

Ostrowski ML, Wheeler TM. Paraganglia of the prostate: Location, frequency, and differentiation from adenocarcinoma. Am J Surg Pathol 18:412–420, 1994.

Srigley JR, Dardick I, Hartwick RWJ, et al. Basal epithelial cells of human prostate gland are not myoepithelial cells: A comparative immunohisto-chemical and ultrastructural study with the human salivary gland. Am J Pathol 136:957–966, 1990.

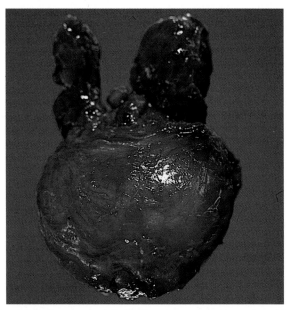

Figure 1–1. Prostate gland. Radical prostatectomy specimen viewed from the anterior aspect, with the apex (*A*), bladder base (*B*), and seminal vesicles (*SV*) visible.

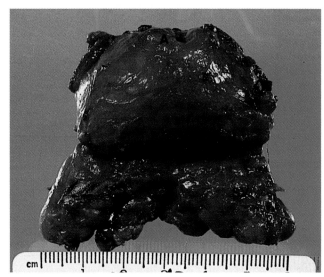

Figure 1–2. Prostate gland. Prostatectomy specimen viewed from the posterior aspect. Note the smooth posterior surface with an intact thin fibrous connective tissue covering (*A*, apex; *SV*, seminal vesicles).

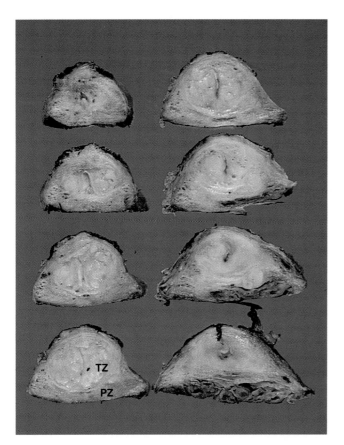

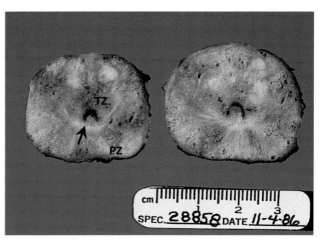

Figure 1–4. Prostate gland. Cross sections through the region of the verumontanum highlighting the fibrous band or so-called surgical capsule (*arrow*) which separates the transition zone (*TZ*) from the peripheral zone (*PZ*).

Figure 1–3. Prostate gland. Serial cross sections beginning at the apical end (*upper left*) and extending to the bladder base (*lower right*). Note the demarcation of the transition zone (*TZ*) from the peripheral zone (*PZ*).

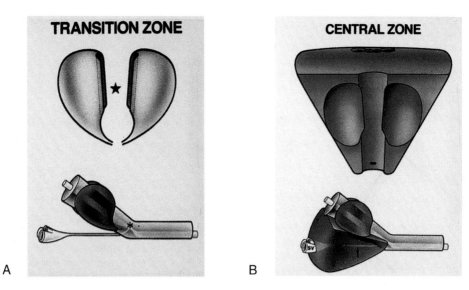

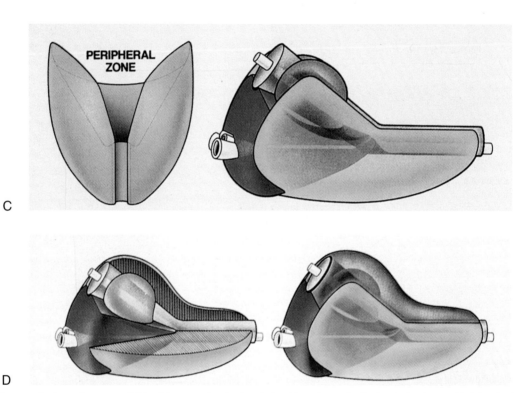

Figure 1–5. Prostate gland, zonal anatomy. *A*, Transition zone showing its relationship to the urethra in the proximal one half of the gland. *B*, Central zone, demonstrating its relationship to the urethra and ejaculatory ducts. *C*, Peripheral zone, with its relationship to the urethra, transition zone, and central zone. *D*, Depiction of all three zones with the anterior fibromuscular stroma depicted. *Blue*, transition zone; *red*, central zone; *yellow*, peripheral zone; *green*, anterior fibromuscular stroma. (From Lee F, Torp-Pedersen ST, Siders DB, et al. Transrectal ultrasound in the diagnosis and staging of prostate cancer. Radiology 170:610, 611, 1989.)

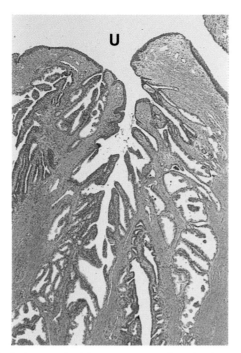

Figure 1–6. Prostate gland. Verumontanum region with ejaculatory duct, prostatic duct, and acini entering into the urethra (*U*).

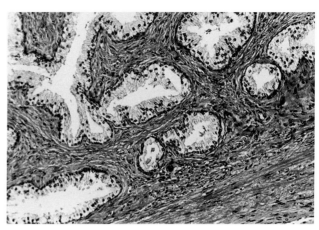

Figure 1–7. Prostate gland. Distal duct with associated acini. Note that the distal duct and acini have an identical double cell layer lining with tall columnar secretory cells and basal cells having minimal cytoplasm.

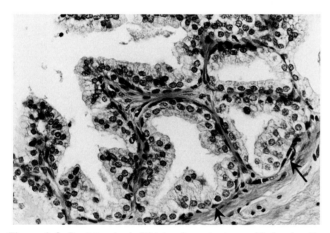

Figure 1–8. Prostate gland. Distal acinar structure with basal cells (*arrows*) and tall columnar secretory cells.

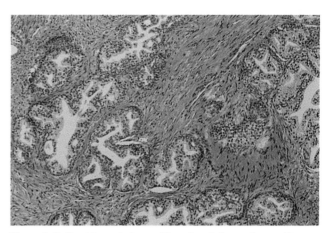

Figure 1–9. Prostate, central zone. Normal central zone tissue with complex, irregularly shaped glands and dense fibromuscular stroma.

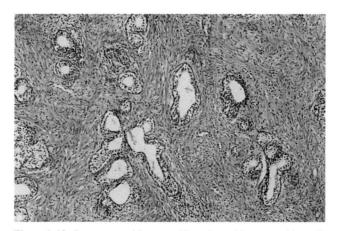

Figure 1–10. Prostate, transition zone. Normal transition zone with small, more uniform glands and a less dense fibromuscular stroma than in the central zone. Note that this pattern is almost never seen in pathologic material, as hyperplastic changes begin very early at a microscopic level.

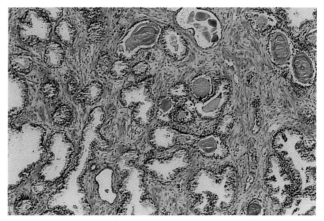

Figure 1–11. Prostate, peripheral zone. Normal peripheral zone tissue with ducts and acini. The glands are more complex in shape than in the transition zone but less so than in the central zone. The stroma is looser and the smooth muscle bundles are more widely separated.

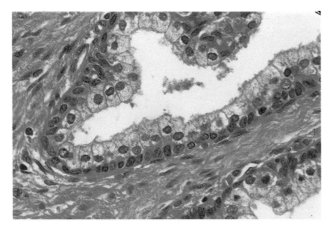

Figure 1–12. Prostate, normal histology. Normal prostatic acini with clearly visible basal cells. The basal cells have scant cytoplasm and round to slightly elongated nuclei compressed between the secretory cell layer and the basal lamina.

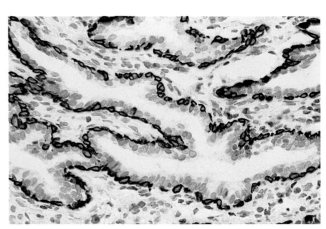

Figure 1–13. Prostate, normal histology. Immunohistochemical stain for high-molecular-weight cytokeratin showing the complete basal cell layer around the ducts and acini. Note the complete absence of immunoreactivity in the secretory cells, a useful diagnostic feature of this antibody.

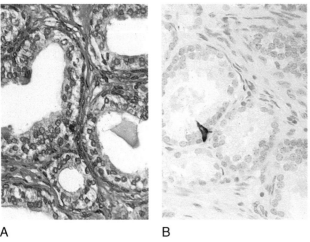

A   B

Figure 1–14. Prostate, normal histology. Normal prostatic glandular tissue (*A*). Immunohistochemical stain for chromogranin (*B*) showing a single pyramidal neuroendocrine cell within one of the acini.

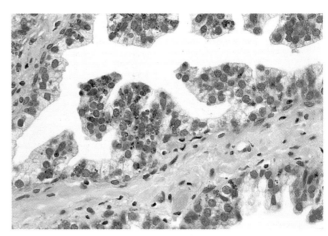

Figure 1–15. Prostate, normal histology. Prostatic epithelium containing abundant pigment. This pigment can be found within the glandular element throughout the prostate gland.

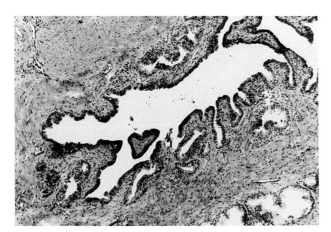

Figure 1–16. Prostate, ejaculatory duct. Histology of the normal ejaculatory duct with the characteristic open lumen and small acinar structures around the periphery.

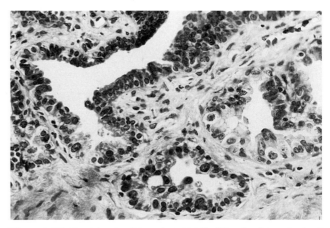

Figure 1–17. Prostate, ejaculatory duct. Detail of the ejaculatory duct and the associated small acinar structures. Note the presence of cells having enlarged, hyperchromatic, atypical nuclei, some of which contain small nucleoli.

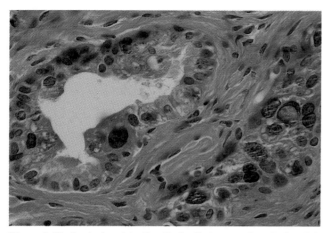

Figure 1–18. Seminal vesicle. Detail of cells in normal seminal vesicle with characteristic large, hyperchromatic nuclei and abundant lipofuscin pigment. These features are similar to those in the ejaculatory duct. See Figure 1–30 for a low-power photomicrograph of the seminal vesicle structure.

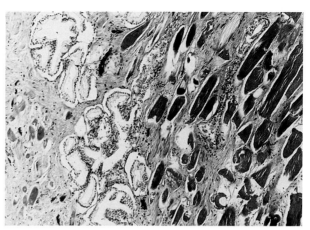

Figure 1–19. Prostate, normal histology. Anterior aspect of the prostate gland with normal acinar elements present within skeletal muscle bundles. The demonstration of glandular elements in skeletal muscle does not indicate prostate carcinoma and the presence of malignant glands in skeletal muscle does not necessarily indicate extraprostatic extension of carcinoma.

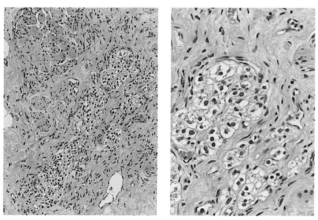

Figure 1–20. Prostate, normal histology. Paraganglion tissue, which can be found within the prostatic stroma or in the periprostatic fibroadipose tissue. These structures should not be mistaken for adenocarcinoma.

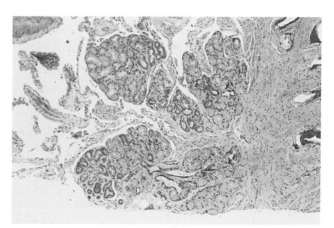

Figure 1–21. Cowper's gland. Normal structure of Cowper's gland with lobular architecture and surrounding loose fibrous connective tissue. This example is present in a needle biopsy specimen.

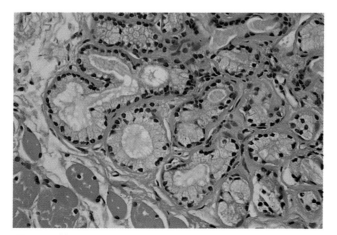

Figure 1–22. Cowper's gland. Detail of Cowper's gland showing ducts and acinar structures lined by a double cell layer with the inner cells being mucin-secreting. These should not be confused with adenocarcinoma.

■ Reporting and Handling of Specimens

Transurethral Resectates

- Specimen weight should be recorded.
- Grossly suspicious chips (yellow) should be sampled.
- Many sampling strategies have been advocated.
- College of American Pathologists recommends embedding first 12 g in total (six to eight cassettes), then one cassette for each additional 10 g.
- If carcinoma is found, and it involves less than 5% of the sample, the remainder should be examined (the 5% is significant for staging purposes; see Staging of Prostate Cancer, Chapter 4).
- For cases with adenocarcinoma, the pathology report should include:
  - Histologic type.
  - Histologic grade (Gleason score; see Chapter 4).
  - Quantification of tumor; we report both the number of involved chips and an estimation of the percentage of tissue involved.
  - Extent of invasion (perineural, vascular, periprostatic tissues).
- If high-grade prostatic intraepithelial neoplasia is present without cancer:
  - Embed all tissue (if not already done).
  - Obtain deeper levels on involved blocks.
  - Report in the diagnosis.

Needle Biopsies

- Number of cores, length of each core, and orientation (if designated) should be recorded for each.
- Tissue should be submitted in total for histologic examination.
- If carcinoma is present in the biopsy, report should include:
  - Histologic type.
  - Histologic grade (Gleason score).
  - Some measure of amount of tumor present (both length of tumor in millimeters per core and estimated percentage of core involved by tumor have been advocated).
  - Extent of tumor (perineural invasion, vascular invasion, involvement of periprostatic tissue [fat] or adjacent organs [seminal vesicle]).
  - All the above should be reported for each site biopsied.
- If high-grade prostatic intraepithelial neoplasia is present without carcinoma:
  - Obtain deeper levels on involved biopsies.
  - Report in diagnosis.
- Low-grade prostatic intraepithelial neoplasia does not need to be reported in diagnosis.
- In "negative" biopsies note that:
  - "Hyperplasia" is rarely present as the biopsies are usually from the peripheral zone; hyperplasia is almost exclusively a transition zone lesion (in patients with pronounced hyperplasia the transition zone compresses the peripheral zone and may be sampled).
  - Chronic prostatitis should be reported because it can elevate the serum PSA; this diagnosis should not be made if appropriate criteria are not present (see Chapter 2).
  - Granulomatous prostatitis should be reported because it can also elevate PSA and produce a suspicious-feeling gland.

Radical Prostatectomies

- Gland should be properly oriented prior to processing.
- Gland weight and specimen dimensions should be recorded.
- The entire external surface should be marked with India ink; we use color coding (e.g., posterior—black, left—yellow, right—green) to aid in orientation but this is not essential if careful documentation of origin of blocks is maintained.
- If fresh tissue is required for research purposes, the gland can be processed as described below (recommended sampling methods are provided in the references below).
- If fresh tissue is not required, fixation in 10% neutral buffered formalin overnight will make sectioning and identification of gross tumor easier.
- The apical margin can be handled in two ways:
  - A thin "shave" margin, 1 to 2 mm thick (any tumor in the microscopic section is then considered "positive").
  - The distal 1 cm is amputated and then processed with sections perpendicular to the true surgical margin (submitted as a cone biopsy or as a series of sections from left to right); tumor at the inked surface is considered positive.
  - We prefer the second method.
- The bladder base margin can be handled in a similar fashion, either as a shave or as sections perpendicular to the surface.
- The remainder of the prostate is serially sectioned perpendicular to the posterior (rectal) surface at 3- to 4-mm intervals.
- Tumor recognition can be difficult in fresh tissue; helpful clues include:
  - Yellow or gray-white color.
  - Loss of the spongy texture of normal prostate.
  - Firmness on palpation.
  - Comparison of one side with the other helps highlight differences.
- In fixed specimens:
  - Tumor is gray-white.
  - Has a more solid appearance.
- Submission of the cross sections as large whole-mount blocks aids in tumor mapping and volume determinations, but is not necessary for the documentation of important pathologic findings.
- Embedding the specimen in total using "quarters" provides the same information.
- Significant pathologic findings, including all features needed for tumor staging (see Chapter 4), can be determined by using a logical sampling method without resorting to complete embedding.
- One possible scheme is detailed below:
  - The apical segment (distal 1 cm) should be examined in total.
  - The posterolateral quarters from the proximal sections (cross sections closest to bladder base) should be submitted in all cases.

- If tumor is grossly visible, all quarters containing tumor should be embedded.
- If tumor is not grossly apparent, alternate sections from the posterolateral quarters should be submitted (orientation of the remaining wet tissue should be preserved in case additional sections are required).
- Three sections from the anterior one half taken at the distal, middle, and proximal thirds.
- The bladder base margin embedded in total (e.g., as two shave sections, left and right).
- The seminal vesicle bases (left and right).
- Pelvic lymph nodes should be submitted in total for histologic evaluation (if frozen sections are requested, selective sampling is adequate).
- The pathology report should include:
  - Histologic type.
  - Histologic grade (Gleason score); should be based on major tumor nodule.
  - Location of main tumor nodule.
  - Size or volume of main tumor nodule; percentage of gland involved.
  - Presence of multicentricity.
  - Presence or absence of capsular penetration and location.
  - Presence or absence of seminal vesicle invasion (left, right, or both).
  - Perineural or vascular invasion.
  - Status of inked surgical margins (sites and extent of positivity when present).
- Lymph node status; if positive, number positive; location, size, presence, or absence of extranodal extension.

References

Association of Directors of Anatomic and Surgical Pathology: Ad hoc committee report: Recommendations for the reporting of resected prostate specimens. Hum Pathol 27:321–323, 1996.

Ayala AG, Ro JY, Babaian R, et al. The prostatic capsule: Does it exist? Its importance in the staging and treatment of prostatic carcinoma. Am J Surg Pathol 13:21–27, 1989.

Epstein JI, Pizov G, Walsh PC. Correlation of pathologic findings with progression after radical retropubic prostatectomy. Cancer 71:3582–3593, 1993.

Hall GS, Kramer CE, Epstein JI. Evaluation of radical prostatectomy specimens: A comparative analysis of sampling methods. Am J Surg Pathol 16:315–324, 1992.

Henson DE, Hutter RVP, Farrow G. Practice protocol for the examination of specimens removed from patients with carcinoma of the prostate gland: A publication of the Cancer Committee, College of American Pathologists. Arch Pathol Lab Med 118:779–783, 1994.

Humphrey PA, Walther PJ. Adenocarcinoma of the prostate: Tissue sampling considerations. Am J Clin Pathol 99:746–759, 1993.

Ohori M, Scardino PT, Lapin SL, et al. The mechanism and prognostic significance of seminal vesicle involvement by prostate cancer. Am J Surg Pathol 17:1252–1261, 1993.

Sakr WA, Grignon DJ, Schomer KL, et al. Evaluating the radical prostatectomy specimen II: Documentation of pathologic stage with limited sampling. J Urol Pathol (in press).

Sakr WA, Grignon DJ, Visscher DW, et al. Evaluating the radical prostatectomy specimen I: A protocol for establishing prognostic parameters and defining genetic abnormalities. J Urol Pathol 3:355–364, 1995.

Wheeler TM, Lebovitz RM. Fresh tissue harvest for research from prostatectomy specimens. Prostate 25:274–279, 1994.

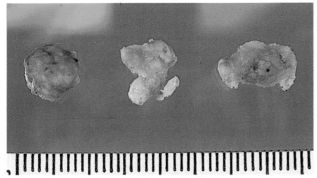

Figure 1–23. Prostate, adenocarcinoma. Prostate chips from a transurethral resection showing small yellow areas. These corresponded to foci of low-grade adenocarcinoma.

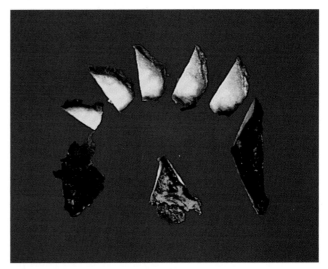

Figure 1–24. Prostate, apex. Prostatic apex processed using the cone method. Note the presence of carcinoma in the sections, extending close to the inked apical margin.

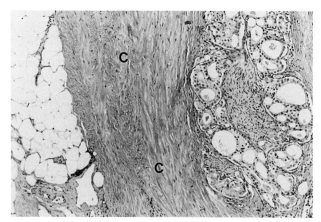

Figure 1–25. Adenocarcinoma. Prostatic adenocarcinoma (Gleason grade 4), showing perineural invasion. The tumor is confined to the prostate gland with no extension into the capsule (*C*) or periprostatic adipose tissue.

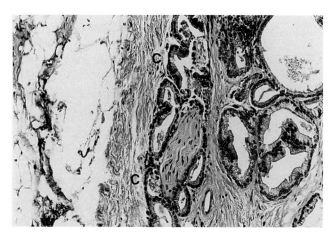

Figure 1–26. Adenocarcinoma. The carcinoma (Gleason grade 3) is invading the capsule (*C*) along a nerve tract, but has not extended through the capsule into periprostatic connective tissue. This tumor is considered to be confined to the prostate (stage T2).

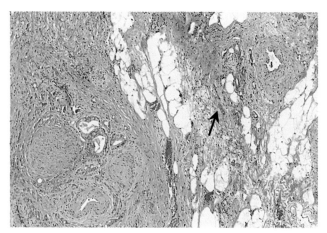

Figure 1–27. Adenocarcinoma. Prostatic adenocarcinoma (Gleason grade 3) with focal extension through the capsule into the periprostatic fibroadipose connective tissue (*arrow*). This is classified as stage T3.

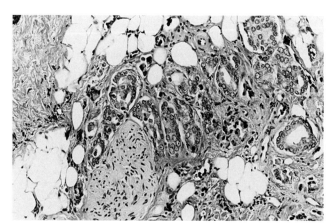

Figure 1–28. Adenocarcinoma. The tumor (Gleason grade 4) is extensively involving nerve and fibroadipose tissue beyond the prostate capsule. This is stage T3.

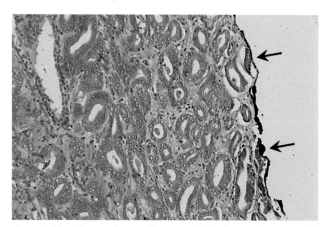

Figure 1–29. Adenocarcinoma. Gleason grade 3 adenocarcinoma extending to the inked surgical resection margin (*arrows*). This would be classified as a positive surgical margin.

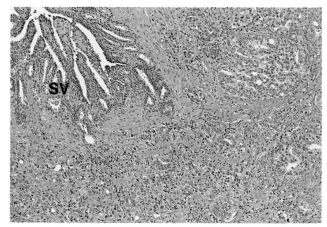

Figure 1–30. Adenocarcinoma. Prostatic adenocarcinoma (Gleason grade 4) extensively invading the muscular wall of the seminal vesicle (*SV*). Note the structure of the seminal vesicle with a central duct surrounded by small acinar structures.

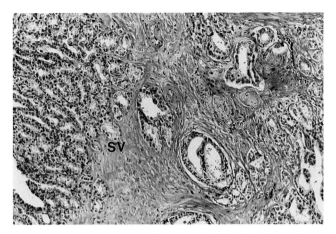

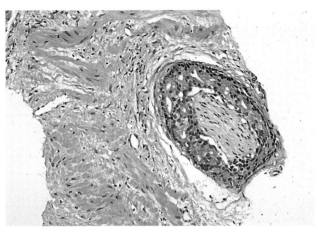

Figure 1–31. Adenocarcinoma. Gleason score 7 (4 + 3) adenocarcinoma invading the muscular wall of the seminal vesicle (*SV*). Note the structure of the seminal vesicle with multiple small acini.

Figure 1–32. Adenocarcinoma. Needle biopsy of the prostate gland demonstrating prostatic adenocarcinoma (Gleason grade 4) circumferentially surrounding a peripheral nerve fiber. This does not indicate extracapsular extension in a needle biopsy.

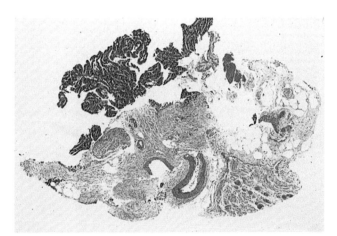

Figure 1–33. Adenocarcinoma. Gleason grade 4 adenocarcinoma present in fibroadipose tissue in a needle biopsy specimen. Fragmentation of tumor is seen at the *top* of the figure; however, glandular elements are present within the tissue of the biopsy. This almost certainly indicates extraprostatic extension in this case; but occasionally small amounts of adipose tissue can be seen within the prostate gland beneath the capsule.

CHAPTER 2

Benign Conditions

■ **Metaplasias**

Transitional Cell Metaplasia

CLINICAL

- No clinical symptoms or significance

GROSS

- None (histologic abnormality)

MICROSCOPIC

- Transitional epithelium normally extends from urethra into proximal ducts.
- Transitional epithelium involving distal ducts and acini is considered metaplastic.
- Ovoid or polygonal epithelial cells oriented perpendicular to basement membrane.

- May be complete replacement of gland space or with residual lumen.
- No nuclear pleomorphism; nuclear grooves can be seen.

SPECIAL STAINS AND IMMUNOHISTOCHEMISTRY

- Mucin-positive cells can be present.
- Positive staining with high-molecular-weight cytokeratin.

DIFFERENTIAL DIAGNOSIS

- Basal cell hyperplasia
- Squamous cell metaplasia
- Prostatic intraepithelial neoplasia (PIN)
- Transitional cell carcinoma

Reference

McNeal JE. Prostate. In Sternberg SS (ed). *Histology for Pathologists.* New York, Raven Press, 1992.

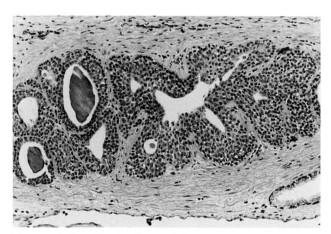

Figure 2–1. Transitional cell metaplasia. Transitional cell metaplasia involving prostatic ducts and acini. Note the stratification, with cells having slightly elongated nuclei arranged perpendicular to the basement membrane.

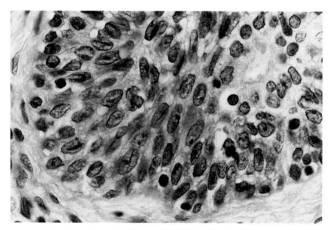

Figure 2–2. Transitional cell metaplasia. Detail of cells highlighting the characteristic nuclear features with several of the nuclei containing grooves.

Squamous Metaplasia

CLINICAL

- No clinical symptoms; no known clinical significance
- Associated with:
  - Infarcts
  - Hormone therapy (estrogens, androgen ablation)
  - Radiation therapy

GROSS

- None (histologic abnormality)

MICROSCOPIC

- Squamous differentiation indicated by keratin production or intercellular bridges.
- May be associated with infarct.
- With infarcts, nuclear atypia can be present.

SPECIAL STAINS AND IMMUNOHISTOCHEMISTRY

- Positive for high-molecular-weight cytokeratin.
- Focal prostatic acid phosphatase (PAP) positivity can be seen.

DIFFERENTIAL DIAGNOSIS

- Transitional cell metaplasia
- Basal cell hyperplasia
- Squamous cell carcinoma
- Transitional cell carcinoma with squamous differentiation
- Adenocarcinoma with squamous differentiation (post therapy)

References

Bostwick DG, Egbert BM, Fajardo LF. Radiation injury of the normal and neoplastic prostate. Am J Surg Pathol 6:541–551, 1982.

Franks LM. Estrogen-treated prostate cancer: The variation in responsiveness of tumor cells. Cancer 13:490–501, 1960.

Lager DJ, Goeken JA, Kemp JD, et al. Squamous metaplasia of the prostate: An immunohistochemical study. Am J Clin Pathol 90:597–601, 1988.

Mostofi FK, Morse WH. Epithelial metaplasia in "prostatic infarction." Arch Pathol 51:340–345, 1951.

Mucinous Metaplasia

CLINICAL

- None (histologic abnormality)

GROSS

- None (histologic abnormality)

MICROSCOPIC

- Presence of mucin-secreting cells in normal and non-neoplastic prostate epithelium
- Has been described in normal ducts and acini; usual hyperplasia, atrophy, basal cell hyperplasia, transitional cell metaplasia, and sclerosing adenosis

SPECIAL STAINS AND IMMUNOHISTOCHEMISTRY

- Stain positive for intracytoplasmic acid (alcian blue and mucicarmine) and neutral (periodic acid–Schiff, PAS) mucin

DIFFERENTIAL DIAGNOSIS

- Mucinous adenocarcinoma

Reference

Grignon DJ, O'Malley FP. Mucinous metaplasia in the prostate gland. Am J Surg Pathol 17:287–290, 1993.

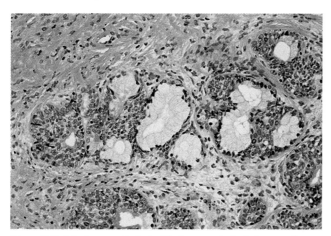

Figure 2–3. Mucinous metaplasia. Mucinous metaplasia in normal prostatic glands in association with transitional cell metaplasia. The mucin-secreting cells are tall and columnar with basally located nuclei.

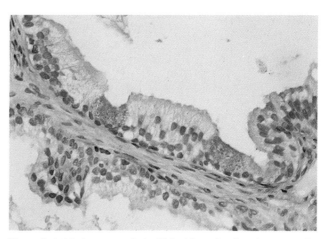

Figure 2–4. Mucinous metaplasia. Alcian blue stain of mucinous metaplasia in a hyperplastic gland. Note the interspersed mucin-positive cells between the normal mucin-negative secretory and basal cells.

Paneth Cell–Like Metaplasia

CLINICAL

- Microscopic change; no known clinical significance

GROSS

- None (histologic abnormality)

MICROSCOPIC

- Cells with large eosinophilic granules that may be seen in normal or hyperplastic prostatic epithelium and adenocarcinoma.
- In normal and hyperplastic cells the granules are exocrine in type; in carcinoma cells the granules are neuroendocrine in type.
- Can be identified in up to 10% of adenocarcinomas.

SPECIAL STAINS AND IMMUNOHISTOCHEMISTRY

- In benign epithelium can be PAS-positive diastase-resistant; in carcinoma, PAS-negative.
- Benign cells with granules are prostate-specific antigen (PSA)- and PAP-positive; alpha$_1$-antichymotrypsin also positive.
- Benign cells with granules are chromogranin-, neuron-specific enolase (NSE)-, and serotonin-negative.
- Carcinoma cells with granules are PSA-, PAP-, chromogranin-, serotonin-, and NSE-positive.

DIFFERENTIAL DIAGNOSIS

- Other cytoplasmic inclusions (viral particles, protozoans, melanin pigment, or crystalloids).

References

Adlakha H, Bostwick DG. Paneth cell-like change in prostatic adenocarcinoma represents neuroendocrine differentiation: Report of 30 cases. Hum Pathol 25:135–139, 1994.

Frydman CP, Bleiweiss IJ, Unger PD, et al. Paneth cell-like metaplasia of the prostate gland. Arch Pathol Lab Med 116:274–276, 1992.

Weaver MG, Abdul-Karim FW, Srigley JR. Paneth cell-like change and small cell carcinoma of the prostate: Two divergent forms of prostatic neuroendocrine differentiation. Am J Surg Pathol 16:1013–1016, 1992.

Weaver MG, Abdul-Karim FW, Srigley JR, et al. Paneth cell-like change of the prostate gland: A histological, immunohistochemical and electron microscopic study. Am J Surg Pathol 16:62–68, 1992.

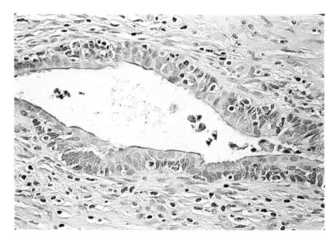

Figure 2–5. Paneth cell–like metaplasia. Normal prostatic gland showing filling of the cytoplasm of some secretory cells by coarse eosinophilic granules. (See also Figure 4–24.)

■ Inflammatory Conditions

Acute Prostatitis

CLINICAL

- Fever and chills, low back and perineal pain, dysuria.
- Swollen, boggy, tender prostate.
- Pathogenesis is bacterial, usually gram-negative (*Escherichia coli* most common).
- Urine cultures usually positive.
- Treated by antibiotics; biopsy or resection not indicated.

GROSS

- Enlarged, swollen, and soft

MICROSCOPIC

- Sheets of neutrophils with abscess formation.
- Ducts packed with neutrophils and necrotic debris.
- Focal acute inflammation is not "acute prostatitis" but usually represents a nonspecific finding without a clinical correlate; it may be seen as part of chronic prostatitis or in association with ruptured ducts, the latter often in association with hyperplasia.
- Reactive atypia in glandular epithelium, including prominent nucleoli.

SPECIAL STAINS AND IMMUNOHISTOCHEMISTRY

- Not applicable

DIFFERENTIAL DIAGNOSIS

- Chronic prostatitis
- Granulomatous prostatitis
- Adenocarcinoma

Reference

Meares EM Jr. Prostatitis and related disorders. In Walsh PC, Retik AB, Stamey TA, Vaughan ED Jr (eds). *Campbell's Urology*, ed 6. Philadelphia, WB Saunders, 1992, pp 807–822.

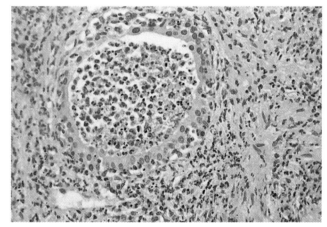

Figure 2–6. Acute prostatitis. Focus of acute prostatitis with a duct showing partial necrosis of the lining and filling of the lumen by neutrophils and cellular debris. The surrounding stroma shows mixed acute and chronic inflammation.

Chronic Prostatitis

CLINICAL

- Variable symptomatology can include irritative voiding symptoms, pelvic pain, hemospermia, recurrent urinary tract infections.
- Asymptomatic bacteriuria.
- Organisms may be identified on urine culture.
- Bacterial and nonbacterial (?*Chlamydia*).
- Recurrences are frequent following treatment.
- Histology correlates poorly with clinical findings.

GROSS

- Normal or enlarged

MICROSCOPIC

- Lymphocytic infiltrates are common in prostate tissue and should not be interpreted as chronic prostatitis.
- Diagnosis is limited to cases with:
  - Neutrophils and lymphocytes in lumina and epithelium.
  - Chronic inflammatory infiltrate, including plasma cells.
- Even with these criteria there is poor clinical correlation—a definitive diagnosis requires clinical correlation.

- Often associated with atrophy.
- Acinar epithelium may show atypia, including presence of nucleoli.

SPECIAL STAINS AND IMMUNOHISTOCHEMISTRY

- If adenocarcinoma seriously considered, high-molecular-weight cytokeratin will mark basal cells.

DIFFERENTIAL DIAGNOSIS

- Granulomatous prostatitis
- Lymphoma
- Adenocarcinoma

References

Gorelick JI, Senterfit LB, Vaughan ED Jr. Quantitative bacterial tissue cultures from 209 prostatectomy specimens: Findings and implications. J Urol 139:57–60, 1988.

Nielsen ML, Asnaes S, Hattel T. Inflammatory changes in the noninfected prostate gland: A clinical, microbiological and histological investigation. J Urol 110:423–426, 1973.

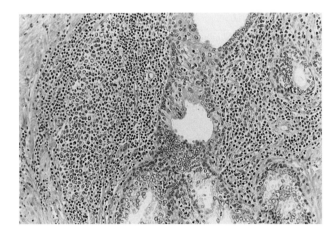

Figure 2–7. Chronic prostatitis. Diffuse chronic inflammatory infiltrate surrounding prostatic ducts with extension of lymphocytes into the ductal epithelium.

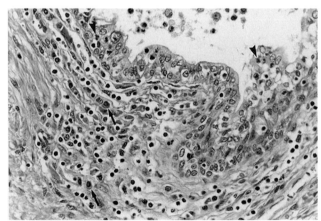

Figure 2–8. Chronic prostatitis. Detail of inflammatory infiltrate showing mixed chronic inflammation which includes plasma cells (*arrows*). Also note the presence of lymphocytes and neutrophils (*arrowheads*) within the epithelial lining. Reactive atypia is present in the epithelial cells, including small nucleoli in several.

Granulomatous Prostatitis

CLASSIFICATION

- Nonspecific
- Post–transurethral resection
- Post–BCG (bacille Calmette-Guérin) therapy
- Infectious
- Allergic (eosinophilic)
- Malacoplakia
- Miscellaneous

Nonspecific Granulomatous Prostatitis

CLINICAL

- Obstructive symptoms.
- Recurrent infections.
- Wide age range (majority 50–70 years).
- Digital rectal examination may be normal, or nodular and hard and suspicious of carcinoma.
- Pathogenesis believed to be related to duct obstruction with accumulation of secretions, rupture, and tissue response to the leaked material; often associated with hyperplasia.

GROSS

- Variably enlarged, nodular, or irregular

MICROSCOPIC

- Mixture of histiocytes, lymphocytes, plasma cells, eosinophils, neutrophils, and giant cells.

- Eosinophils may be abundant (does not indicate "eosinophilic prostatitis").
- Giant cells frequently associated with extravasated secretions or concretions.
- Term "granulomatous prostatitis" somewhat of a misnomer; the cells are usually arranged in sheets without formation of discrete granulomas.
- Histiocytes may be vacuolated, mimicking signet ring cells.

SPECIAL STAINS AND IMMUNOHISTOCHEMISTRY

- Large cells stain with histiocytic markers and are negative for epithelial markers (cytokeratin, PSA, PAP).

DIFFERENTIAL DIAGNOSIS

- Poorly differentiated prostatic adenocarcinoma
- Infectious granulomatous prostatitis
- Allergic (eosinophilic) granulomatous prostatitis

References

Epstein JI, Hutchins GM. Granulomatous prostatitis: Distinction among allergic, non-specific, and post transurethral resection lesions. Hum Pathol 15:818–825, 1984.

Kelalis PP, Harrison EG Jr. Granulomatous prostatitis: A mimic of carcinoma of the prostate. JAMA 191:111–113, 1965.

Stillwell TJ, Engen DE, Farrow GM. The clinical spectrum of granulomatous prostatitis: A report of 200 cases. J Urol 138:320–323, 1987.

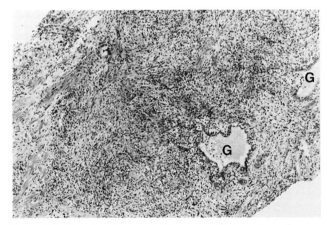

Figure 2–9. Granulomatous prostatitis, nonspecific type. Area of granulomatous prostatitis in a needle biopsy specimen. At low power the focus is cellular with a mixed inflammatory infiltrate and a few scattered residual glands (*G*). Note that true "granuloma" formation is not present.

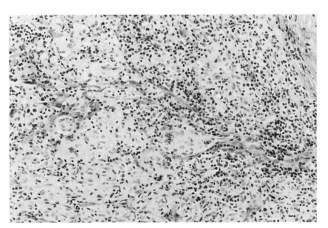

Figure 2–10. Granulomatous prostatitis, nonspecific type. Polymorphous inflammatory infiltrate with epithelioid histiocytes, lymphocytes, and eosinophils.

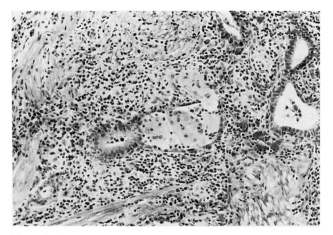

Figure 2–11. Granulomatous prostatitis, nonspecific type. Focus of granulomatous prostatitis with residual glands, some of which are ruptured with giant cells surrounding concretions. The infiltrate is polymorphous with many eosinophils included.

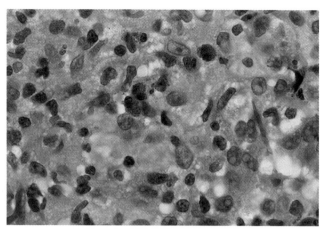

Figure 2–12. Granulomatous prostatitis, nonspecific type. Detail of cellular composition in nonspecific granulomatous prostatitis with epithelioid histiocytes and eosinophils.

Post–Transurethral Resection Granulomas

CLINICAL

- May be found up to 5 years following transurethral resection and cautery
- No clinical significance

GROSS

- None (histologic abnormality)

MICROSCOPIC

- Resemble rheumatoid nodules
- Central zone of fibrinoid necrosis
- Rim of palisaded epithelioid histiocytes
- Variable numbers of multinucleated giant cells
- Eosinophils may be present

SPECIAL STAINS AND IMMUNOHISTOCHEMISTRY

- Stains for microorganisms are negative.

DIFFERENTIAL DIAGNOSIS

- Infectious granulomas (fungi, acid-fast bacilli)

References

Castrillon JV, Maurino MLG, Carcavilla CB, et al. Palisading lower urinary tract granuloma. Br J Urol 62:489–491, 1988.
Mies C, Balogh K, Stadecker M. Palisading prostate granulomas following surgery. Am J Surg Pathol 8:217–221, 1984.

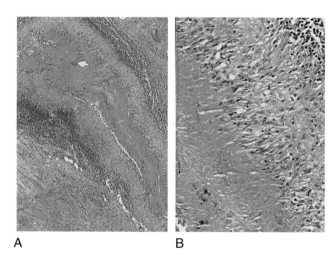

A   B

Figure 2–13. Granulomatous prostatitis, post–transurethral resection. *A,* Geographic nodule with central fibrinoid necrosis and a surrounding zone of histiocytes with an outer rim of chronic inflammatory cells. *B,* Detail of granuloma with central fibrinoid necrosis and palisading of histiocytes at the periphery.

Post–BCG Treatment Granulomas

CLINICAL

- Treatment of urothelial cancer frequently includes instillation of BCG into the bladder.
- Development of histologic granulomatous prostatitis in up to 100%.
- In a small number, prostate becomes hard and nodular, simulating carcinoma.

GROSS

- Normal or enlarged (nodular or diffuse) and hard; necrosis may be present

MICROSCOPIC

- Diffuse, discrete granulomas
- With or without caseating necrosis

SPECIAL STAINS AND IMMUNOHISTOCHEMISTRY

- Acid-fast bacilli can be identified (rarely).
- Fungal stains negative.
- It is not necessary to do special stains if history of BCG instillation available.

DIFFERENTIAL DIAGNOSIS

- Other infectious granulomas
- Sarcoidosis

Reference

Oates RD, Stilmant MM, Fredlund MC, et al. Granulomatous prostatitis following bacillus Calmette-Guérin immunotherapy of bladder cancer. J Urol 140:751–754, 1988.

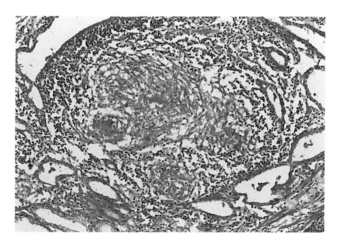

Figure 2–14. Granulomatous prostatitis, post–BCG therapy. Prostate tissue with numerous well-formed granulomas including giant cells characteristic of changes associated with treatment of bladder cancer using BCG (bacille Calmette-Guérin) instillation.

Infectious Granulomatous Prostatitis

CLINICAL

- Exhaustive spectrum of organisms has been reported:
  - Bacterial (tuberculosis, brucellosis, syphilis)
  - Fungal (cryptococcosis, coccidioidomycosis, blastomycosis, histoplasmosis, paracoccidioidomycosis)
  - Parasitic (schistosomiasis, echinococcosis, enterobiasis)
  - Viral (herpes)
- Unusual infections often associated with immunocompromised state

GROSS

- No specific findings; may see hyperemia, areas of necrosis, or infarction

MICROSCOPIC

- Granulomatous inflammation
- With or without necrosis
- Eosinophils (parasitic)

SPECIAL STAINS AND IMMUNOHISTOCHEMISTRY

- As appropriate to identify the offending agent

DIFFERENTIAL DIAGNOSIS

- Nonspecific granulomatous prostatitis
- Post–BCG therapy
- Sarcoidosis

References

Alexis R, Domingo J. Schistosomiasis and adenocarcinoma of the prostate: A morphologic study. Hum Pathol 17:757–760, 1986.

Lief M, Sarfarazi F. Prostatic cryptococcosis in acquired immunodeficiency syndrome. Urology 28:318, 1986.

Schwartz J. Mycotic prostatitis. Urology 19:1–5, 1982.

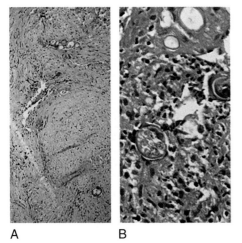

Figure 2–15. Granulomatous prostatitis, coccidioidomycosis. *A,* Granulomatous prostatitis induced by infection with coccidioidomycosis. *B,* The organisms are demonstrated in the high-power photomicrograph.

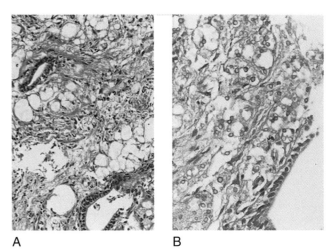

Figure 2–16. Granulomatous prostatitis, cryptococcal. *A,* Involvement of the prostate gland by cryptococcal infection in a human immunodeficiency virus (HIV)-positive patient. *B,* The organisms are highlighted in the mucicarmine stain.

Allergic (Eosinophilic) Prostatitis

CLINICAL

- Younger patients
- History of asthma or allergy
- Peripheral eosinophilia
- May have associated systemic syndromes (e.g., Churg-Strauss syndrome, polyarteritis nodosa)

GROSS

- No characteristic features

MICROSCOPIC

- Intense eosinophilic infiltrate
- With or without fibrinoid necrosis
- With or without vasculitis
- Diagnosis requires appropriate clinical history

SPECIAL STAINS AND IMMUNOHISTOCHEMISTRY

- Not applicable

DIFFERENTIAL DIAGNOSIS

- Nonspecific granulomatous prostatitis
- Infectious granulomatous prostatitis
- Post–transurethral resection granulomas

References

Epstein JI, Hutchins GM. Granulomatous prostatitis: Distinction among allergic, non-specific, and post transurethral resection lesions. Hum Pathol 15:818–825, 1984.
Yonker RA, Katz P. Necrotizing granulomatous vasculitis with eosinophilic infiltrates limited to the prostate. Am J Med 77:362–364, 1984.

Malacoplakia

CLINICAL

- Obstructive symptoms and fever
- Older men (>50 years)
- Urine cultures positive for *E. coli*

GROSS

- Enlarged and indurated
- Discrete soft yellow plaques

MICROSCOPIC

- Sheetlike replacement of tissue by histiocytes with clear-to-eosinophilic cytoplasm (Hansemann cells).
- Admixed lymphocytes and plasma cells.
- Intra- and extracellular, round, target-like structures (Michaelis-Gutmann bodies).
- In older lesions cells may become spindle-shaped.

SPECIAL STAINS AND IMMUNOHISTOCHEMISTRY

- Michaelis-Gutmann bodies best demonstrated with calcium stains (von Kossa)
- Also stain with PAS and iron stains
- Fungal (silver) stains negative

DIFFERENTIAL DIAGNOSIS

- Nonspecific granulomatous prostatitis
- Poorly differentiated adenocarcinoma

References

Altaffer LF, Enghardt M. Malakoplakia of prostate gland. Urology 24:196–198, 1984.
Shimizu S, Takimoto Y, Niimura T, et al. A case of prostatic malacoplakia. J Urol 126:277–279, 1981.

Miscellaneous

- A wide range of other conditions that can result in granuloma formation can involve the prostate:
- Sarcoidosis
- Autoimmune disease
- Wegener's granulomatosis
- Benign lymphocytic angiitis and granulomatosis
- Foreign body

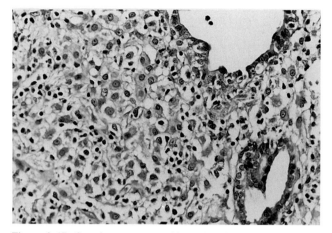

Figure 2–17. Granulomatous prostatitis, malacoplakia. Diffuse replacement of the prostatic stroma by histiocytes with intermingled chronic inflammatory cells. Michaelis-Gutmann bodies are difficult to recognize in routine stains in many cases.

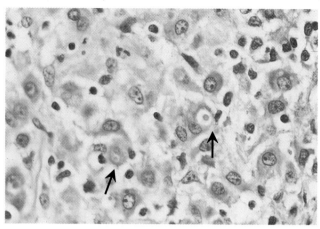

Figure 2–18. Granulomatous prostatitis, malacoplakia. Detail of histiocytes in malacoplakia with recognizable Michaelis-Gutmann bodies (*arrows*). See also Chapter 14, Figures 14–7 and 14–8, for other photomicrographs of malacoplakia.

■ Prostatic Xanthoma

CLINICAL

- Usually an incidental finding
- Can produce a palpable nodule

GROSS

- Lesions up to 5 cm in diameter described
- May have a yellow color mimicking carcinoma

MICROSCOPIC

- Relatively well-demarcated sheets of pale cells.
- Cells have clear-to-foamy cytoplasm with well-defined cell borders.
- Nuclei are small without pleomorphism or prominent nucleoli.
- Other inflammatory cells usually present but few in number.

SPECIAL STAINS AND IMMUNOHISTOCHEMISTRY

- Cells are positive with histiocytic markers.
- Cells are negative for cytokeratin, PSA, and PAP.

DIFFERENTIAL DIAGNOSIS

- Granulomatous prostatitis
- Prostatic adenocarcinoma, particularly clear cell type of transition zone origin, and the high-grade hypernephroid pattern
- Metastatic clear cell carcinoma
- Malignant lymphoma

Reference

Sebo TJ, Bostwick DG, Farrow GM, et al. Prostatic xanthoma: A mimic of prostatic adenocarcinoma. Hum Pathol 25:386–389, 1994.

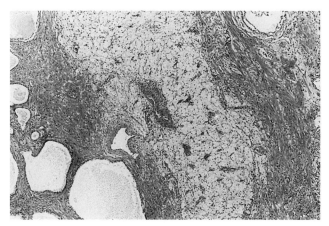

Figure 2–19. Prostatic xanthoma. Relatively well circumscribed aggregate of foamy histiocytes within prostatic stroma. Note the relative absence of other inflammatory cells in the surrounding tissue.

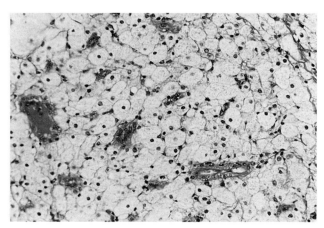

Figure 2–20. Prostatic xanthoma. Detail of cells in prostatic xanthoma with foamy histiocytes having small, round, uniform nuclei.

■ Prostatic Infarction

CLINICAL

- Occurs in the setting of nodular prostatic hyperplasia
- Asymptomatic or urinary retention and gross hematuria

GROSS

- Variable size, up to 5 cm
- Central pale zone with surrounding hyperemia

MICROSCOPIC

- Central coagulative necrosis and hemorrhage.
- Congestion around periphery.
- Immediately adjacent glands show reactive atypia, which can be marked, with large nucleoli in epithelial cells.
- Squamous metaplasia and immature squamous metaplasia.
- Central fibrous scar with hemosiderin in older lesions.

SPECIAL STAINS AND IMMUNOHISTOCHEMISTRY

- High-molecular-weight cytokeratin: positive

DIFFERENTIAL DIAGNOSIS

- Squamous cell carcinoma
- Prostatic carcinoma

References

Lager DJ, Goeken JA, Kemp JD, et al. Squamous metaplasia of the prostate: An immunohistochemical study. Am J Clin Pathol 90:597–601, 1988.

Mostofi FK, Morse WH. Epithelial metaplasia in "prostatic infarction." Arch Pathol 51:340–345, 1951.

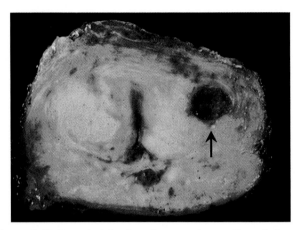

Figure 2–21. Prostatic infarction. Gross specimen with well-circumscribed red-brown infarct within the transition zone of the prostate gland (*arrow*). As in this case, infarcts are typically associated with nodular prostatic hyperplasia.

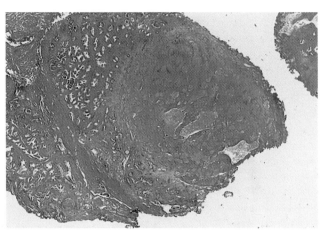

Figure 2–22. Prostatic infarction. Focus of infarction in a transurethral resection specimen. The infarct partially involves a hyperplastic nodule with a central area of ischemic necrosis.

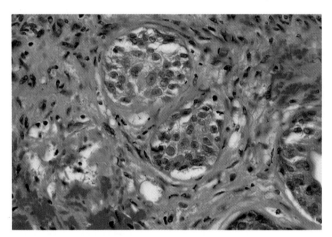

Figure 2–23. Prostatic infarction. Immature squamous metaplasia in prostatic gland immediately adjacent to a prostatic infarct. Note the nuclear atypia with prominent nucleoli. This should not be mistaken for carcinoma.

■ Atrophy

CLINICAL

- Asymptomatic
- Pathogenesis unknown but local ischemia and compression (secondary to nodular hyperplasia), inflammation, and nutritional deficiency are postulated to have a role

GROSS

- No characteristic gross findings; can be seen in association with normal or hyperplastic tissue

MICROSCOPIC

- Four basic patterns: simple (lobular), cystic, sclerotic, and postatrophic hyperplasia.
- Simple (lobular) atrophy: small uniform glands, lined by flattened cells with scant cytoplasm, arranged in a lobular pattern around a central duct. Nuclei are hyperchromatic and nucleoli are generally inconspicuous. Identifying a double cell layer is often difficult because of flattening of the epithelium.
- Cystic atrophy: similar except the acini surrounding the central duct become cystically dilated.
- Sclerotic atrophy: the acini are more irregular in shape, often angulated, and are embedded in a dense, hyalinized stroma. The lining epithelium is similar to that described under simple atrophy. The architecture is lobular and non-infiltrative.
- Postatrophic hyperplasia: architecture similar to simple or sclerotic atrophy. The lining epithelial cells have larger nuclei, which may contain small nucleoli. Although increased compared to usual atrophy, the cytoplasm is still scant and basophilic when compared to adenocarcinoma. Occasionally the cytoplasm is clear. A lobular, non-infiltrative architecture is maintained.
- In many cases of atrophy an inflammatory infiltrate is present which consists of lymphocytes and plasma cells.

SPECIAL STAINS AND IMMUNOHISTOCHEMISTRY

- High-molecular-weight cytokeratin highlights the basal cells, confirming the benign nature.

DIFFERENTIAL DIAGNOSIS

- Adenocarcinoma
- Atypical adenomatous hyperplasia
- Sclerosing adenosis
- Seminal vesicle

References

Cheville JC, Bostwick DG. Postatrophic hyperplasia of the prostate: A histologic mimic of prostatic adenocarcinoma. Am J Surg Pathol 19:1068–1076, 1995.

McNeal JE. Regional morphology and pathology of the prostate. Am J Clin Pathol 49:347–357, 1968.

Srigley JR. Small-acinar patterns in the prostate gland with emphasis on atypical adenomatous hyperplasia and small-acinar carcinoma. Semin Diagn Pathol 5:254–272, 1988.

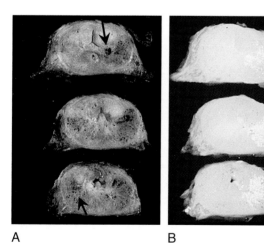

A   B

Figure 2–24. Atrophy. (*A*), Cross sections of the prostate gland demonstrating cystic atrophy (*arrows*). The accompanying specimen radiographs (*B*) show the abundant calcifications within the areas of atrophy.

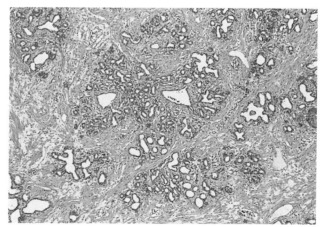

Figure 2–25. Atrophy. Lobular atrophy with multiple lobular units involved. Note the consistent presence of an ectatic central duct surrounded by small glandular units.

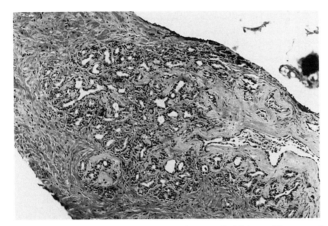

Figure 2–26. Atrophy. Lobular atrophy in a needle biopsy with a central duct surrounded by sclerotic stroma and numerous small glands around the periphery. The sclerotic central duct and lobular arrangement are important clues to distinguish this from adenocarcinoma.

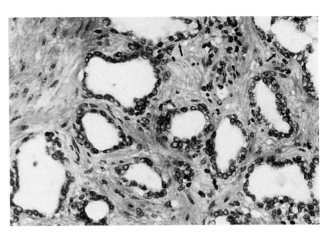

Figure 2–27. Atrophy. Detail of cells in the small glands of atrophy (same case as Figure 2–26). Note the hyperchromatic nuclei with scant cytoplasm and double cell layer, which is only apparent focally (*arrows*).

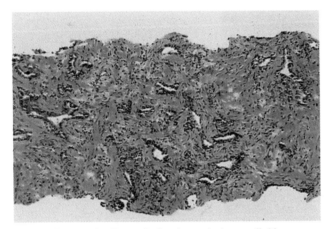

Figure 2–28. Atrophy. Focus of sclerotic atrophy in a needle biopsy specimen. Note the ectatic appearance of the glands with an angulated or branching architecture. The apparent hyperchromasia of the lining cells is due to the absence of cytoplasm.

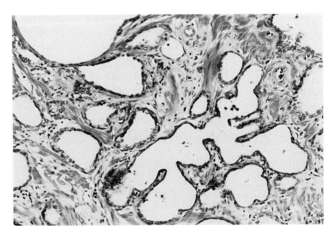

Figure 2–29. Atrophy. Detail of ectatic glands and other small acinar structures with flattened epithelium.

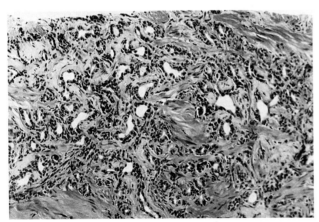

Figure 2–30. Atrophy. Focus of atrophy with apparent secondary proliferation of small glandular units with many of the cells having more abundant cytoplasm than that present in typical areas of atrophy. Note the focal sclerosis around some of the glands and the ectatic lumina, useful features in the distinction from adenocarcinoma.

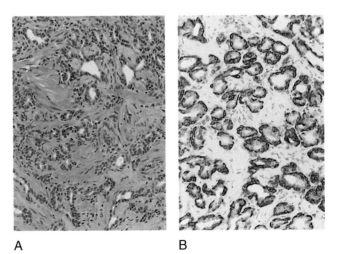

A   B

Figure 2–31. Atrophy. *A*, Atrophy with postatrophic hyperplasia (same case as Figure 2–30). *B*, Positive staining for high-molecular-weight cytokeratin confirms the benign nature of this process.

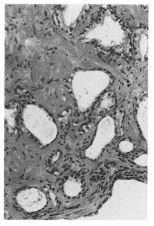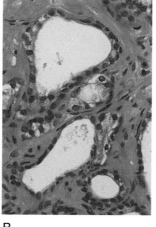

A   B

Figure 2–32. Atrophy. Focus of so-called postatrophic hyperplasia with the cells having increased amounts of pale-to-clear cytoplasm. Note the lobular architecture and the sclerotic background (low- [*A*] and high-power [*B*] photomicrographs).

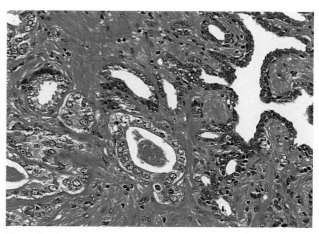

Figure 2–33. Atrophy. Focus of atrophy (*right*) infiltrated by Gleason grade 3 adenocarcinoma. Note the more abundant cytoplasm, open nuclei, and prominent nucleoli in the malignant glands compared with the atrophic glands.

▪ Hyperplasias

Benign (Nodular) Prostatic Hyperplasia (BPH)

CLINICAL

- Increasing frequency with age.
- Very common after age 60.
- Obstructive symptomatology.
- Pathogenesis poorly understood but considered to be hormonally related.
- Treatment includes medical and surgical approaches (transurethral resection of prostate [TURP], prostatectomy). Other new approaches include laser and cryoablation methods.

GROSS

- Almost exclusively localized to transition zone (periurethral) and periurethral glands.
- Variably sized nodules, from millimeters to several centimeters.
- Bulging and frequently multilobulated fresh cut surface.
- Infarcts may be present.
- Compression (atrophy) of peripheral zone.

MICROSCOPIC

- Well-circumscribed, nonencapsulated, expansile nodules.
- Both epithelial and stromal components participate in varying proportions.
- Glandular element generally made up of large, complex, irregularly shaped glands with undulating profile.
- Invaginations ("papillae") have central fibrovascular core.

- Double cell layer (secretory and basal cells).
- Some piling-up and pseudostratification of secretory cells often present but not associated with nuclear enlargement or nucleoli.
- Stroma consists of fibroblasts and smooth muscle cells.

SPECIAL STAINS AND IMMUNOHISTOCHEMISTRY

- High-molecular-weight cytokeratin highlights basal cells.

DIFFERENTIAL DIAGNOSIS

- Normal tissue
- Prostatic intraepithelial neoplasia
- Variants of nodular hyperplasia (basal cell hyperplasia, clear cell cribriform hyperplasia)
- Stromal nodules, fibroadenoma-like and phyllodes-like lesions
- Adenocarcinoma

References

Berry SJ, Coffey DS, Walsh PC, et al. The development of human benign prostatic hyperplasia with age. J Urol 132:474–479, 1984.

Gleason DF. Atypical hyperplasia, benign hyperplasia and well differentiated adenocarcinoma of the prostate. Am J Surg Pathol 9(suppl):53–67, 1985.

McNeal JE. Origin and evolution of benign prostatic enlargement. Invest Urol 15:340–345, 1978.

Price H, McNeal JE, Stamey TA. Evolving patterns of tissue composition in benign prostatic hyperplasia as a function of specimen size. Hum Pathol 21:578–585, 1990.

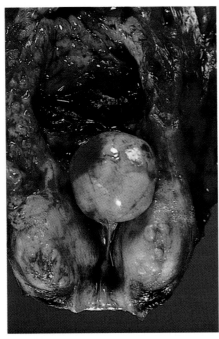

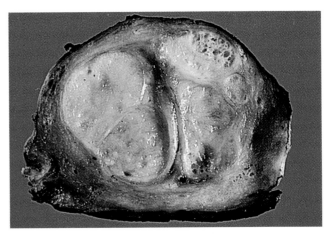

Figure 2–35. Nodular prostatic hyperplasia. Cross section of prostate showing large hyperplastic nodules filling the transition zone and compressing and distorting the urethra. Note the multinodularity and the focal area of cystic change in one of the nodules.

Figure 2–34. Nodular prostatic hyperplasia. Typical gross appearance of nodular prostatic hyperplasia with involvement of the transition zone ("lateral lobes") bilaterally. This photograph also illustrates hyperplasia involving the median lobe producing a ball valve type of obstruction.

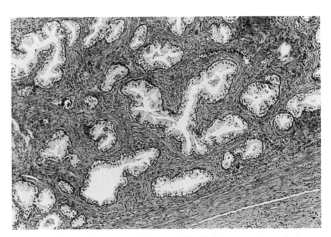

Figure 2–37. Nodular prostatic hyperplasia. Peripheral portion of a hyperplastic nodule composed of roughly equal parts of epithelium and stroma. Note the increased cellularity of the stroma within the nodule compared with that of the adjacent prostatic tissue.

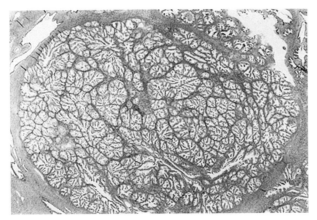

Figure 2–36. Nodular prostatic hyperplasia. Well-circumscribed hyperplastic nodule composed of complex glands. In this focus there is only a minor stromal component.

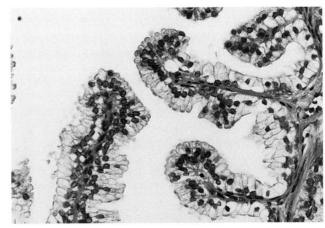

Figure 2–38. Nodular prostatic hyperplasia. Detail of the cellular component of nodular hyperplasia. Note the inward folding of the stroma producing a papillary architecture and the presence of a double cell layer.

Basal Cell Hyperplasia

CLINICAL

- Almost always seen as part of nodular prostatic hyperplasia (BPH)
- Obstructive symptoms or asymptomatic
- Usually encountered in transurethral resections (transition zone)

GROSS

- No specific gross features; may see bulging nodules similar to those of nodular hyperplasia (prostatectomy specimens)

MICROSCOPIC

- Relatively well-circumscribed nodules which usually merge with typical hyperplastic nodules
- Proliferation of basaloid cells, often oriented toward the basement membrane, with (incomplete) or without (complete) preservation of the lumen (and luminal secretory cells).
- Cells have scant basophilic cytoplasm and oval-to-spindle-shaped hyperchromatic nuclei. Nuclear grooves are absent. Nucleoli are usually absent, although in rare cases nucleoli may be prominent.
- Scattered microcalcifications are present in about one half of cases.
- The stroma is also hypercellular owing to proliferating fibroblasts and myofibroblasts.

SPECIAL STAINS AND IMMUNOHISTOCHEMISTRY

- The lumen may contain acidic mucin (alcian blue– and mucicarmine-positive).
- The cells stain positive for high-molecular-weight cytokeratin.
- PSA and PAP stain residual luminal secretory cells in the incomplete form, but the basal cells are nonreactive.

DIFFERENTIAL DIAGNOSIS

- Transitional cell metaplasia
- Squamous metaplasia
- Prostatic intraepithelial neoplasia
- Adenoid basal cell tumor, adenoid cystic carcinoma
- Basal cell carcinoma
- Transitional cell carcinoma
- Adenocarcinoma

References

Cleary KR, Choi HY, Ayala AG. Basal cell hyperplasia of the prostate. Am J Clin Pathol 80:850–854, 1983.

Deveraj LT, Bostwick DG. Atypical basal cell hyperplasia of the prostate: Immunophenotypic profile and proposed classification of basal cell proliferations. Am J Surg Pathol 17:645–659, 1993.

Grignon DJ, Ro JY, Ordonez NG, et al. Basal cell hyperplasia, adenoid basal cell tumor, and adenoid cystic carcinoma of the prostate gland: An immunohistochemical study. Hum Pathol 19:1425–1433, 1988.

van de Voorde W, Baldewijns M, Lauweryns J. Florid basal cell hyperplasia of the prostate. Histopathology 24:341–348, 1994.

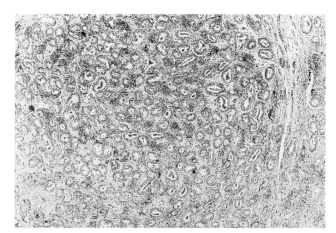

Figure 2–39. Basal cell hyperplasia. Part of a nodule of basal cell hyperplasia with the majority of the glands having persistent lumina (incomplete form). Note also the cellularity of the stroma, an active component of this process.

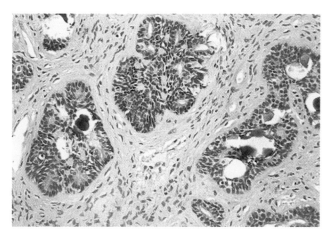

Figure 2–40. Basal cell hyperplasia. An area of basal cell hyperplasia with irregularly shaped and complex acini, some with persistent lumina. Note the presence of microcalcifications, a frequent finding in this process.

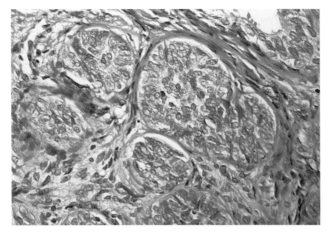

Figure 2–41. Basal cell hyperplasia. Detail of cells in basal cell hyperplasia (complete form) with open nuclei and scant cytoplasm. Nucleoli can be seen in this process and occasionally mitoses are present. This pattern has been referred to as "atypical basal cell hyperplasia" by some authors.

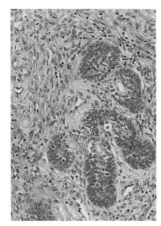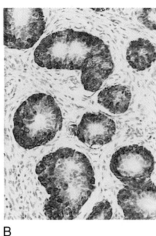

A   B

Figure 2–42. Basal cell hyperplasia. Focus of basal cell hyperplasia (*A*) with corresponding staining for high-molecular-weight cytokeratin (*B*). Note the negative staining of the residual secretory layer in this example of the incomplete form.

Clear Cell Cribriform Hyperplasia

CLINICAL

- No specific symptoms
- Typically seen as part of BPH and may be associated with obstruction

GROSS

- Always associated with BPH, therefore bulging nodules may be seen

MICROSCOPIC

- Always associated with usual hyperplasia and may make up an entire nodule or only part of a nodule.
- Acini are distended by proliferating cells arranged in a cribriform or papillary-cribriform architecture.
- Cells are cuboidal to columnar with abundant clear cytoplasm and small, round-to-oval hyperchromatic nuclei. Nuclei may be somewhat larger at the periphery. Nucleoli are absent or inconspicuous and mitoses are not seen.

- An intact basal cell layer is present at the periphery.
- Central necrosis is not seen.

SPECIAL STAINS AND IMMUNOHISTOCHEMISTRY

- Acidic mucin is usually absent.
- High-molecular-weight cytokeratin highlights basal cell layer.
- The clear cells are PSA- and PAP-positive.

DIFFERENTIAL DIAGNOSIS

- Usual prostatic hyperplasia (BPH)
- Prostatic intraepithelial neoplasia
- Cribriform adenocarcinoma

References

Ayala AG, Srigley JR, Ro JY, et al. Clear cell cribriform hyperplasia of prostate. Am J Surg Pathol 10:665–671, 1986.
Frauenhoffer EE, Ro JY, El-Naggar AK, et al. Clear cell cribriform hyperplasia of the prostate: Immunohistochemical and flow cytometric study. Am J Clin Pathol 95:446–453, 1991.

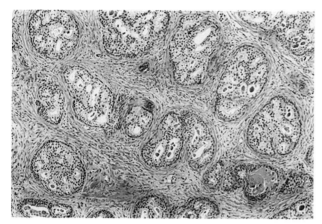

Figure 2–43. Clear cell cribriform hyperplasia. Nodule of clear cell cribriform hyperplasia with variably sized, sharply circumscribed islands of epithelial cells having a cribriform architecture. Note the cellularity of the stroma. Many of the lumina contain secretions.

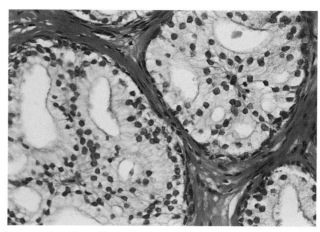

Figure 2–44. Clear cell cribriform hyperplasia. Detail of cells showing the small, uniform, round nuclei and abundant clear cytoplasm.

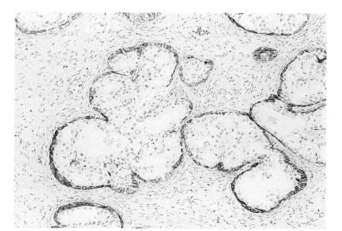

Figure 2–45. Clear cell cribriform hyperplasia. Section stained for high-molecular-weight cytokeratin demonstrating an intact basal cell layer around the cribriform islands.

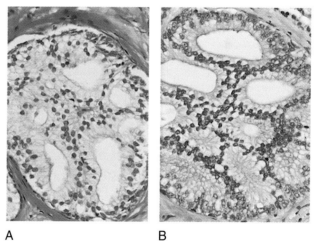

A   B

Figure 2–46. Clear cell cribriform hyperplasia. Comparison of clear cell cribriform hyperplasia (*A*) with cribriform adenocarcinoma (*B*). Note that the nuclei in the adenocarcinoma are larger and contain prominent nucleoli. The cytoplasm in carcinoma tends to have more intense staining.

Sclerosing Adenosis

CLINICAL

- Asymptomatic

GROSS

- No gross features; an incidental finding in transurethral resection or prostatectomy specimens

MICROSCOPIC

- Poorly circumscribed proliferation of variably sized and shaped glands in a cellular stroma. Although the acini may extend outward from the lesion, infiltration of surrounding structures is not seen.
- Glands show considerable variation in size and shape and may be round, compressed, and slitlike, angulated, or large and irregular (resembling normal glands).
- Although a double cell layer is present, it may be difficult to recognize in many of the glands.
- Glands are surrounded by a thick basement membrane.
- Luminal cells have medium-to-large open nuclei with fine chromatin, usually with inconspicuous nucleoli, although prominent nucleoli may occasionally be seen.
- The stroma is typically cellular with plump spindle-shaped cells arranged haphazardly or in small fascicles (an important and integral component of the lesion).
- Luminal secretions, including acidic mucin (alcian blue–

and mucicarmine-positive), and the presence of prostatic crystalloids have been described.

SPECIAL STAINS AND IMMUNOHISTOCHEMISTRY

- Acid mucin may be present in the lumen.
- High-molecular-weight cytokeratin stains the basal cells and some of the spindle cells.
- Some of the basal and spindle cells also stain with muscle-specific actin and S-100 protein indicating myoepithelial differentiation. This is unique to this lesion.

DIFFERENTIAL DIAGNOSIS

- Postatrophic hyperplasia
- Atypical adenomatous hyperplasia
- Adenocarcinoma

References

Grignon DJ, Ro JY, Srigley JR, et al. Sclerosing adenosis of the prostate gland: A lesion showing myoepithelial differentiation. Am J Surg Pathol 16:383–391, 1992.

Jones EC, Clement PB, Young RH. Sclerosing adenosis of the prostate gland: A clinicopathologic and immunohistochemical study of 11 cases. Am J Surg Pathol 15:1171–1180, 1991.

Sakamoto N, Tsuneyoshi M, Enjoji M. Sclerosing adenosis of the prostate: Histopathologic and immunohistochemical analysis. Am J Surg Pathol 15:660–667, 1991.

Young RH, Clement BB. Sclerosing adenosis of the prostate. Arch Pathol Lab Med 111:363–366, 1987.

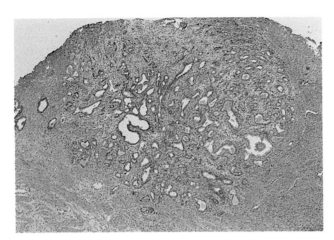

Figure 2–47. Sclerosing adenosis. Focus of sclerosing adenosis in a transurethral resection specimen. Note that the nodule is relatively circumscribed but not encapsulated. Even at low magnification the mixed stromal and epithelial elements are readily apparent.

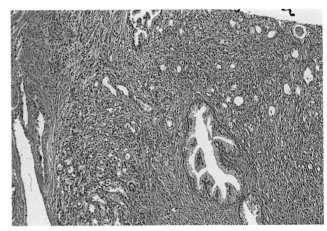

Figure 2–48. Sclerosing adenosis. Another example of sclerosing adenosis with the impression of marked cellularity. This is due to the presence of both small acinar structures and a cellular stroma. Note also the presence of large, obviously benign glands within the lesion.

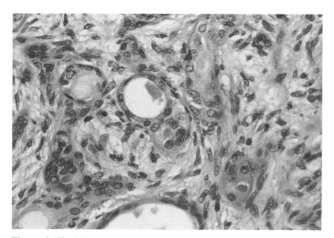

Figure 2–49. Sclerosing adenosis. Detail of glandular and stromal elements with relatively uniform acini and, in this case, a loose stromal component.

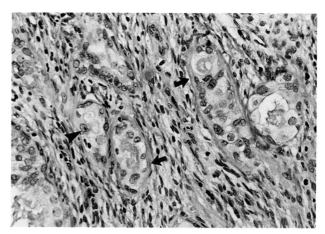

Figure 2–50. Sclerosing adenosis. Detail of stromal and glandular components. Note that the acini appear to have a single cell layer with the basal and myoepithelial cells being inconspicuous. The lining cells may contain nucleoli (*arrowhead*). The glands are surrounded by a thick basement membrane (*arrows*), a feature not seen in adenocarcinoma. The stroma is cellular with spindle-shaped cells.

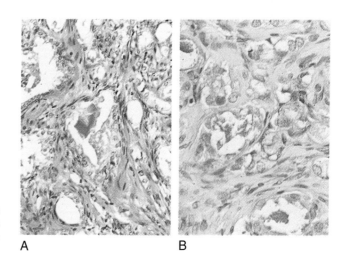

A   B

Figure 2–51. Sclerosing adenosis. Sclerosing adenosis may demonstrate the presence of crystalloids (*A*) and can also contain acidic mucin (*B*, alcian blue stain). Although these features are characteristic of adenocarcinoma, they are not specific.

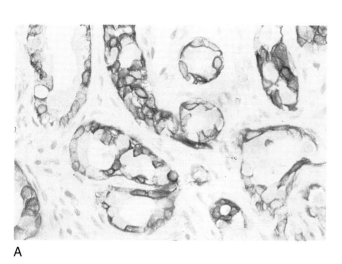

A

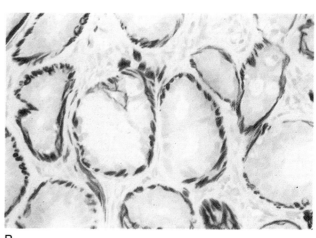

B

Figure 2–52. Sclerosing adenosis. Immunohistochemical stain demonstrating positive reactivity of the basal cells for high-molecular-weight cytokeratin (*A*) and smooth muscle actin (*B*). These cells show features of both basal cells and myoepithelial cells.

Verumontanum Mucosal Gland Hyperplasia

CLINICAL

- Incidental finding in radical prostatectomy specimens (14%)
- No known clinical symptoms or significance

GROSS

- None (histologic abnormality)

MICROSCOPIC

- Single or multiple foci, less than 1 mm in diameter.
- Expansile growth pattern.
- Back-to-back microacini with double cell layer.
- Nucleoli inconspicuous.
- Glands contain numerous corpora amylacea.

SPECIAL STAINS AND IMMUNOHISTOCHEMISTRY

- Cells are PSA- and PAP-positive.
- High-molecular-weight cytokeratin highlights basal cell layer.

DIFFERENTIAL DIAGNOSIS

- Atypical adenomatous hyperplasia
- Nephrogenic adenoma
- Basal cell hyperplasia
- Mesonephric hyperplasia
- Prostatic adenocarcinoma

Reference

Gagucas RJ, Brown RW, Wheeler TM. Verumontanum mucosal gland hyperplasia. Am J Surg Pathol 19:30–36, 1995.

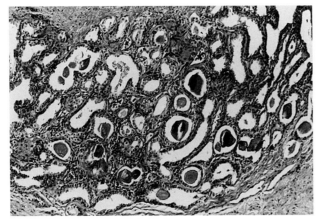

Figure 2–53. Verumontanum gland hyperplasia. Proliferation of small and irregular glands in the region of the verumontanum. Many of the acini contain concretions.

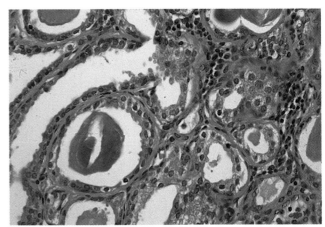

Figure 2–54. Verumontanum gland hyperplasia. Detail of components of verumontanum gland hyperplasia. The acini have a double cell layer and nucleoli are inconspicuous.

■ Miscellaneous Conditions

Nephrogenic Adenoma

CLINICAL

- Infrequently involves the prostatic urethra
- Almost always a history of prior surgery or instrumentation

GROSS

- At cystoscopy, the urologist may see a small papillary or polypoid lesion and suspect transitional cell carcinoma.

MICROSCOPIC

- Histologically, there is both an exophytic papillary and a glandular component. The papillae are covered by a single layer of cuboidal or hobnail cells; this component may be absent in prostatic urethral lesions.
- The glandular component consists of small, closely packed tubules surrounded by a prominent basement membrane. The tubules may become dilated and even cystic. The stroma is frequently edematous, but desmoplasia is absent. Variable degrees of inflammation may be associated.
- The cells have from scant-to-abundant eosinophilic or clear cytoplasm. Nuclei tend to be round and uniform with inconspicuous nucleoli, although occasional prominent nucleoli may be seen. Mitoses are infrequent, but can be present.
- Some tubules may have only a single recognizable lining cell producing a signet ring–like appearance.
- The adjacent urothelium may show ulceration, cystitis cystica, or cystitis glandularis.

SPECIAL STAINS AND IMMUNOHISTOCHEMISTRY

- The cytoplasm may stain for mucin and glycogen.
- The cells are nonreactive for PSA and PAP.

DIFFERENTIAL DIAGNOSIS

- Prostatic adenocarcinoma
- Clear cell carcinoma of urethra

References

Bhagavan BS, Tiamso EM, Wenk RE, et al. Nephrogenic adenoma of the urinary bladder and urethra. Hum Pathol 12:907–916, 1981.
Malpica A, Ro JY, Troncoso P, et al. Nephrogenic adenoma of the prostatic urethra involving the prostate gland: A clinicopathologic and immunohistochemical study of eight cases. Hum Pathol 25:390–395, 1994.

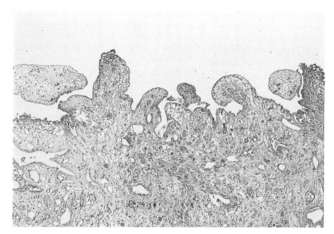

Figure 2–55. Nephrogenic adenoma. Involvement of the prostatic urethra with an exophytic papillary component at the surface and a tubular component in the underlying stroma.

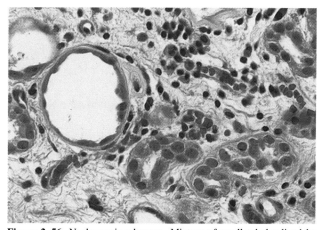

Figure 2–56. Nephrogenic adenoma. Mixture of small tubules lined by cuboidal cells, and ectatic tubules lined by flattened epithelial cells. Note the distinct basal lamina surrounding all the tubules.

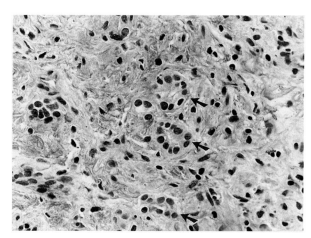

Figure 2–57. Nephrogenic adenoma. Small, round, uniform tubular structures scattered in the stroma (*arrows*). The lining cells are cuboidal and some have small inconspicuous nucleoli.

Urethral Polyp with Prostatic-Type Epithelium

CLINICAL

- Young males (third to fourth decade); cases have been reported in elderly.
- Present with hematuria or hemospermia.
- At cystoscopy, small exophytic papillary or polypoid lesion in region of verumontanum or, less often, membranous urethra.

GROSS

- Small, polypoid, or papillary lesion

MICROSCOPIC

- Papillary or glandular pattern, or both
- Covered by prostatic (double layer, columnar secretory epithelial cells) and transitional epithelium
- Prostatic glands in underlying stroma

SPECIAL STAINS AND IMMUNOHISTOCHEMISTRY

- Prostatic-type epithelium is PSA- and PAP-positive, confirming its prostatic origin.

DIFFERENTIAL DIAGNOSIS

- Papillary transitional cell neoplasm
- Nephrogenic adenoma
- Ductal (endometrioid) adenocarcinoma

References

Craig JR, Hart WR. Benign polyps with prostatic-type epithelium of the urethra. Am J Clin Pathol 63:343–347, 1975.
Eglen DE, Pontius EE. Benign prostatic epithelial polyp of the urethra. J Urol 131:120–122, 1984.

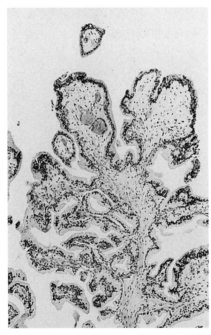

Figure 2–58. Urethral polyp with prostatic-type epithelium. Polypoid growth extending into the urethra with prostatic-type glands within the stroma.

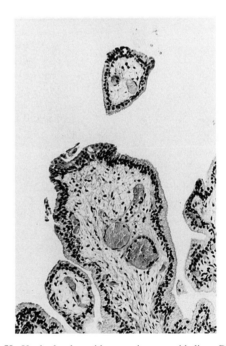

Figure 2–59. Urethral polyp with prostatic-type epithelium. Detail of the surface epithelium having a double cell layer, with the outer surface being tall and columnar. Histologically, this is identical to normal prostatic-type epithelium and these cells do stain positively with prostate-specific antigen and prostatic acid phosphatase.

Inverted Papilloma

CLINICAL

- Present with hematuria
- Cystoscopically, a small submucosal nodule which can result in an exophytic polypoid lesion
- Infrequent in prostatic urethra

GROSS

- Small, submucosal, or exophytic polypoid lesion

MICROSCOPIC

- Anastomosing cords of benign transitional epithelium without cytologic atypia or mitoses
- Overlying urethral transitional epithelium normal or atrophic.

- Glandular or trabecular types
- No exophytic papillary component
- No infiltrative growth at periphery

SPECIAL STAINS AND IMMUNOHISTOCHEMISTRY

- PSA- and PAP-negative

DIFFERENTIAL DIAGNOSIS

- Transitional cell carcinoma
- Squamous cell carcinoma

Reference

DeMeester LJ, Farrow GM, Utz TC. Inverted papilloma of the urinary bladder. Cancer 36:505–513, 1975.

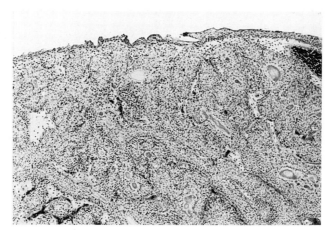

Figure 2–60. Inverted papilloma. Inverted papilloma of the prostatic urethra showing the characteristic downward growth of anastomosing trabeculae of transitional epithelium. Many of the islands have central lumina with a lining of columnar, mucin-secreting cells. The overlying epithelium is histologically normal.

Mesonephric Hyperplasia

CLINICAL

- Rare lesion
- No clinical symptoms

GROSS

- No gross lesions (microscopic finding)

MICROSCOPIC

- Lobular arrangement of small tubular structures lined by a single-layered epithelium.
- Cells are cuboidal with minimal cytoplasm, resulting in an "atrophic" appearance.
- Some tubules dilated with eosinophilic secretions.
- Other tubules are irregular with apparent tufting of epithelium.

- Tubules can be associated with nerve and ganglion tissue in periprostatic fat.

SPECIAL STAINS AND IMMUNOHISTOCHEMISTRY

- PSA and PAP: negative
- High-molecular-weight cytokeratin: positive

DIFFERENTIAL DIAGNOSIS

- Prostatic adenocarcinoma
- Atypical adenomatous hyperplasia
- Sclerosing adenosis
- Nephrogenic adenoma

Reference

Gikas PW, Del Buono EA, Epstein JI. Florid hyperplasia of mesonephric remnants involving prostate and periprostatic tissue: Possible confusion with adenocarcinoma. Am J Surg Pathol 17:454–460, 1993.

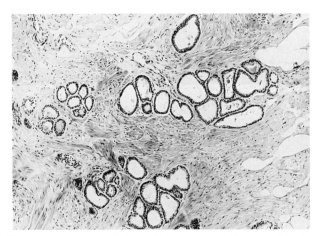

Figure 2–61. Mesonephric hyperplasia. Scattered collections of tubular structures within the fibromuscular stroma. The tubules have dilated lumina.

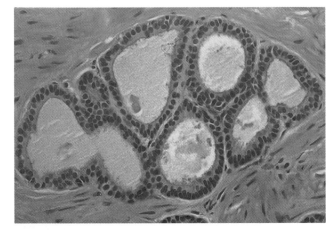

Figure 2–62. Mesonephric hyperplasia. The tubular structures are lined by a single layer of cuboidal cells with scant cytoplasm.

Blue Nevus and Melanosis

CLINICAL

- Wide age spectrum (20–80 years).
- Most have had obstructive symptoms related to nodular prostatic hyperplasia (BPH).
- Black color may be apparent at the time of resection, raising the possibility of malignant melanoma.

GROSS

- Tissue may have a black color.

MICROSCOPIC

- The term *blue nevus* is applied when pigment is confined to the dendritic cells in the stroma and *melanosis* when the glandular cells also contain melanin pigment.
- Pigmented spindle cells with dendritic processes are present in the stroma and in association with acini.

- Pigment may also be seen in the acinar epithelium and has been described in carcinomatous cells when associated with melanosis.

SPECIAL STAINS AND IMMUNOHISTOCHEMISTRY

- Pigment stains with Fontana-Masson and Lillie's ferrous iron stains for melanin.
- Spindle cells are S-100 protein–positive.

DIFFERENTIAL DIAGNOSIS

- Pigmented (nonmelanotic) prostatic epithelium
- Malignant melanoma

References

Aguilar M, Gaffney EF, Finnerty DP. Prostatic melanosis with involvement of benign and malignant epithelium. J Urol 128:825–827, 1982.

Ro JY, Grignon DJ, Ayala AG, et al. Blue nevus and melanosis of the prostate: Electron-microscopic and immunohistochemical studies. Am J Clin Pathol 90:530–535, 1988.

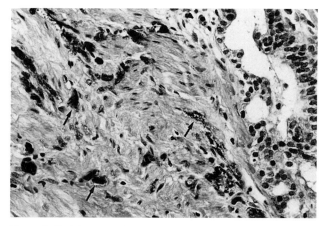

Figure 2–63. Blue nevus. Blue nevus involving the prostate gland, with numerous dendritic cells containing abundant melanin pigment scattered throughout the stroma (*arrows*). The heavy pigmentation obscures the nuclear detail of these cells.

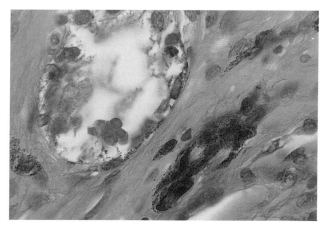

Figure 2–64. Blue nevus. Example of a blue nevus with associated melanosis. There are dendritic cells within the stroma and in addition the prostatic epithelial cells contain granular, brown, melanin pigment.

CHAPTER 3

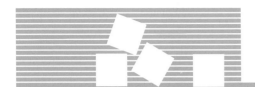

Putative Premalignant Lesions

■ Atypical Adenomatous Hyperplasia

CLINICAL

- No clinical symptoms attributable.
- Part of nodular prostatic hyperplasia (BPH).
- Has been speculated to be a precursor lesion for adeno-carcinoma arising in the transition zone; to date evidence of a premalignant potential is lacking.
- Risk, if any, of progression to cancer unknown.
- The term "adenosis" is used interchangeably by some, although the majority of urologic pathologists favor use of *atypical adenomatous hyperplasia*.

GROSS

- None (histologic abnormality)

MICROSCOPIC

- Well-circumscribed proliferation of small glands in association with the usual hyperplastic nodules of BPH.
- An infiltrative pattern is absent.
- Glands become increasingly uniform at periphery.
- Glandular contours are more variable than the more uniform, rigid, round glands of adenocarcinoma.
- Double cell layer at least focally apparent in routine (hematoxylin and eosin [H&E]) sections.
- Cells show no cytologic atypia and nucleoli are usually absent or inconspicuous.
- Acid mucin and crystalloids can be seen, but much less frequently than with adenocarcinoma.

SPECIAL STAINS AND IMMUNOHISTOCHEMISTRY

- High-molecular-weight cytokeratin demonstrates partial basal cell layer.

DIFFERENTIAL DIAGNOSIS

- Adenocarcinoma (well-differentiated)
- Sclerosing adenosis
- Usual (nodular) hyperplasia
- Mesonephric hyperplasia

References

Bostwick DG, Algaba F, Amin MB, et al. Consensus statement on terminology: Recommendation to use atypical adenomatous hyperplasia in place of adenosis of the prostate. Am J Surg Pathol 18:1069–1070, 1994.

Bostwick DG, Qian J. Atypical adenomatous hyperplasia of the prostate: Relationship with carcinoma in 217 whole-mount radical prostatectomies. Am J Surg Pathol 19:506–518, 1995.

Bostwick DG, Srigley J, Grignon DJ, et al. Atypical adenomatous hyperplasia of the prostate: Morphologic criteria for its distinction from well-differentiated carcinoma. Hum Pathol 24:819–832, 1993.

Gaudin PB, Epstein JI. Adenosis of the prostate: Histologic features in transurethral resection specimens. Am J Surg Pathol 18:863–870, 1994.

Gleason DF. Atypical hyperplasia, benign hyperplasia and well-differentiated adenocarcinoma of the prostate. Am J Surg Pathol 9(suppl):53–67, 1985.

McNeal JE. Origin and development of carcinoma in the prostate. Cancer 23:24–34, 1969.

■ Prostatic Intraepithelial Neoplasia (PIN)

CLINICAL

- Widely accepted as the likely precursor lesion for most cases of prostatic adenocarcinoma.
- High-grade PIN is present in over 80% of prostate glands harboring adenocarcinoma.
- High-grade PIN has been reported to produce hypoechoic lesions on ultrasound and to be associated with elevated serum prostate-specific antigen (PSA) in some cases; both of these reports are, however, controversial and not uniformly accepted.
- Its presence in biopsies or transurethral resections indicates a high likelihood of adenocarcinoma being present. Most authors currently recommend re-biopsy in patients with high-grade PIN in biopsy material.

GROSS

- Not associated with a grossly visible lesion

MICROSCOPIC

- Low-grade PIN (grade 1) is characterized by crowded, piled-up epithelial cells in architecturally normal ducts and acini. Individual cells have marked variation in nuclear size; nucleoli are absent or inconspicuous.

- The diagnosis of low-grade PIN is limited by problems of reproducibility, and separation from simple hyperplasia is difficult. For these reasons, and because it is not a marker for carcinoma, making this diagnosis is not recommended. Its presence is not an indication for re-biopsy.
- High-grade PIN (grades 2 and 3) is characterized by the proliferation of highly atypical cells having more uniformly enlarged nuclei than low-grade PIN. Prominent nucleoli (similar to adenocarcinoma) are present in many of the cells and are essential to the diagnosis.
- High-grade PIN is associated with four architectural patterns: tufted, micropapillary, cribriform, and flat.
- The basal cell layer may be complete or incomplete in high-grade PIN, but at least some basal cells are present.

SPECIAL STAINS AND IMMUNOHISTOCHEMISTRY

- Acid mucin can be found in the lumina of glands involved by high-grade PIN.
- Staining for high-molecular-weight cytokeratin highlights remaining basal cells.
- The atypical cells stain for PSA and prostatic acid phosphatase (PAP).

DIFFERENTIAL DIAGNOSIS

- Nodular prostatic hyperplasia (BPH)
- Transitional cell metaplasia
- Basal cell hyperplasia
- Clear cell cribriform hyperplasia
- Cribriform adenocarcinoma
- Ductal (endometrioid) adenocarcinoma
- Urothelial carcinoma

References

Amin MB, Ro JY, Ayala AG. Precursor lesions of prostate adenocarcinoma: Fact or fancy? Mod Pathol 6:476–483, 1993.

Amin MB, Ro JY, Ayala AG. Prostatic intraepithelial neoplasia: Relationship to adenocarcinoma of the prostate. Pathol Annu 29(2):1–30, 1994.

Bostwick DG, Amin MB, Dundore P, et al. Architectural patterns of high grade prostatic intraepithelial neoplasia. Hum Pathol 24:298–310, 1993.

Bostwick DG, Brawer MK. Prostatic intra-epithelial neoplasia and early invasion in prostate cancer. Cancer 61:555–561, 1987.

Epstein JI, Grignon DJ, Humphrey PA, et al. Interobserver reproducibility in the diagnosis of prostatic intraepithelial neoplasia. Am J Surg Pathol 19:873–886, 1995.

McNeal JE, Bostwick DG. Intraductal dysplasia: A premalignant lesion of the prostate. Hum Pathol 17:64–71, 1986.

Troncoso P, Babaian RJ, Ro JY, et al. Prostatic intraepithelial neoplasia and invasive adenocarcinoma in cystoprostatectomy specimens. Urology 24 (suppl):52–56, 1989.

Weinstein MH, Epstein JI. Significance of high grade prostatic intraepithelial neoplasia on needle biopsy. Hum Pathol 24:624–629, 1993.

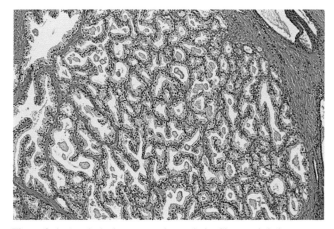

Figure 3–1. Atypical adenomatous hyperplasia. Characteristic low-power appearance of atypical adenomatous hyperplasia with complex, irregular glands typical of the usual type of hyperplasia at left with progressively smaller glands toward the right side of the nodule. Note the sharp circumscription.

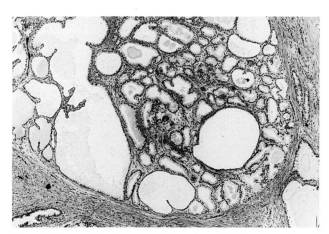

Figure 3–2. Atypical adenomatous hyperplasia. Portion of a nodule of atypical adenomatous hyperplasia with small, uniform, round glands in association with regular and dilated glands more typical of the usual hyperplasia.

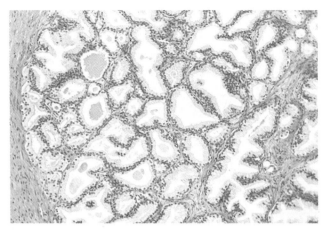

Figure 3–3. Atypical adenomatous hyperplasia. Nodule of atypical adenomatous hyperplasia with more uniform small glands at the periphery *(left)* and obviously benign glandular component toward the right.

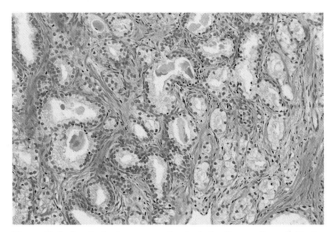

Figure 3–4. Atypical adenomatous hyperplasia. Focus of atypical adenomatous hyperplasia with many of the glands having an obvious double cell layer even at low power, but with other smaller glands with pale-staining cytoplasm of the lining cells interspersed. There are also crystalloids within this focus.

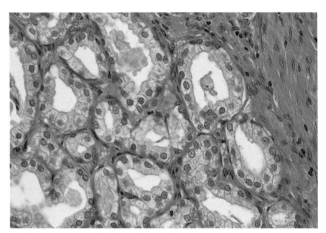

Figure 3–5. Atypical adenomatous hyperplasia. Detail of small glands at periphery of a focus of atypical adenomatous hyperplasia (upper right corner of Figure 3–1). A double cell layer is apparent in some of the acini but not in all.

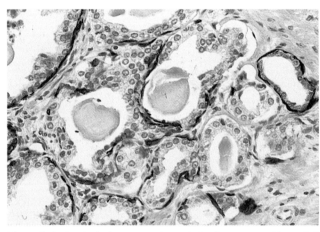

Figure 3–6. Atypical adenomatous hyperplasia. Same area as Figure 3–5 stained for high-molecular-weight cytokeratin demonstrating the presence of an incomplete basal cell layer around many of the acini.

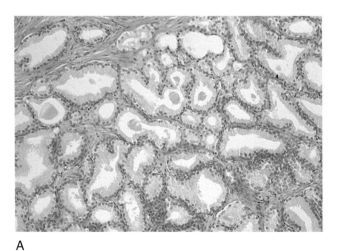

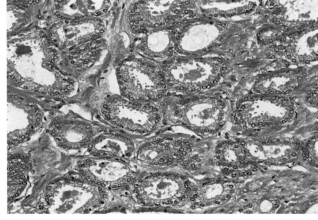

A   B

Figure 3–7. Atypical adenomatous hyperplasia. Comparative photomicrograph of atypical adenomatous hyperplasia *(A)* and Gleason grade 2 adenocarcinoma *(B)*. The malignant glands are more uniform and the cytoplasm has greater eosinophilia.

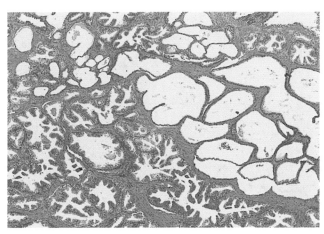

Figure 3–8. Prostatic intraepithelial neoplasia. At low magnification, areas of high-grade PIN are readily recognized by the basophilic appearance of the lining of the complex, irregularly shaped glands *(lower left)*. These foci stand out from the adjacent normal glands in which the lining epithelium has a very pale appearance.

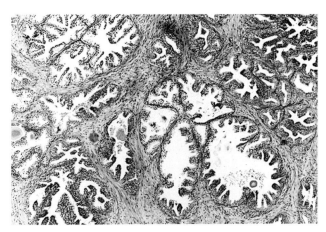

Figure 3–9. Prostatic intraepithelial neoplasia. The area of high-grade PIN *(right)* stands out from the benign tissue *(left)* because of the nuclear enlargement and crowding with increased basophilia of the cytoplasm.

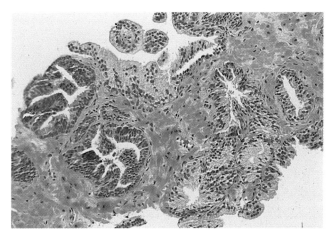

Figure 3–10. Prostatic intraepithelial neoplasia. Focus of high-grade PIN in a needle biopsy specimen. The cellularity and basophilia of the lining epithelium stands out even at low magnification *(lower left)*.

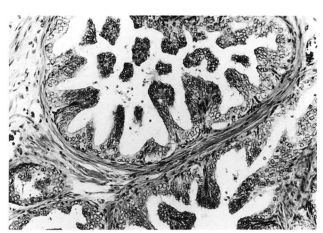

Figure 3–11. Prostatic intraepithelial neoplasia. Micropapillary pattern of high-grade PIN with papillary structures having a fine central fibrovascular core with a covering of atypical cells having enlarged nuclei and prominent nucleoli.

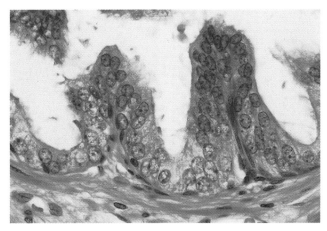

Figure 3–12. Prostatic intraepithelial neoplasia. Detail of micropapillary type of high-grade PIN with cells having enlarged nuclei and prominent nucleoli.

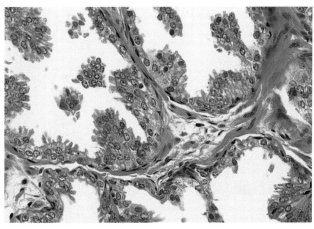

Figure 3–13. Prostatic intraepithelial neoplasia. Tufted pattern of high-grade PIN with areas of piling-up of the atypical cells producing small tuft-like projections into the glandular lumina.

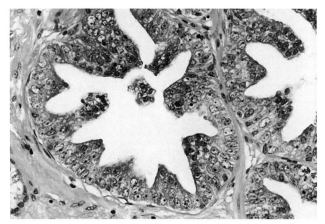

Figure 3–14. Prostatic intraepithelial neoplasia. Detail of the cellular elements in a focus of high-grade PIN having a tufted architectural pattern.

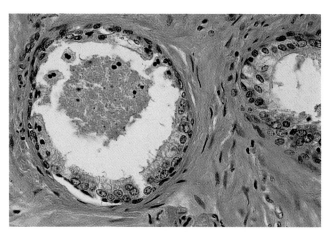

Figure 3–15. Prostatic intraepithelial neoplasia. Focus of high-grade PIN involving dilated glandular spaces. The atypical cells are present as a single or double cell layer producing a flat pattern of growth.

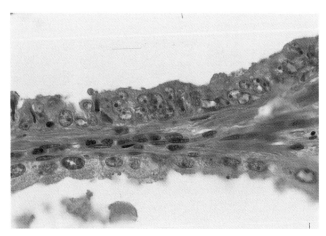

Figure 3–16. Prostatic intraepithelial neoplasia. Detail of the individual cells making up this flat pattern of high-grade PIN.

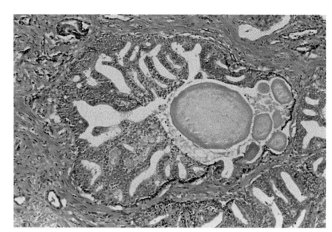

Figure 3–17. Prostatic intraepithelial neoplasia. Large gland involved by high-grade PIN producing a cribriform pattern. Note the presence of concretions within the involved gland. There is also an infiltrative adenocarcinoma (Gleason grade 3) in the surrounding fibrous stroma.

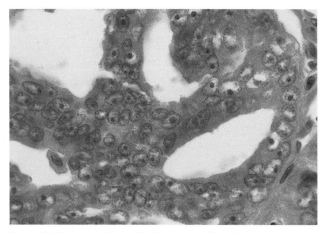

Figure 3–18. Prostatic intraepithelial neoplasia. Detail of the cellular composition from an area of a cribriform pattern of high-grade PIN.

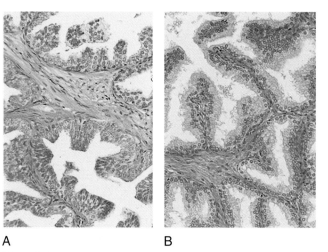

A   B

Figure 3–19. Prostatic intraepithelial neoplasia. Comparative photograph of high-grade PIN (*A*) with nodular prostatic hyperplasia (*B*). Note the basophilia of the cytoplasm, the nuclear crowding and atypia, and the tufted architecture in PIN.

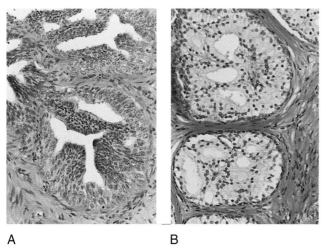 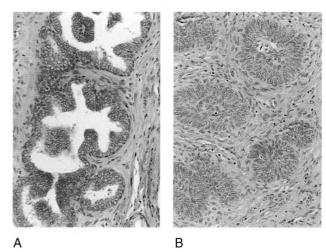

A   B   A   B

Figure 3–20. Prostatic intraepithelial neoplasia. Comparative photomicrographs of high-grade PIN (*A*) and clear cell cribriform hyperplasia (*B*). High-grade PIN is characterized by marked basophilia with enlargement and atypia of the nuclei.

Figure 3–21. Prostatic intraepithelial neoplasia. Comparison of high-grade PIN (*A*) with basal cell hyperplasia (*B*). The glands of high-grade PIN have a complex shape with more pronounced nuclear atypia.

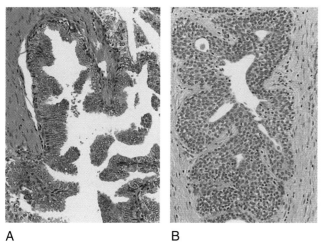 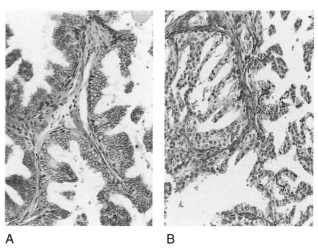

A   B   A   B

Figure 3–22. Prostatic intraepithelial neoplasia. Photomicrographs contrasting the characteristic features of high-grade PIN (*A*) with transitional cell metaplasia (*B*). The cells of high-grade PIN show a considerably greater nuclear atypia and complex tufted pattern compared with the smoother contours of the glands involved by transitional metaplasia.

Figure 3–23. Prostatic intraepithelial neoplasia. Comparison of high-grade PIN (*A*) with the normal glands of the central zone (*B*). The latter are complex in shape, but the cells have uniform, round nuclei and a pale eosinophilic cytoplasm.

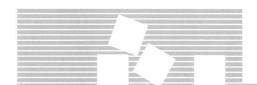

CHAPTER 4

Carcinoma of the Prostate

■ Adenocarcinoma

CLINICAL

- Prostate cancer is the most common malignancy occurring in men and the second leading cause of cancer deaths; over 317,000 new cases are expected in 1996 with about 41,400 related deaths.
- Early prostate cancer is asymptomatic, with obstructive symptoms usually not being produced until later in the disease course. Presently, increasing numbers of men are being diagnosed through testing (and screening) with serum prostate-specific antigen (PSA) and ultrasound-guided biopsies.
- Many patients are still initially diagnosed because of symptoms related to metastases, most often bone pain with radiographs revealing osteoblastic bone metastases.
- On digital rectal examination, the tumor may be nonpalpable or the prostate may have an isolated, hard nodule or diffuse firm irregularity. Asymmetry is a useful feature for identifying cancer.
- Treatment depends on the patient's age and general health status, the tumor stage, and the histologic grade.

STAGING OF PROSTATE CANCER (TNM)

Primary Tumor (T)
T1   Nonpalpable cancer
    T1a Five percent or less of TURP tissue
    T1b More than 5% of TURP tissue
    T1c Nonpalpable, nonvisible cancer detected by biopsy (elevated PSA)
T2   Palpable or visible cancer confined within the capsule
    T2a Involves 50% or less of one lobe
    T2b Involves more than 50% of one lobe
    T2c Involves both lobes
T3   Local extracapsular extension
    T3a Unilateral extracapsular extension
    T3b Bilateral extracapsular extension
    T3c Seminal vesicle invasion
T4   Invasion of adjacent organs and tissues
    T4a Invasion of bladder neck, rectum, or external sphincter
    T4b Invasion of levator muscle or pelvic wall

Regional Lymph Nodes (N)
NX Nodal status unknown
NO No lymph node involvement
N1 Single regional lymph node, 2 cm or less in greatest dimension
N2 Single regional lymph node, 2 to 5 cm, or multiple lymph nodes 5 cm or less
N3 Single regional lymph node, more than 5 cm

Distant Metastases (M)
MX Status unknown
MO No distant metastases
M1a Nonregional lymph nodes
M1b Bone
M1c Other sites

- Staging system is clinical; no separate pathologic system is presently available.
- In the radical prostatectomy specimen, T1 as an entity does not exist.
- It is possible to have positive surgical margins in T2 lesions if the resection specimen does not include extraprostatic tissue.
- Subdivision of T2 lesions is difficult because of the multifocal nature of prostate cancer; from a practical perspective, all pathologic stage T2 cancers with negative surgical margins have an excellent prognosis.
- Definition of extracapsular extension is not possible where a defined capsule does not exist—the anterior portion of the gland.
- Seminal vesicle invasion is defined by involvement of the muscularis.

GROSS

- In transurethral resection specimens, foci of adenocarcinoma may have a bright-yellow appearance, although gross evaluation is not reliable in identifying the tumor (see Chapter 1, Fig. 1–23).
- In radical prostatectomy specimens, tumor identification can be extremely difficult in the unfixed specimen. Areas of cancer may be yellow, but more often are gray-tan and

poorly defined. The tumor tends to have less of the spongy appearance of normal tissue. Palpation may be most valuable in localizing the tumor.

- In fixed specimens, the carcinoma tends to be firm and gray-white with a more solid appearance than uninvolved tissue.
- The tumor is typically multifocal, and gross evaluation generally underestimates the extent of disease.

MICROSCOPIC

- The vast majority of prostate cancers are adenocarcinomas (>95%).
- Most adenocarcinomas are composed predominantly or significantly of small glands (usual acinar type).
- The glands may be related to one another in a variety of architectural patterns (see descriptions below under Grading).
- Several special types (variants) of adenocarcinoma are recognized: mucinous, signet ring, ductal (endometrioid), carcinoid-like; small cell and sarcomatoid are described separately below.

Diagnostic Criteria

- For well-differentiated adenocarcinoma (Gleason grades 1, 2, and the small acinar pattern of 3), the criteria established by Gleason are those most widely accepted and applied.
- These criteria are that the lesion be composed of (1) *a relatively uniform proliferation* of (2) *small glands* lined by a (3) *single-layered epithelium* with at least some cells containing (4) *prominent nucleoli.*
- At scanning magnification, foci of well-differentiated adenocarcinoma can be suspected when the following features are seen (rule of three too's):
  - Too many glands (crowded).
  - Too small and uniform.
  - Too clear.

- The small glands of adenocarcinoma have a distinct appearance compared with adjacent benign glandular elements.
- Nucleoli by themselves are not diagnostic of cancer. Nucleoli can be seen in prostatitis, atrophy (especially postatrophic hyperplasia), sclerosing adenosis, atypical basal cell hyperplasia, atypical adenomatous hyperplasia, and prostatic intraepithelial neoplasia.
- Depending on how the term "prominent nucleoli" is defined, all adenocarcinomas may not fulfill these criteria. Most consider prominent nucleoli to be 1.25 to 1.5 μm in diameter.
- The nucleoli are not necessarily present in all cells; in low-grade cancers they may be apparent in only a few cells. Good histologic preparations of adequately fixed tissues are a prerequisite for evaluation of these lesions.
- Cell shape is cuboidal or tall columnar and always there is abundant cytoplasm in contrast to atrophy where cells usually have little cytoplasm.

References

Bostwick DG, Myers RP, Oesterling JE. Staging of prostate cancer. Semin Surg Oncol 10:60–72, 1994.

Bostwick DG, Srigley J, Grignon D, et al. Atypical adenomatous hyperplasia of the prostate: Morphologic criteria for its distinction from well-differentiated adenocarcinoma. Hum Pathol 24:819–832, 1993.

Gleason DF. Atypical hyperplasia, benign hyperplasia and well-differentiated adenocarcinoma of the prostate. Am J Surg Pathol 9(suppl):53–67, 1985.

Kelemen PR, Buschmann RJ, Weisz-Carrington P. Nucleolar prominence as a diagnostic variable in prostatic carcinoma. Cancer 65:1017–1020, 1990.

Kramer CE, Epstein JI. Nucleoli in low grade prostate cancer and adenosis. Hum Pathol 24:618–623, 1993.

Schroder FH, Hermanek P, Denis L, et al. The TNM classification of prostate cancer. Prostate 4(suppl):7–26, 1992.

Srigley JR. Small acinar patterns in the prostate gland with emphasis on atypical adenomatous hyperplasia and small-acinar carcinoma. Semin Diagn Pathol 5:254–272, 1988.

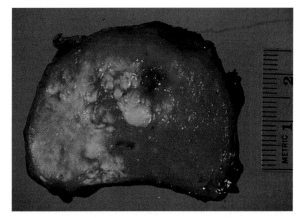

Figure 4–1. Adenocarcinoma. Cross section of the prostate gland showing extensive involvement of the left side of the gland, including both the peripheral zone and the transition zone, by prostatic adenocarcinoma. In this example, the tumor has a distinctive yellow color and, particularly in the transition zone region, is acquiring a somewhat nodular architecture.

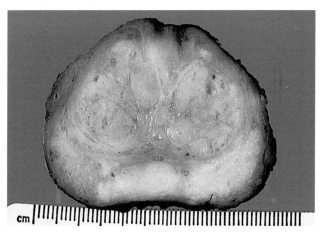

Figure 4–2. Adenocarcinoma. Cross section through the prostate gland showing a large peripheral zone adenocarcinoma involving the posterior and right posterior aspects of the gland. In this example the tumor has a gray-white color.

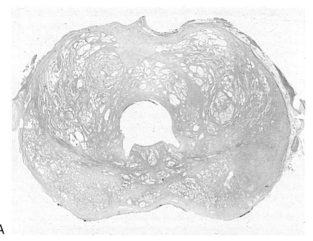
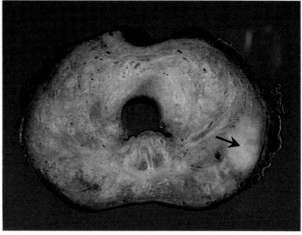

Figure 4–3. Adenocarcinoma. Gross photograph of a cross section of the prostate (*B*) showing a peripherally located nodule of adenocarcinoma *(arrow)*. Note the ejaculatory ducts in the verumontanum region. A whole-mount section (*A*) shows the corresponding area of small gland adenocarcinoma.

Helpful Features

PROSTATIC CRYSTALLOIDS

- Sharp-edged, brightly eosinophilic, needle-to-rectangular-to-rhomboid-shaped structures.
- Found in a large number of small acinar adenocarcinomas.
- Presence in a gland is not diagnostic of cancer, but does indicate a high likelihood that cancer is nearby.
- Crystalloids have also been described in sclerosing adenosis and atypical adenomatous hyperplasia.

References

Del Rosario AD, Bui HX, Abdulla M, et al. Sulfur-rich prostatic intraluminal crystalloids: A surgical pathologic and electron probe x-ray microanalytic study. Hum Pathol 24:1159–1167, 1993.

Ro JY, Ayala AG, Ordonez NG, et al. Intraluminal crystalloids in prostatic adenocarcinoma: Immunohistochemical, electron microscopic, and x-ray microanalytic studies. Cancer 57:2397–2407, 1986.

Ro JY, Grignon DJ, Troncoso P, et al. Intraluminal crystalloids in whole-organ sections of prostate. Prostate 13:233–239, 1988.

ACID MUCIN

- In H&E-stained sections it appears as wispy, basophilic material.
- Acid mucin (detected by alcian blue at pH 2.5) is frequently present in the lumen of small acinar adenocarcinoma.
- The presence of acid mucin is not restricted to adenocarcinoma, but can occasionally be found in atrophy, sclerosing adenosis, atypical adenomatous hyperplasia, prostatic intraepithelial neoplasia, and even usual hyperplasia.
- Intracytoplasmic mucin is not usually present in prostatic adenocarcinoma.

References

Epstein JI, Fynheer DA. Acid mucin in the prostate: Can it differentiate adenosis from adenocarcinoma? Hum Pathol 23:1321–1325, 1992.

Goldstein N, Qian J, Bostwick DG. Mucin expression in atypical adenomatous hyperplasia of the prostate. Hum Pathol 26:887–891, 1995.

Humphrey PA. Mucin in severe dysplasia in the prostate. Surg Pathol 4:137–143, 1991.

Ro JY, Grignon DJ, Troncoso P, et al. Mucin in prostatic adenocarcinoma. Semin Diagn Pathol 5:273–283, 1988.

PERINEURAL INFILTRATION

- A characteristic feature of prostate adenocarcinoma when present.
- Considered to be an important route by which tumor transgresses the prostatic capsule to invade periprostatic tissue.
- Since benign glands can be seen apposed to nerves, care must be taken in using this finding as a diagnostic criterion for malignancy.
- Invasion into the substance of a nerve or circumferential growth of the glands in a wreathlike fashion around a nerve would be unique to carcinoma.

References

Bastacky SI, Walsh PC, Epstein JI. Relationship between perineural tumor invasion on needle biopsy and radical prostatectomy capsular penetration in clinical Stage B adenocarcinoma of the prostate. Am J Surg Pathol 17:336–341, 1993.
Carstens PHB. Perineural glands in normal and hyperplastic prostates. J Urol 123:686–688, 1980.
McIntire TL, Franzini DA. The presence of benign prostatic glands in perineural spaces. J Urol 135:507–509, 1986.

COLLAGENOUS MICRONODULES

- A histologic feature associated with mucin production by prostatic adenocarcinoma.
- The nodules are composed of fibrillar eosinophilic material and are not found in benign conditions.

Reference

Bostwick DG, Wollan P, Adlakha K. Collagenous micronodules in prostate cancer: A specific but infrequent diagnostic finding. Arch Pathol Lab Med 119:444–447, 1995.

HIGH-MOLECULAR-WEIGHT CYTOKERATIN (HMWK)

- Expression of HMWK is restricted to prostatic basal cells; it is not present in secretory cells.
- Several studies have documented the usefulness of this test in confirming the absence of basal cells in cancer, and the presence of basal cells in benign small acinar lesions.
- The clone most frequently used is 34βE12 (CK903, a catalogue number, has frequently been used to refer to a specific commercially available antibody).
- The presence of "positive" cells in a small-gland lesion excludes the diagnosis of adenocarcinoma.
- While the absence of staining supports a diagnosis of cancer, it should not be considered diagnostic (lack of reactivity can be a technical problem). As with all antibodies, appropriate controls are essential for correct interpretation. In almost all biopsy specimens where this antibody is utilized, benign glandular elements will be present providing a valuable inbuilt control.

References

Brawer MK, Peehl DM, Stamey TA, et al. Keratin immunoreactivity in benign and neoplastic human prostate. Cancer Res 45:3665–3669, 1985.
Hedrick L, Epstein JI. Use of keratin 903 as an adjunct in the diagnosis of prostate carcinoma. Am J Surg Pathol 13:389–396, 1989.
O'Malley FP, Grignon DJ, Shum DT. Usefulness of immunoperoxidase staining with high-molecular-weight cytokeratin in the differential diagnosis of small-acinar lesions of the prostate. Virchows Arch [A] 417:191–196, 1990.
Wojno KJ, Epstein JI. The utility of basal cell–specific anti-cytokeratin antibody (34βE12) in the diagnosis of prostate cancer: Review of 228 cases. Am J Surg Pathol 19:251–260, 1995.

Grading

- Grading of prostatic adenocarcinoma has repeatedly been shown to correlate significantly with tumor stage and patient survival.

- Numerous grading systems have been proposed for prostatic adenocarcinoma. The most widely used are the Gleason, World Health Organization (Mostofi), and M.D. Anderson Cancer Center systems.
- Although numerous articles have been written detailing the advantages and disadvantages of the various systems, the Gleason system has become the most widely accepted system used in clinical decision-making.
- Grading of needle biopsy specimens has been shown to be a reliable indicator of grade when compared with radical prostatectomy specimens. Most errors are represented by undergrading on the needle biopsy.
- All prostate cancers should have a Gleason grade assigned, including needle biopsies containing limited material.

GLEASON GRADING SYSTEM

- This system, first proposed by Gleason in 1966, is based on the architectural growth pattern of the tumor and as such is based on the low-power impression of the tumor growth.
- The range of architectural histologic patterns is grouped into five grade categories.
- These are viewed as a continuum and so differences in individual grading are not unexpected.
- In the original Veterans Administration Cooperative Urological Research Group (VACURG) studies, tumors behaved more like the "average" grade than the worst.
- Because of this Gleason developed a "score" equal to the grade of the predominant pattern added to the grade of the second most prevalent pattern (e.g., 4 + 3 = 7).
- Most carcinomas show at least two patterns with a full spectrum present in some (particularly evident in radical prostatectomy specimens).
- In occasional cases, the two major patterns are from the low and high ends of the spectrum (e.g., 2 + 5 = 7).
- When reporting prostate cancers, both grades and the final score should be given even if only a single pattern is present (e.g., 3 + 3 = 6). This avoids potential confusion where only a single number is provided.
- In our experience, undergrading of prostate cancer is much more common than overgrading.
- Gleason grading of all prostate cancers is important in the therapeutic decision-making process which can range from no treatment ("watchful waiting") for low-grade cancers to the assumption that metastases are almost certainly present (high-grade cancers).
- Grouping of grades has been done differently by various groups.
- All concur that Gleason scores 8 to 10 constitute the "poorly differentiated," highly aggressive category.
- Recent studies indicate that Gleason score 7 cancers do not belong with Gleason score 5 and 6 tumors as an "intermediate" category.
- Some authorities consider any tumor harboring a Gleason grade 4 element to be potentially aggressive.
- Gleason score 2 to 4 carcinomas are almost exclusively of transition zone origin, have a low malignant potential, and are very uncommon in the needle biopsy or radical prostatectomy group of patients.

Grade 1

- Closely packed, uniform, round glands arranged in a nodule with pushing borders.
- Separation of glands at the periphery from the main collection by more than one gland diameter indicates a component of at least grade 2.
- This is a very uncommon pattern except in transition zone adenocarcinomas and is almost never seen in needle biopsy specimens.

Grade 2

- Similar to grade 1 except glands show more variability in shape and are separated by more stroma.
- Most glands are separated by less than one average gland diameter.
- At the periphery, a less circumscribed appearance is present, although infiltration into stroma and between benign glands is not seen.
- This pattern is common in transition zone adenocarcinomas, but much less frequent in peripheral zone cancers.
- The presence of even a few well-formed malignant glands in a needle biopsy (often interspersed among benign elements) indicates a grade 3 pattern and is not indicative of grades 1 or 2.

Grade 3

- Includes three distinct architectural patterns.
- Most common are well-formed, relatively uniform glands growing in an infiltrative manner; growth between benign glands is a useful clue to this grade.
- The glands may show an angulated pattern or can be compressed.
- The glands are separated by more than one gland diameter (a variable feature).
- The tumor cells in this pattern tend to have more basophilic cytoplasm and larger nucleoli than seen in grades 1 and 2.
- In the second pattern the glands are small with inconspicuous or even absent lumina.
- The glands are still separate without fusion into cords or chains (a grade 4 pattern).

- Finally, grade 3 includes papillary and cribriform patterns.
- The islands have smooth, rounded, pushing-type edges without stromal infiltration.

Grade 4

- The most common grade 4 pattern consists of small acinar structures, some with well-formed lumina, fusing into cords or chains; this pattern is frequently undergraded as 3.
- Grade 4 also includes papillary-cribriform tumors where the edges are more irregular with an invasive appearance; many, though not all, endometrioid carcinomas fall into this category.
- The hypernephroid pattern, characterized by nests of cells with abundant clear cytoplasm and small, hyperchromatic nuclei, is considered to be grade 4.
- The acini may also fuse into more solid sheets with the appearance of back-to-back glands without intervening stroma.

Grade 5

- This includes two major patterns.
- Carcinomas with little or no evidence of glandular differentiation fall into this grade category; these can range from infiltrating single cells (including signet ring cell carcinoma) to solid sheets of tumor cells.
- Papillary-cribriform carcinomas with central necrosis (comedocarcinoma pattern).

References

Bostwick DG. Gleason grading of prostatic needle biopsies: Correlation with grade in 316 matched prostatectomies. Am J Surg Pathol 18:796–803, 1994.

Epstein JI, Pizov G, Walsh PC. Correlation of pathologic findings with progression after radical retropubic prostatectomy. Cancer 71:3582–3593, 1993.

Gleason D. Classification of prostatic carcinomas. Cancer Chemother Rep 50:125–128, 1966.

Gleason DF. Histologic grading of prostatic carcinoma. In Bostwick DG (ed). *Pathology of the Prostate.* New York, Churchill Livingstone, 1990.

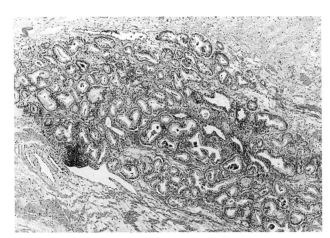

Figure 4–4. Adenocarcinoma. Low-power appearance of a Gleason grade 2 adenocarcinoma. The presence of closely packed, relatively uniform glands should raise the possibility of adenocarcinoma. Confirmation of the diagnosis requires evaluation at high magnification to fulfill the diagnostic criteria.

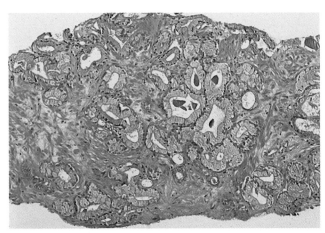

Figure 4–5. Adenocarcinoma. Focus of adenocarcinoma in a needle biopsy specimen. The relatively uniform, crowded small glands should raise the possibility of malignancy. In this case the tumor cells are tall and columnar with basally located nuclei (Gleason grade 3).

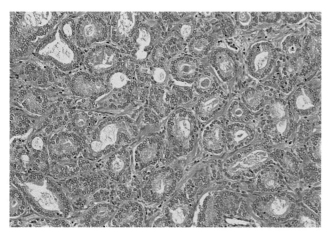

Figure 4–6. Adenocarcinoma. The crowded, uniform, small glands indicate the diagnosis of adenocarcinoma. High-power examination to fulfill the diagnostic criteria is required. This photomicrograph could be from either a Gleason grade 2 or a Gleason grade 3 adenocarcinoma.

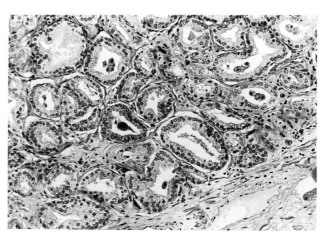

Figure 4–7. Adenocarcinoma. Edge of a nodule of a Gleason grade 2 adenocarcinoma showing a single cell layer and prominent nucleoli in many of the cells.

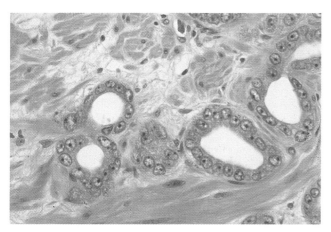

Figure 4–8. Adenocarcinoma. Focus of Gleason grade 3 adenocarcinoma showing the single cell layer and prominent nucleoli in individual cells.

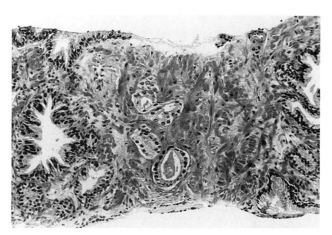

Figure 4–9. Adenocarcinoma. Small focus of a Gleason grade 3 adenocarcinoma in a needle biopsy. The small collection of uniform, round glands between the benign glandular elements on either side should immediately raise the possibility of adenocarcinoma.

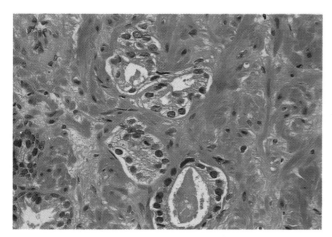

Figure 4–10. Adenocarcinoma. Detail of glands from Figure 4–9 showing a single cell layer and individual cells having prominent nucleoli. This small focus does fulfill the diagnostic criteria for adenocarcinoma.

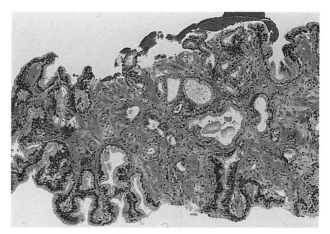

Figure 4–11. Adenocarcinoma. Small focus of Gleason grade 3 adenocarcinoma in a needle biopsy specimen. The presence of uniform, small glands interspersed among benign complex glandular elements should raise the possibility of malignancy.

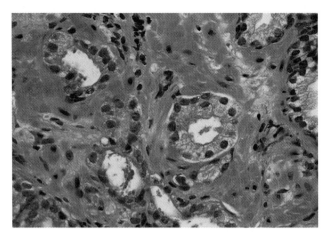

Figure 4–12. Adenocarcinoma. Detail of the small glands seen in Figure 4–11; the glands are lined by a single layer of epithelium with individual cells having prominent nucleoli. This fulfills the criteria for adenocarcinoma.

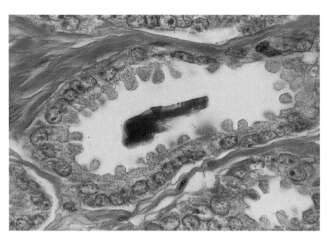

Figure 4–13. Adenocarcinoma. High-power image of prostatic crystalloid. Note the sharp edges, the intense eosinophilic staining, and the glassy "birefringent" appearance. (These structures are in fact not birefringent under polarized microscopy.)

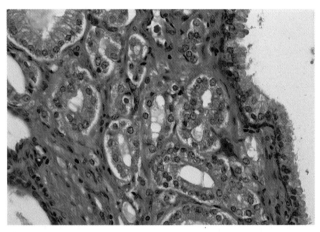

Figure 4–14. Adenocarcinoma. Gleason grade 3 adenocarcinoma with well-formed glands infiltrating between benign glandular elements. Note the presence of wispy bluish staining material within the glandular lumina. This corresponds to acidic-type mucin.

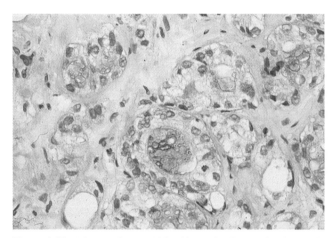

Figure 4–15. Adenocarcinoma. Alcian blue stain of prostatic adenocarcinoma demonstrating positivity of the luminal secretions.

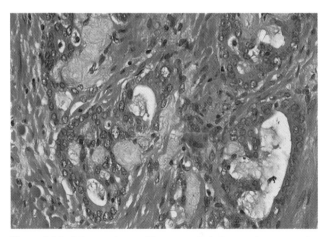

Figure 4–16. Adenocarcinoma. Gleason grade 4 adenocarcinoma containing multiple pink collagenous micronodules. Note also the presence of abundant basophilic mucin in the glandular lumina.

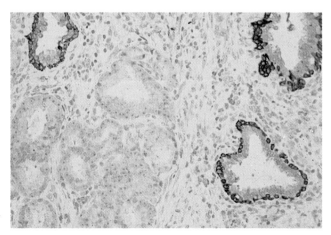

Figure 4–17. Adenocarcinoma. Prostatic adenocarcinoma stained for high-molecular-weight cytokeratin. The stain highlights the normal basal cell layer in the benign glands but shows a complete absence of staining in the adenocarcinoma.

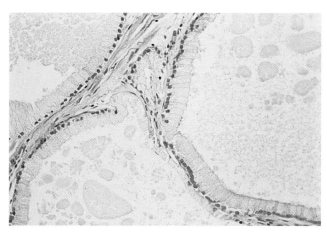

Figure 4–18. Adenocarcinoma. Example of a prostatic adenocarcinoma with cystic dilation of the malignant acini. The malignant cells have a tall columnar appearance with basally located nuclei and pale-staining cytoplasm (see Figure 4–19).

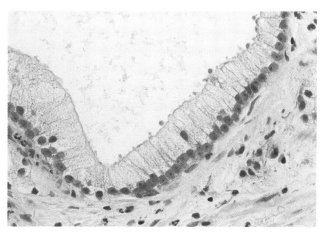

Figure 4–19. Adenocarcinoma. Detail of the cellular lining from a focus of cystic prostatic adenocarcinoma. The individual cells have basally located nuclei with prominent nucleoli (see Figure 4–18).

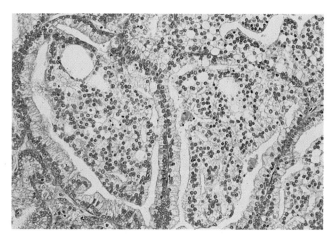

Figure 4–20. Adenocarcinoma. An unusual pattern of prostatic adenocarcinoma with a passing resemblance to clear cell cribriform hyperplasia. The cells, however, have large nuclei with prominent nucleoli.

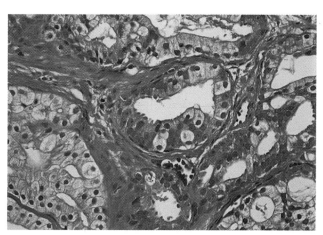

Figure 4–21. Adenocarcinoma. Photomicrograph of a Gleason grade 4 adenocarcinoma in which some of the cells have pale-staining cytoplasm (light cells), whereas others have more eosinophilic cytoplasm (dark cells).

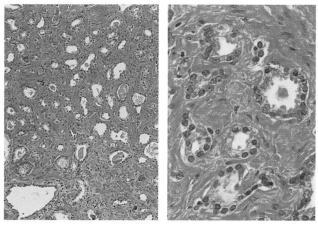

Figure 4–22. Adenocarcinoma. Gleason grade 3 adenocarcinoma in which the small glands have a somewhat ectatic appearance. The glands are lined by a single-layered epithelium with individual cells having prominent nucleoli.

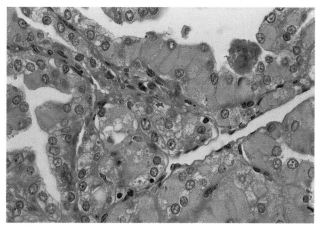

Figure 4–23. Adenocarcinoma. Gleason grade 4 adenocarcinoma in which many of the tumor cells have abundant eosinophilic cytoplasm producing an "apocrine-like" appearance.

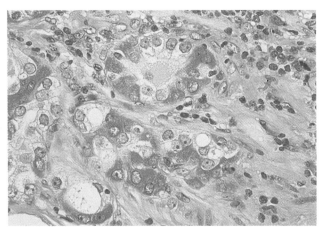

Figure 4–24. Adenocarcinoma. Prostatic adenocarcinoma containing many cells with abundant coarse eosinophilic granules (Paneth-like cells). These cells correspond to neuroendocrine differentiation.

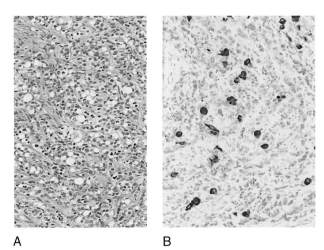

A   B

Figure 4–25. Adenocarcinoma. Gleason score 9 (4 + 5) adenocarcinoma showing numerous chromogranin-positive (*B*) neuroendocrine cells. In this case the neuroendocrine cells do not have a Paneth cell-like morphology on the hematoxylin and eosin–stained section (*A*).

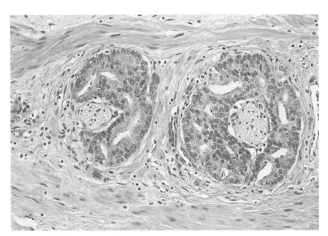

Figure 4–26. Adenocarcinoma. Perineural invasion by a prostatic adenocarcinoma (Gleason grade 4) producing a wreathlike appearance circumferentially around the nerve fibers.

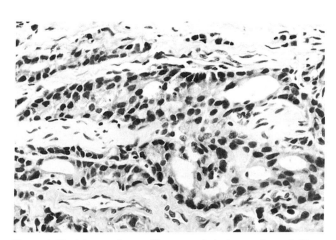

Figure 4–27. Adenocarcinoma. Gleason grade 4 adenocarcinoma infiltrating around and within the substance of a peripheral nerve fiber.

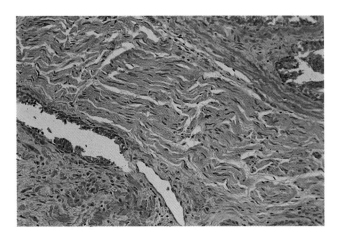

Figure 4–28. Normal gland. Benign prostatic glands adjacent to peripheral nerve fiber. Care must be taken not to overdiagnose as perineural invasion by carcinoma.

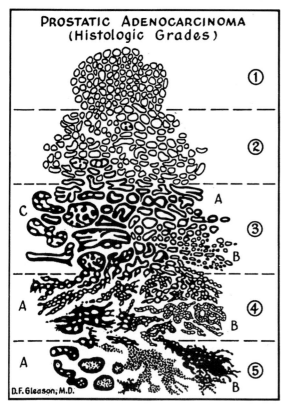

Figure 4–29. Diagrammatic representation of the Gleason grading system.

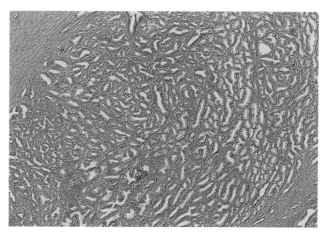

Figure 4–30. Gleason grade 1 adenocarcinoma. This circumscribed nodule is composed of relatively uniform glands sharply demarcated from the adjacent stroma. In our practice we would assign a Gleason score of 3 (1 + 2) to a similar nodule because of the variability of the gland shape as well as the presence of greater than one gland diameter of stroma between some glands within the tumor. In our experience Gleason grade 1 adenocarcinomas are extraordinarily rare and we practically never assign this as a pure grade.

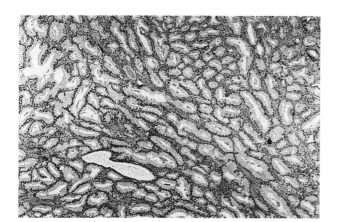

Figure 4–31. Gleason grade 1 adenocarcinoma. This photomicrograph shows the detail of the glandular tumor seen in Figure 4–30.

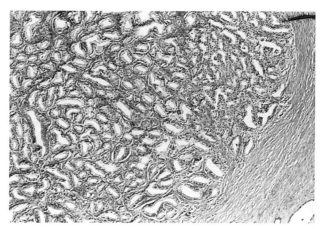

Figure 4–32. Gleason grade 2 adenocarcinoma. This circumscribed nodule of adenocarcinoma is composed of relatively uniform glands but with some branching and irregularity. In some areas there is stroma greater than one gland in diameter in width between adjacent glands.

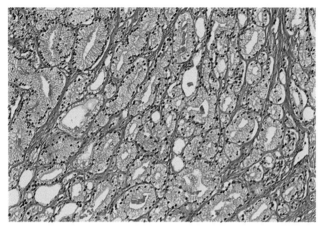

Figure 4–33. Gleason grade 2 adenocarcinoma. This tumor is composed of relatively uniform glands lined by cells having abundant pale-to-clear cytoplasm. This pattern is typical of the low-grade carcinomas originating in the transition zone.

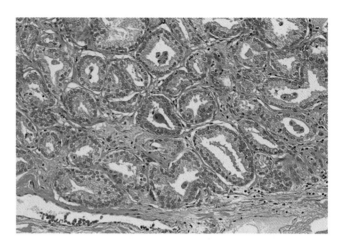

Figure 4–34. Gleason grade 2 adenocarcinoma. This tumor is composed of relatively uniform glands having more basophilic-staining cytoplasm than the tumor shown in Figure 4–33. Gleason grade 2 adenocarcinomas may have cytoplasmic characteristics more typical of grade 3 tumors as in this case.

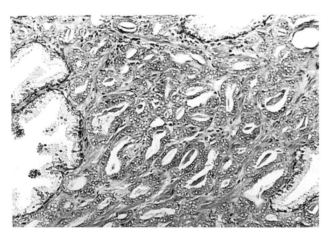

Figure 4–35. Gleason grade 3 adenocarcinoma. This tumor is composed of well-formed small glands which are diffusely infiltrating between benign glandular elements. The presence of a small acinar adenocarcinoma between normal glandular structures indicates at least a grade 3 pattern.

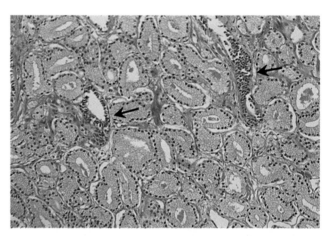

Figure 4–36. Gleason grade 3 adenocarcinoma. Another example of a tumor with well-formed glands infiltrating between residual benign glandular elements *(arrows)*.

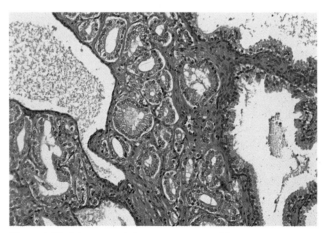

Figure 4–37. Gleason grade 3 adenocarcinoma. This tumor is also composed of well-formed glands infiltrating between benign glandular elements. Note the presence of basophilic secretions (acid mucin) within the glandular lumina.

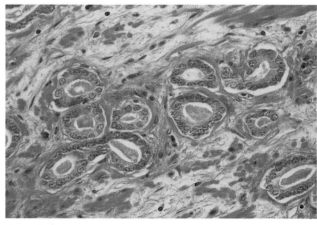

Figure 4–38. Gleason grade 3 adenocarcinoma. High-power photomicrograph showing well-formed glands containing eosinophilic material, with the lining epithelial cells having prominent nucleoli. This could also have originated from a Gleason grade 2 adenocarcinoma.

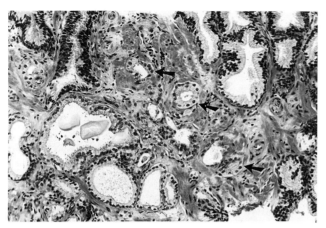

Figure 4–39. Gleason grade 3 adenocarcinoma. Scattered, well-formed glands *(arrows)* infiltrating between benign glandular elements. This photomicrograph is from a needle biopsy specimen.

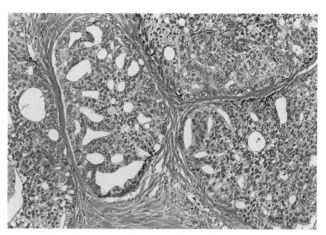

Figure 4–40. Gleason grade 3 adenocarcinoma. This illustrates the cribriform pattern of Gleason grade 3 adenocarcinoma. The tumor nests are sharply circumscribed with round, punched-out holes.

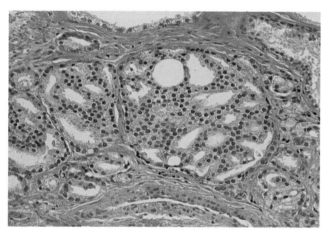

Figure 4–41. Gleason grade 3 adenocarcinoma. Another example of a cribriform pattern of Gleason grade 3 adenocarcinoma. An infiltrative grade 3 small acinar component is present also.

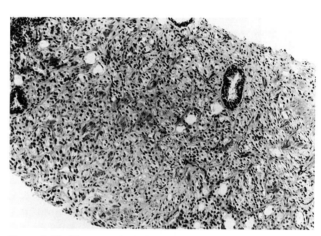

Figure 4–42. Gleason grade 4 adenocarcinoma. This needle biopsy specimen is diffusely permeated by a small acinar adenocarcinoma. Only a minority of the glands contain central lumina and there is fusion between many of the glandular structures.

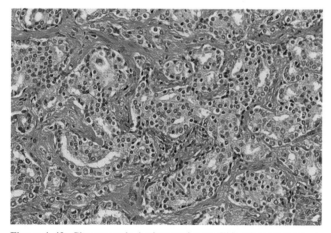

Figure 4–43. Gleason grade 4 adenocarcinoma. This adenocarcinoma is showing prominent fusion of the small acini producing a complex architectural pattern. This should not be confused with Gleason grade 3 adenocarcinoma in which the acini are separated by stroma.

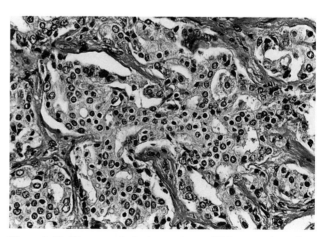

Figure 4–44. Gleason grade 4 adenocarcinoma. High-power photomicrograph of same case illustrated in Figure 4–43. Note the fusion of the small acini into a complex architectural pattern.

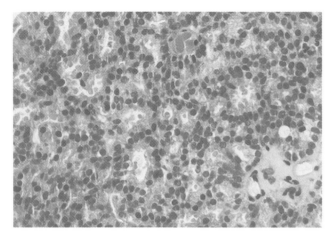

Figure 4–45. Gleason grade 4 adenocarcinoma. This tumor is composed of a solid sheet of fused glands without intervening stroma. This pattern should not be confused with a Gleason grade 3 cribriform pattern.

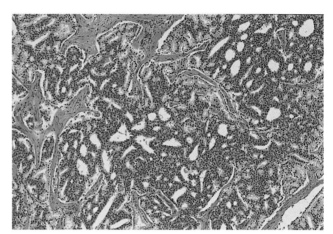

Figure 4–46. Gleason grade 4 adenocarcinoma. Complex papillary cribriform architecture with large irregularly outlined nests. This should not be confused with Gleason grade 3 cribriform adenocarcinoma.

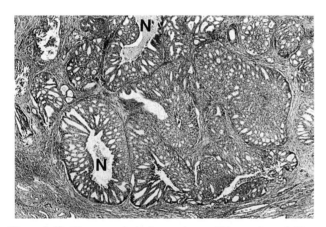

Figure 4–47. Gleason grade 4 adenocarcinoma. This complex cribriform architecture corresponds to a Gleason grade 4 adenocarcinoma. Although there are a few small islands that are well-circumscribed, the overall pattern is most compatible with a grade 4 neoplasm. The focal necrosis *(N)* indicates a minor grade 5 component in this case.

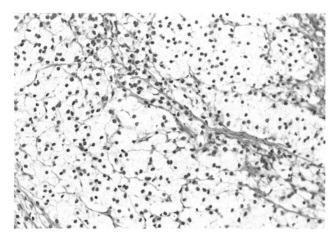

Figure 4–48. Gleason grade 4 adenocarcinoma. This tumor shows the hypernephroid pattern with cells having abundant clear cytoplasm and small uniform nuclei. This pattern could be confused with granulomatous prostatitis or prostatic xanthoma.

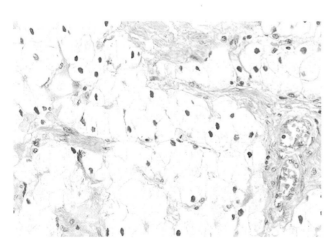

Figure 4–49. Gleason grade 4 adenocarcinoma. Another example of the hypernephroid pattern of prostate carcinoma. Despite the low-grade appearance of the nuclei, this is a high-grade pattern.

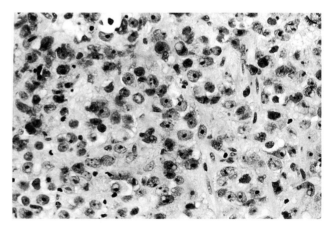

Figure 4–50. Gleason grade 5 adenocarcinoma. High-power photomicrograph from a Gleason grade 5 adenocarcinoma. Note that despite the high-grade architecture, the nuclei are relatively uniform and contain a single prominent nucleolus. This is a useful feature in differentiating this lesion from transitional cell carcinoma.

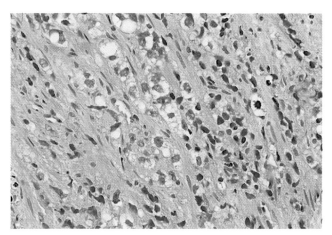

Figure 4–51. Gleason grade 5 adenocarcinoma. In this case the tumor is composed of infiltrating single cells with no evidence of glandular differentiation.

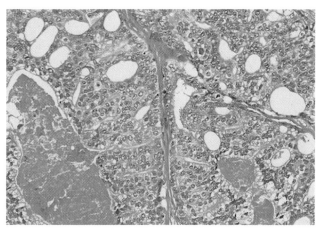

Figure 4–52. Gleason grade 5 adenocarcinoma. In this case comedonecrosis is seen within the center of this complex papillary cribriform pattern. The presence of comedonecrosis indicates a Gleason grade 5 tumor.

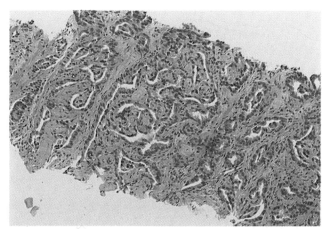

Figure 4–53. Gleason score 7 adenocarcinoma. This needle biopsy shows a predominant Gleason grade 4 pattern with infiltrating fused glands and a minor Gleason grade 3 element with individual small acinar formation *(right).*

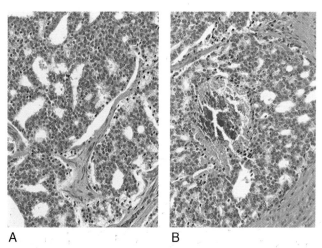

A   B

Figure 4–54. Gleason score 9 adenocarcinoma. This tumor shows a complex cribriform grade 4 pattern **(A)** with areas of comedonecrosis **(B,** grade 5). This combination is a relatively common finding.

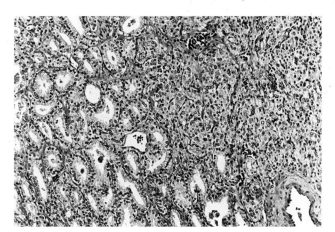

Figure 4–55. Gleason score 8 adenocarcinoma. This unusual tumor shows a well-formed Gleason grade 3 small gland component *(left)* merging with a poorly differentiated grade 5 component *(right),* which shows no glandular differentiation.

■ Special Types of Prostate Carcinoma

Mucinous Variant

CLINICAL

- Contrary to early reports, these tumors are now considered to be a variant of usual prostatic adenocarcinoma.
- Mucinous carcinoma is associated with elevated serum PSA, a similar pattern of metastases (including bone), and hormone sensitivity.
- Pure mucinous carcinoma is extremely rare.

GROSS

- May have a glistening, mucinous cut surface

MICROSCOPIC

- Characterized by mucin lakes containing tumor cells, often arranged in cribriform masses or incomplete glands.
- Virtually always associated with a typical acinar type of adenocarcinoma.
- Diagnosis of mucinous adenocarcinoma is restricted to cases with at least 25% of the tumor volume made up of the extracellular mucin lakes.
- This pattern is considered to be Gleason grade 4.

SPECIAL STAINS AND IMMUNOHISTOCHEMISTRY

- The mucin is positive with PAS, mucicarmine, and alcian blue; cytoplasmic mucin is usually not present.
- The tumor cells are PSA- and prostatic acid phosphatase (PAP)-positive by immunohistochemistry.
- Carcinoembryonic antigen (CEA) is negative.

DIFFERENTIAL DIAGNOSIS

- Mucinous carcinomas of bladder and rectum
- Cowper's gland adenocarcinoma
- Metastatic adenocarcinoma

References

Amin MB, Ro JY, Ayala AG. Clinical significance of histologic variants of adenocarcinoma of prostate. Cancer Bull 45:403–410, 1994.

Epstein JI, Lieberman PH. Mucinous adenocarcinoma of the prostate gland. Am J Surg Pathol 9:299–308, 1985.

Ro JY, Grignon DJ, Ayala AG, et al. Mucinous adenocarcinoma of the prostate: Histochemical and immunohistochemical studies. Hum Pathol 21:593–600, 1990.

Teichman JMH, Shabaik A, Demby AM. Mucinous adenocarcinoma of the prostate and hormone sensitivity. J Urol 151:701–702, 1994.

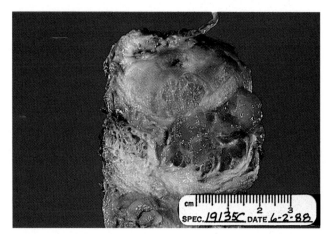

Figure 4–56. Mucinous adenocarcinoma. This gross photograph of a radical prostatectomy specimen shows extensive involvement of the gland by a mucin-producing adenocarcinoma. Large globules of glistening mucinous material are evident.

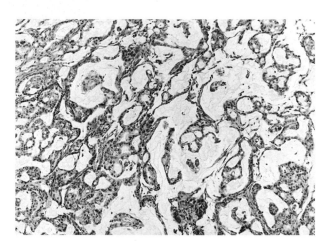

Figure 4–57. Mucinous adenocarcinoma. This adenocarcinoma shows abundant mucin production within the glandular lumina as well as in an extraglandular location. This is a Gleason grade 4 pattern.

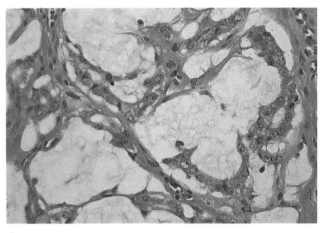
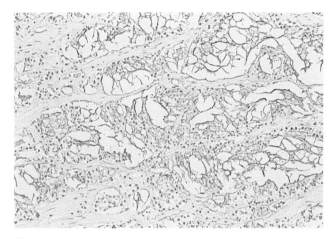

A   B

Figure 4–58. Mucinous adenocarcinoma. High-power photomicrograph of mucinous carcinoma (*A*) with positive staining for acid mucin (*B*, Alcian blue, pH 2.5).

Signet Ring Cell Carcinoma

CLINICAL

- Similar presentation to usual prostatic adenocarcinoma.
- Patients frequently present with an advanced stage; the tumor is associated with a poor prognosis.

GROSS

- No specific gross features

MICROSCOPIC

- Diagnosis restricted to cases with at least 25% signet ring cells.
- Cells have a cytoplasmic vacuole displacing the nucleus resulting in the typical signet ring appearance.
- Tumor cells diffusely permeate the prostatic stroma.
- Almost always associated with other patterns of poorly differentiated adenocarcinoma.
- The signet ring cells have been shown by electron microscopy to contain cytoplasmic vacuoles and intracytoplasmic lumina.

SPECIAL STAINS AND IMMUNOHISTOCHEMISTRY

- Mucin stains do not stain the cytoplasmic vacuoles in the majority of cases, a useful differential diagnostic feature.
- Tumor cells are positive for PSA and PAP.
- CEA: negative.

DIFFERENTIAL DIAGNOSIS

- Signet ring cell carcinoma from other sites
- Vacuolated lymphocytes and smooth muscle cells
- Granulomatous prostatitis (nonspecific type)

References

Alguacil-Garcia A. Artifactual changes mimicking signet ring cell carcinoma in transurethral prostatectomy specimens. Am J Surg Pathol 10:795–800, 1985.

Catton PA, Hartwick RWJ, Srigley JR. Prostate cancer presenting with malignant ascites: Signet-ring cell variant of prostatic adenocarcinoma. Urology 39:495–497, 1992.

Guerin D, Hasan N, Keen CE. Signet ring cell differentiation in adenocarcinoma of the prostate: A study of five cases. Histopathology 22:367–371, 1993.

Ro JY, El-Naggar A, Ayala AG, et al. Signet-ring cell carcinoma of the prostate. Am J Surg Pathol 12:453–460, 1988.

Segawa T, Kakehi Y. Primary signet ring cell adenocarcinoma of the prostate: A case report and literature review. Acta Urol Jpn 39:565–568, 1993.

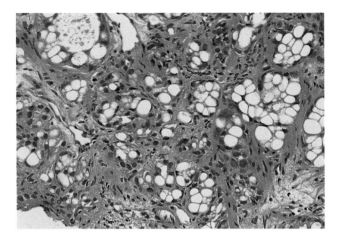

Figure 4–59. Signet ring cell carcinoma. Prostatic carcinoma with prominent signet ring differentiation. This is considered to be a Gleason grade 5 pattern.

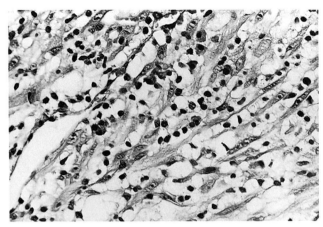

Figure 4–60. Signet ring cell carcinoma. This is the typical pattern of signet ring cell carcinoma seen in the prostate gland with an infiltrating poorly differentiated carcinoma showing signet ring morphology in a minority of the tumor cells (Gleason grade 5).

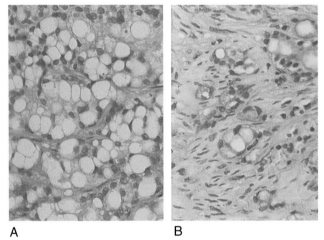

A   B

Figure 4–61. Signet ring cell carcinoma. In most cases of signet ring cell carcinoma the cytoplasmic vacuole does not stain for mucin (*A*). *B*, In a minority of cases the mucin stain is positive. (Both alcian blue, pH 2.5.)

Ductal (Endometrioid) Carcinoma

CLINICAL

- Clinical presentation in most is similar to usual prostatic adenocarcinoma.
- The tumor may be exophytic into the urethra producing a papillary lesion visible cystoscopically.
- In the latter, patients may present earlier with hematuria or obstruction and can be diagnosed on TURP specimen.
- Has been reported to have lower levels of serum PSA elevation than usual adenocarcinoma.

- Produces osteoblastic bone metastases.
- Originally it was considered to originate from the utricle, a female remnant in the prostate, indicating a likely lack of responsiveness to hormone therapy, a hypothesis now proved not to be true.

GROSS

- May have an exophytic component extending into the urethra, otherwise has no specific gross characteristics

MICROSCOPIC

- Usually, though not always, located primarily in the larger prostatic ducts in the periurethral region.
- Architecturally, grows with a papillary or cribriform pattern; frequently there is a mixture of the two.
- The tumor cells are columnar with pseudostratification and show significant nuclear anaplasia with large nuclei having coarse chromatin and prominent nucleoli.
- Mitoses are frequent.
- In the majority of cases there is an associated small acinar component.
- Most are considered to be Gleason grade 4.
- Comedonecrosis is common in this pattern; when present, this indicates Gleason grade 5.

SPECIAL STAINS AND IMMUNOHISTOCHEMISTRY

- The tumors are PSA- and PAP-positive.
- CEA has been reported to be positive in some cases.

DIFFERENTIAL DIAGNOSIS

- Transitional cell carcinoma
- Prostatic intraepithelial neoplasia
- Secondary involvement of prostate by colon carcinoma

References

Bostwick DG, Kindrachuk RW, Rouse RV. Prostatic adenocarcinoma with endometrioid features. Am J Surg Pathol 9:595–609, 1985.

Christenson WN, Steinberg C, Walsh PC, et al. Prostatic duct adenocarcinoma: Findings at radical prostatectomy. Cancer 67:2118–2124, 1991.

Epstein JI, Woodruff JM. Adenocarcinoma of the prostate with endometrioid features: A light microscopic and immunohistochemical study of 10 cases. Cancer 57:111–119, 1986.

Lee SS. Endometrioid adenocarcinoma of the prostate: A clinicopathologic and immunohistochemical study. J Surg Oncol 55:235–238, 1994.

Ro JY, Ayala AG, Wishnow KI, et al. Prostatic duct adenocarcinoma with endometrioid features: Immunohistochemical and electron microscopic study. Semin Diagn Pathol 5:301–311, 1988.

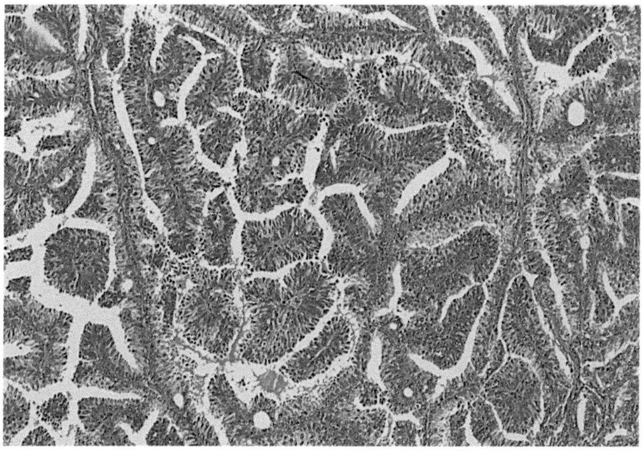

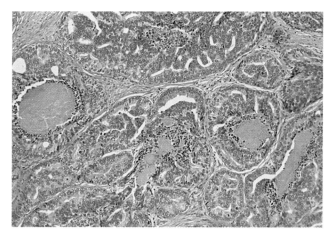

Figure 4–62. Ductal (endometrioid) adenocarcinoma. This papillary architecture is typically associated with carcinomas of ductal origin, although the pattern may be seen peripherally in the gland. This is considered a Gleason grade 4 pattern.

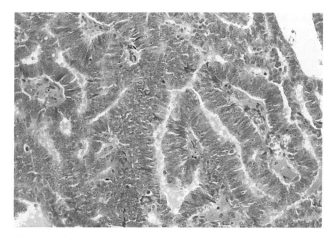

Figure 4–63. Ductal (endometrioid) adenocarcinoma. This photomicrograph illustrates the columnar shape and pseudostratification of the cells characteristic of a type I ductal (endometrioid) adenocarcinoma of the prostate.

Figure 4–64. Ductal (endometrioid) adenocarcinoma. This tumor shows predominantly a complex papillary cribriform pattern with central comedonecrosis (grade 5) pattern. This architecture has been referred to as a type II ductal (endometrioid) adenocarcinoma.

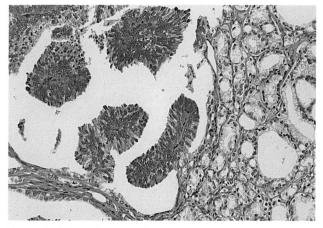

Figure 4–65. Ductal (endometrioid) adenocarcinoma. In most cases of ductal (endometrioid) carcinoma there is an associated small acinar-type adenocarcinoma, as in this case. The Gleason score for this focus would be 7 (4 + 3).

Small Cell Carcinoma

CLINICAL

- Similar signs and symptoms to usual prostate carcinoma.
- Rare cases with paraneoplastic syndromes are reported, including Cushing's syndrome, Eaton-Lambert syndrome, hypercalcemia, syndrome of inappropriate secretion of antidiuretic hormone (SIADH), and hyperglucagonemia.
- May be associated with relatively minor increases in serum PSA.
- Patients usually present with advanced-stage disease.
- Unusual metastatic patterns (e.g., liver involvement) can be present.
- May occur de novo but more often presents with the development of rapid progression without the anticipated increase in PSA level in a patient being followed for known prostate cancer (with or without therapy).

GROSS

- No specific gross features

MICROSCOPIC

- Diagnostic criteria are light-microscopic and the same as for bronchogenic small cell carcinoma.
- Cells may be oat cell or intermediate type.
- In over 50% of cases a typical acinar pattern of adenocarcinoma is associated.

- In some cases of prostatic adenocarcinoma, a carcinoid-like growth pattern without small cell features can be seen.

SPECIAL STAINS AND IMMUNOHISTOCHEMISTRY

- Neuroendocrine markers (neuron-specific enolase [NSE] and chromogranin) positive in many but not all cases
- Other specific neuroendocrine markers (e.g., serotonin, calcitonin, adrenocorticotropic hormone [ACTH], bombesin, etc.) present in some cases
- Cytokeratin positive in most (dotlike pattern)
- PSA and PAP only occasionally positive in small cell component and only in few cells; are positive in acinar areas when present.

DIFFERENTIAL DIAGNOSIS

- Metastatic small cell carcinoma (bladder, lung)
- Malignant lymphoma

References

Oesterling JE, Hauzear CG, Farrow GM. Small cell anaplastic carcinoma of the prostate: A clinical, pathological and immunohistological study of 27 patients. J Urol 147:804–809, 1992.

Ro JY, Tetu B, Ayala AG, et al. Small cell carcinoma of the prostate: II. Immunohistochemical and electron microscopic studies of 18 cases. Cancer 59:977–982, 1987.

Tetu B, Ro JY, Ayala AG, et al. Small cell carcinoma of the prostate: I. A clinicopathologic study of 20 cases. Cancer 59:1803–1809, 1987.

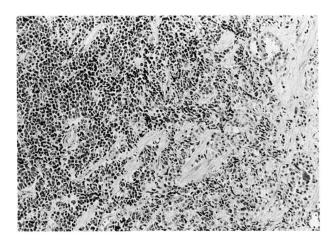

Figure 4–66. Small cell carcinoma. This case illustrates an admixture of small cell carcinoma *(left)* merging with a fused small gland adenocarcinoma *(right)*. The small cell component is made up of sheets of poorly cohesive cells with the characteristic nuclear features.

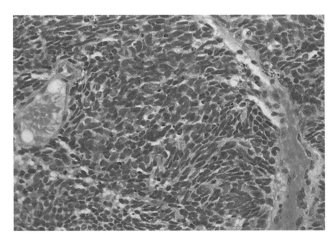

Figure 4–67. Small cell carcinoma. This small cell carcinoma has features of the intermediate cell variant with larger, more elongate nuclei with finely distributed chromatin and absent nucleoli.

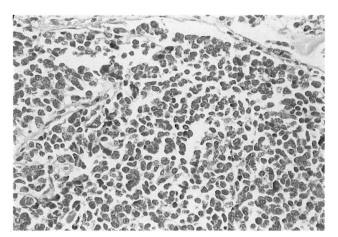

Figure 4–68. Small cell carcinoma. In this case the tumor cells have small hyperchromatic nuclei typical of the oat cell variant of small cell carcinoma.

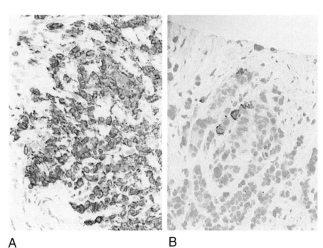

A   B

Figure 4–69. Small cell carcinoma. Immunohistochemical staining shows the majority of cells to be cytokeratin-positive (*A*) with variable reactivity for neuroendocrine markers such as chromogranin (*B*).

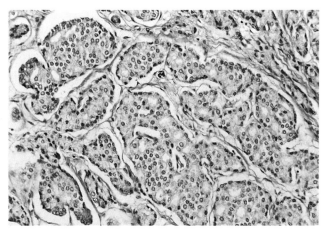

Figure 4–70. Prostatic carcinoma with "carcinoid-like" architecture. Some cases of prostatic carcinoma show features reminiscent of carcinoid tumors. This pattern does not necessarily correspond to the presence of neuroendocrine differentiation. This pattern of fused glands should be considered to represent a grade 4 pattern.

Sarcomatoid Carcinoma

Synonyms

- Carcinosarcoma
- Metaplastic carcinoma
- Spindle cell carcinoma
- Malignant mixed mesodermal tumor
- Carcinoma with pseudosarcomatous stroma

Clinical

- Often elderly patients.
- Almost always associated with previous or concurrent high-grade prostate adenocarcinoma.
- Approximately 50% have a history of prior radiation therapy for prostate cancer.
- Serum PSA may be normal or only slightly elevated.
- Very poor prognosis.

GROSS

- Large, fleshy, variegated gray-white tumors

MICROSCOPIC

- Biphasic tumors with carcinomatous and sarcomatoid components.
- Spindle cells have marked nuclear pleomorphism and frequent mitotic figures.
- Most common patterns are malignant fibrous histiocytoma-like and high-grade sarcoma of no specific type.
- Fibrosarcoma- and leiomyosarcoma-like patterns also seen.
- Heterologous elements such as osteosarcoma, chondrosarcoma, and rhabdomyosarcoma can be present.
- An associated high-grade carcinoma can usually be recognized.

SPECIAL STAINS AND IMMUNOHISTOCHEMISTRY

- Cytokeratin positivity in epithelial component and only focally or absent in sarcomatoid elements

- Carcinoma element PSA- and PAP-positive
- Spindle component vimentin-positive; other markers depend on type of heterologous element(s)

DIFFERENTIAL DIAGNOSIS

- Primary sarcoma
- Phyllodes tumor
- Postoperative spindle cell nodule
- Pseudosarcomatous fibromyxoid tumor

References

Dundore PA, Nascimento AG, Cheville JC, et al. Carcinosarcoma of the prostate: Report of 21 cases. Mod Pathol, in press.

Lauwers GY, Schevchuk M, Armenekas N, et al. Carcinosarcoma of the prostate. Am J Surg Pathol 17:342–349, 1993.

Shannon RL, Ro JY, Grignon DJ, et al. Sarcomatoid carcinoma of the prostate: A clinicopathologic study of 12 cases. Cancer 69:2676–2682, 1992.

Wick MR, Young RH, Malvesta R, et al. Prostatic carcinosarcomas: Clinical, histologic, and immunohistochemical data on two cases, with a review of the literature. Am J Clin Pathol 92:131–139, 1989.

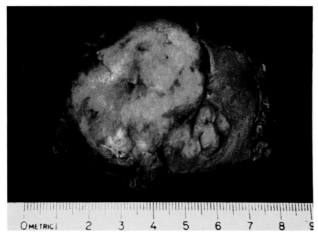

Figure 4–71. Sarcomatoid carcinoma. This gross photograph shows a prostatic carcinoma with extensive sarcomatoid differentiation. Note the gray-white sarcomatous-looking areas apparent even on gross examination.

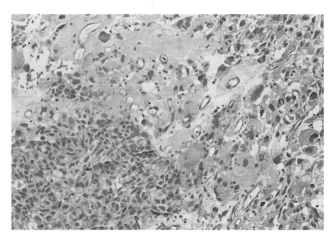

Figure 4–72. Sarcomatoid carcinoma. Mixed pattern with a poorly differentiated carcinomatous component (*bottom left*) merging with an unclassified high-grade sarcoma pattern.

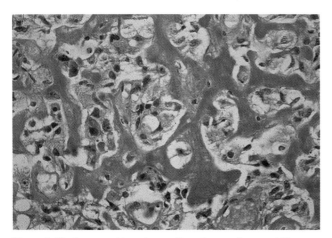

Figure 4–73. Sarcomatoid carcinoma. Heterologous element within a sarcomatoid carcinoma showing an osteosarcomatous growth pattern.

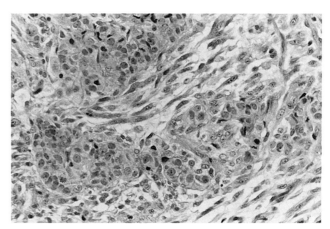

Figure 4–74. Sarcomatoid carcinoma. Transition between the recognizable poorly differentiated carcinomatous component and a malignant spindle cell component.

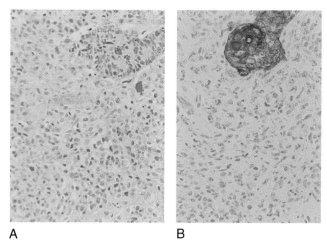

A   B

Figure 4–75. Sarcomatoid carcinoma. Immunohistochemical stain for cytokeratin (*B*) showing positivity within the carcinomatous component and no reactivity within the malignant spindle cell element.

Carcinomas of Transition Zone Origin

CLINICAL

- Approximately 10% to 20% of prostate adenocarcinomas have origin in the transition zone.
- May produce obstructive symptoms early.
- Frequently diagnosed in transurethral resection specimens (account for a high percentage of stage T1a [A1] carcinomas).
- Less aggressive than carcinomas of peripheral zone origin.
- Tend to spread anteriorly and into bladder, rarely involve seminal vesicles and lymph nodes.
- Atypical adenomatous hyperplasia has been proposed as a possible precursor lesion.

GROSS

- Nodular (often associated with prostatic hyperplasia)
- Bright-yellow

MICROSCOPIC

- Most are low-grade, Gleason grades 1 and 2 (McNeal has said that Gleason grades 1 and 2 carcinoma define transition zone origin).
- Arise adjacent to or within hyperplastic nodules (about one third of cases).
- Composed of uniform glands with pale (clear) cytoplasm and small nuclei; nucleoli often difficult to identify.

- May be composed of irregularly shaped glands with papillary infoldings (like BPH) lined by a single layer of tall columnar cells with clear cytoplasm ("tall-cell variant") and basally located nuclei having prominent nucleoli.

SPECIAL STAINS AND IMMUNOHISTOCHEMISTRY

- High-molecular-weight cytokeratin staining shows lack of basal cells.
- Tumor cells are PSA- and PAP-positive.

DIFFERENTIAL DIAGNOSIS

- Atypical adenomatous hyperplasia
- Nodular prostatic hyperplasia

References

Greene DR, Wheeler TM, Egawa S, et al. Relationship between clinical stage and histological zone of origin in early prostate cancer: Morphometric analysis. Br J Urol 68:499–509, 1991.

Lee F, Siders DB, Torp-Pedersen ST, et al. Transrectal ultrasound and pathology comparison: A preliminary study of outer gland (peripheral and central zone) and inner gland (transition zone) cancer. Cancer 67:1132–1142, 1991.

McNeal JE, Price H, Redwine EA, et al. Stage A versus Stage B adenocarcinoma of the prostate: Morphologic comparison and biologic significance. J Urol 139:61–68, 1988.

McNeal JE, Redwine EA, Freiha FS, et al. Zonal distribution of prostatic adenocarcinoma: Correlation with histologic pattern and direction of spread. Am J Surg Pathol 12:897–906, 1988.

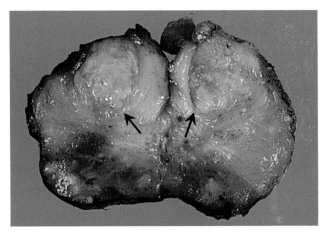

Figure 4–76. Transition zone adenocarcinoma. Cross section of prostate gland illustrating bilateral foci of adenocarcinoma arising in the transition zone. The tumor has a nodular growth pattern with distinctive yellow coloration *(arrows)*.

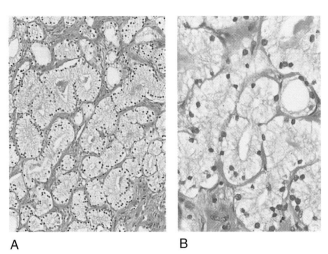

A   B

Figure 4–77. Transition zone adenocarcinoma. These photomicrographs illustrate the characteristic features of a small acinar adenocarcinoma arising in the transition zone. The cells have clear cytoplasm and relatively uniform, small nuclei. Although characteristic of adenocarcinomas arising in the transition zone, this pattern is not entirely specific.

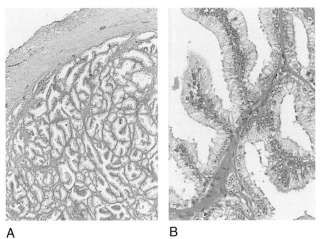

A   B

Figure 4–78. Transition zone adenocarcinoma. *A,* This unusual pattern of adenocarcinoma arising in the transition zone closely mimics nodular prostatic hyperplasia. *B,* At higher power the single cell lining with individual cells having prominent nucleoli can be appreciated.

■ Treatment Effects

Estrogens

CLINICAL

- Treatment with estrogenic agents (diethylstilbestrol) is no longer a commonly applied therapeutic strategy, having been largely supplanted by antiandrogen (total androgen blockade) therapy.

MICROSCOPIC

- Nuclei are shrunken and hyperchromatic (pyknotic) with loss of nucleoli.
- Cytoplasmic vacuolization.
- Squamous metaplasia in normal tissue and less often in the tumor.

SPECIAL STAINS AND IMMUNOHISTOCHEMISTRY

- Reduced expression of PSA and PAP in some cases
- High-molecular-weight cytokeratin negative in carcinoma but may be positive in areas of squamous metaplasia, including malignant glands showing this change

DIFFERENTIAL DIAGNOSIS

- Atrophy
- Granulomatous prostatitis (nonspecific type)

References

Grignon DJ, Sakr WA. Histologic effects of radiation therapy and total androgen blockade on prostate cancer. Cancer 75:1837–1841, 1995.

Grignon DJ, Troster M. Changes in immunohistochemical staining of prostatic adenocarcinoma following diethylstilbestrol therapy. Prostate 7:195–202, 1985.

Schenken JR, Burns EL, Kahle PJ. The effect of diethylstilbestrol and diethylstilbestrol dipropionate on carcinoma of the prostate gland: II. Cytologic changes following treatment. J Urol 48:98–112, 1942.

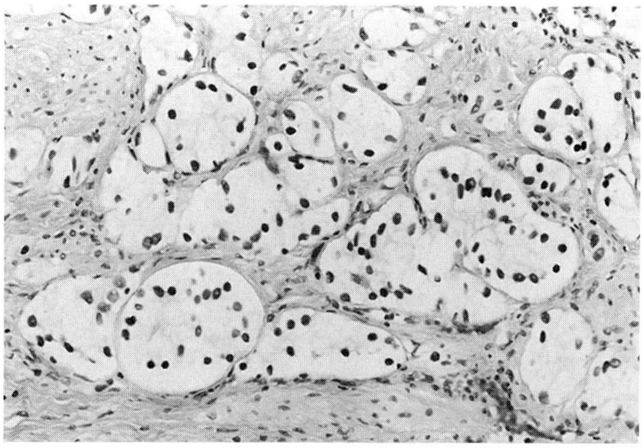

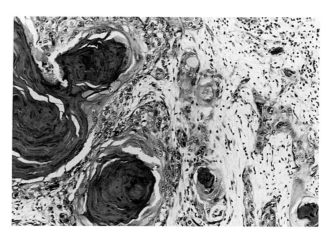

Figure 4–79. Therapy effect. The characteristic effect of estrogen on a small acinar carcinoma is illustrated in this photomicrograph. The tumor cells have ballooned clear cytoplasm and small pyknotic nuclei.

Figure 4–80. Therapy effect. Following estrogen therapy this prostatic carcinoma shows squamous differentiation within the tumor.

Total Androgen Blockade

CLINICAL

- Luteinizing hormone–releasing hormone (LHRH) agonists (e.g., leuprolide) and direct antiandrogens (e.g., flutamide) for total androgen blockade are currently in widespread use.
- Clinical uses include (1) treatment of metastatic disease, (2) cytoreduction prior to radiation therapy, and (3) "downstaging" prior to radical prostatectomy.

MICROSCOPIC

- In normal prostate tissue effects include atrophy, vacuolization of cells, basal cell hyperplasia, squamous and transitional cell metaplasia, and a lymphocytic infiltrate.
- Malignant glands become shrunken with individual cells having clear cytoplasm and small nuclei without nucleoli.

- The tumor may consist only of isolated cells with clear cytoplasm scattered in the stroma (histiocyte-like). Cytokeratin staining may be necessary to identify these as epithelial cells.
- Degree of effect can show considerable variability even in the same patient.
- Application of Gleason grading is problematic; many tumors appear to be higher grade after therapy, reflecting the treatment effects. For prognostic and treatment purposes, the pretreatment grade should be used. We do not grade posttreatment biopsies.

SPECIAL STAINS AND IMMUNOHISTOCHEMISTRY

- High-molecular-weight cytokeratin negative in tumor glands.
- PSA staining reduced and can be negative; PAP is less affected.
- Cytokeratin is positive and useful in identifying single tumor cells.

DIFFERENTIAL DIAGNOSIS

- Atrophy
- Normal tissue with therapy effects
- Inflammatory and stromal cells
- Poorly differentiated carcinoma

References

Armas OA, Aprikian AG, Melamed J, et al. Clinical and pathobiological effects of neoadjuvant total androgen ablation therapy on clinically localized prostatic adenocarcinoma. Am J Surg Pathol 18:979–991, 1994.

Grignon DJ, Sakr WA. Histologic effects of radiation therapy and total androgen blockade on prostate cancer. Cancer 75:1837–1841, 1995.

Murphy WM, Soloway MS, Barrows GH. Pathologic changes associated with androgen deprivation therapy for prostate cancer. Cancer 68:821–828, 1991.

Smith DM, Murphy WM. Histologic changes in prostate carcinomas treated with leuprolide (luteinizing hormone-releasing hormone effect): Distinction from poor tumor differentiation. Cancer 73:1472–1474, 1994.

Tetu B, Srigley JR, Boivin J, et al. Effect of combination endocrine therapy (LHRH agonist and flutamide) on normal prostate and prostatic adenocarcinoma. Am J Surg Pathol 15:111–120, 1991.

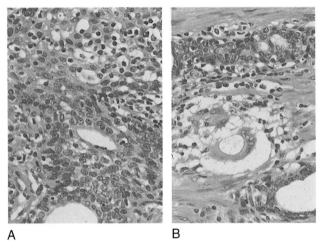

A   B

Figure 4–81. Therapy effect. Normal prostate tissue following antiandrogen treatment showing transitional cell metaplasia (*A*) and giant cell reaction (*B*). Note also the chronic inflammatory infiltrate.

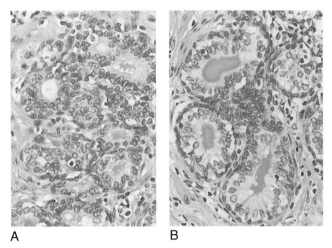

A   B

Figure 4–82. Therapy effect. Normal tissues following antiandrogen therapy showing basal cell hyperplasia and chronic inflammatory infiltrate.

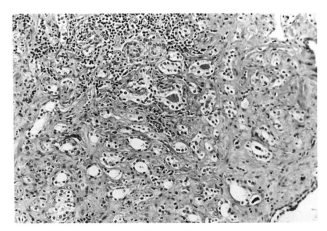

Figure 4–83. Therapy effect. Characteristic morphology of small acinar adenocarcinoma following antiandrogen therapy. The glands are small and shrunken with clearing of the cytoplasm and many nuclei are small and hyperchromatic.

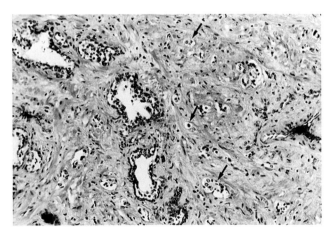

Figure 4–84. Therapy effect. Residual adenocarcinoma following antiandrogen therapy. Note the small shrunken malignant glands and isolated individual tumor cells *(arrows)*. Recognition of this characteristic pattern will aid in identifying tumor in posttreatment biopsy or resection material..

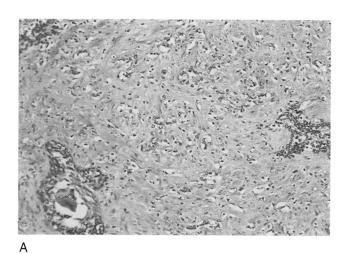 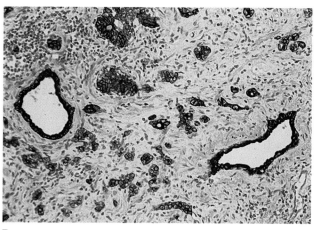

A   B

Figure 4–85. Therapy effect. **A,** Identification of residual tumor following antiandrogen therapy may be difficult. **B,** Immunohistochemical staining for cytokeratin can aid in identifying tumor cells and distinguishing them from histiocytes within the stroma.

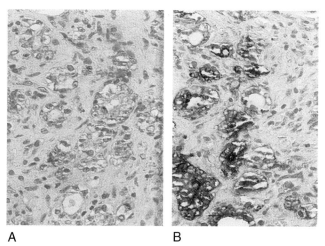

A   B

Figure 4–86. Therapy effect. Following antiandrogen therapy, tumor cells frequently show weak or no immunoreactivity for prostate-specific antigen (*A*), but reactivity of prostatic acid phosphatase (*B*) is usually retained.

Radiation Therapy

CLINICAL

- Significance of needle biopsy findings after radiation therapy (implants or external beam) has been the subject of considerable debate.
- Positive posttherapy biopsies are associated with higher local recurrence rate and reduced survival (compared with patients having negative biopsies).
- A significant proportion of patients (up to 30%) with positive posttherapy biopsies do not develop local or distant failure.

GROSS

- The prostate gland is reduced in size.

MICROSCOPIC

- Normal tissue effects include glandular atrophy with marked cytologic atypia of epithelial cells (secretory and basal).
- Tumor glands may be unchanged, atrophic, or reduced to isolated, single cells.
- Tumor cells often have abundant clear cytoplasm.

- Nuclei may be small and pyknotic or remain large with prominent nucleoli.
- Therapy effects can be variable, even within the same patient.
- Gleason score may increase after therapy, reflecting the treatment effect; we do not grade posttreatment biopsies.

SPECIAL STAINS AND IMMUNOHISTOCHEMISTRY

- High-molecular-weight cytokeratin is negative in tumor; positive staining helps recognize normal glands with radiation effects.
- PCNA (proliferating cell nuclear antigen) has been reported to help distinguish patients with positive biopsies who are unlikely to fail (no positive nuclei)
- Tumor cells are PSA- and PAP-positive.

DIFFERENTIAL DIAGNOSIS

- Normal tissue with radiation effects

References

Bostwick DG, Egbert EM, Fajardo LF. Radiation injury of the normal and neoplastic prostate. Am J Surg Pathol 6:541–548, 1982.

Crook J, Robertson S, Collin G, et al. Clinical relevance of trans-rectal ultrasound biopsy, and serum prostate-specific antigen following external beam radiotherapy for carcinoma of the prostate. Int J Radiat Oncol Biol Phys 27:31–37, 1993.

Crook J, Robertson S, Esche B. Proliferative cell nuclear antigen in postradiotherapy prostate biopsies. Int J Radiat Oncol Biol Phys 30:303–308, 1994.

Siders DB, Lee F. Histologic changes of irradiated prostatic carcinoma diagnosed by transrectal ultrasound. Hum Pathol 23:344–351, 1992.

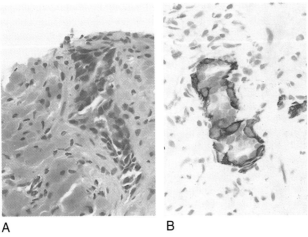

A   B

Figure 4–87. Therapy effect. *A,* Radiation-induced atypia in residual benign glands is characterized by enlarged hyperchromatic nuclei, often with smudging of the chromatin and eosinophilia of the cytoplasm. *B,* Immunohistochemical staining for high-molecular-weight cytokeratin highlights the basal cells, confirming the benign nature of the glands.

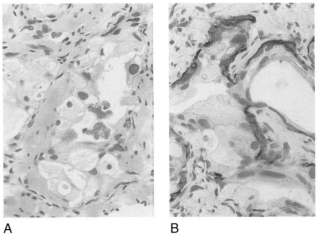

A   B

Figure 4–88. Therapy effect. Radiation-induced atypia in normal glands. In this case the secretory cells have enlarged nuclei with abundant pale-to-vacuolated cytoplasm. The presence of basal cells, highlighted by immunohistochemical staining for high-molecular-weight cytokeratin *(B),* confirms the benign nature of these glands.

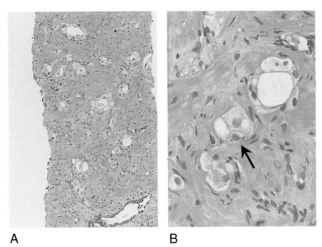

A   B

Figure 4–89. Therapy effect. Post–radiation therapy needle biopsy showing scattered residual malignant glands haphazardly arranged within the stroma *(A).* The tumor cells show clear cytoplasm and have large nuclei, some with prominent nucleoli *(B, arrow).*

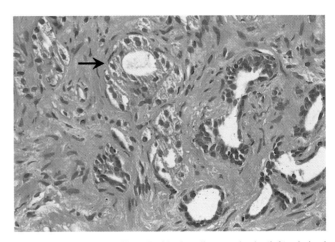

Figure 4–90. Therapy effect. Residual malignant glands *(left)* admixed with atrophic glands *(right)* following external beam radiation therapy. Note the presence of basophilic mucin within the lumen of one of the acini *(arrow).*

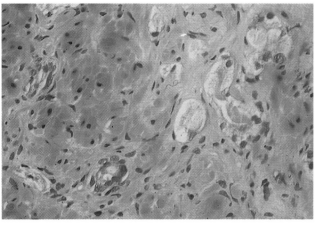

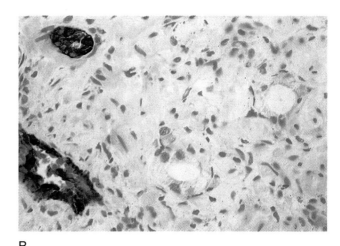

A

B

Figure 4–91. Therapy effect. Composite photomicrographs showing residual isolated tumor cells following radiation therapy. The individual cells have abundant clear cytoplasm. Some nuclei continue to have open chromatin with prominent nucleoli. Immunohistochemical staining for high-molecular-weight cytokeratin (*B*) shows positive staining of the residual benign glands but an absence of reactivity in the residual tumor acini.

Cryotherapy

CLINICAL

• A new modality gaining popularity for the treatment of clinically localized prostate cancer

GROSS

• Little information available on gross features in human prostates following cryotherapy

MICROSCOPIC

• The principal effect of cryotherapy is the induction of ischemic necrosis.
• There is loss of the epithelial elements with replacement by fibrosis.
• Hemosiderin-laden macrophages and calcifications are present.
• Regenerating ducts and acini show basal cell hyperplasia and squamous metaplasia.

• Residual carcinoma, when present, usually demonstrates no treatment effects.

SPECIAL STAINS AND IMMUNOHISTOCHEMISTRY

• Residual normal or neoplastic epithelium is PSA- and PAP-positive.

DIFFERENTIAL DIAGNOSIS

• Prostatic infarction

References

Bahn DK, Lee F, Solomon MH, et al. Prostate cancer: US-guided percutaneous cryoablation. Radiology 194:551–556, 1995.
Onik GM, Cohen JK, Reyes GD, et al. Transrectal ultrasound-guided percutaneous radical cryosurgical ablation of the prostate. Cancer 72:1291–1299, 1993.
Shabaik A, Wilson S, Bidair M, et al. Pathologic changes in prostate biopsies following cryoablation therapy of prostate carcinoma. J Urol Pathol 3:183–193, 1995.

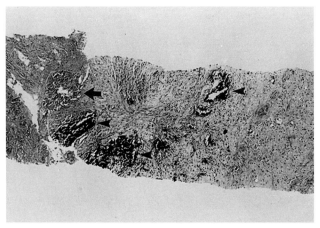

Figure 4–92. Therapy effect. Needle biopsy of prostate gland following cryotherapy. Note the areas of necrosis *(arrow)* and calcification *(arrowheads).*

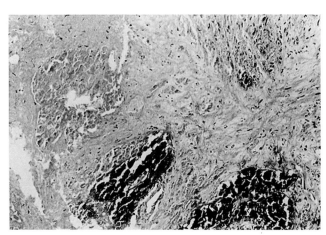

Figure 4–93. Therapy effect. Alterations characteristic of cryotherapy include tissue necrosis *(left)* and calcification (high power of Figure 4–92).

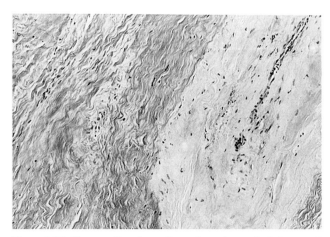

Figure 4–94. Therapy effect. Late effects of cryotherapy include stromal fibrosis and hyalinization. Typically scattered hemosiderin-laden macrophages are also noted.

■ Other Carcinomas

Transitional Cell Carcinoma

CLINICAL

• Three types of prostate involvement: (1) primary origin in prostatic urethra, ducts, or acini; (2) secondary mucosal involvement (reflecting pagetoid spread or multifocality) in patient with prior or synchronous bladder cancer; and (3) direct invasion by a bladder cancer through the bladder wall.

• Mucosal type of involvement present in up to 40% of patients with invasive bladder cancer, especially when associated with carcinoma in situ.

- Staging and treatment depend on degree of involvement (urethra only or ducts and acini) and presence or absence of prostatic stromal invasion.
- For limited involvement, bacille Calmette-Guérin (BCG) immunotherapy remains an option; with more extensive disease and if stromal invasion is present, radical cysto-prostatectomy is indicated.
- Presence of stromal invasion is a poor prognostic sign.

GROSS

- Depends on degree of involvement

MICROSCOPIC

- Papillary transitional cell carcinoma can occur in the prostatic urethra and rarely involves proximal ducts.
- In the vast majority of cases, involvement is by transitional cell carcinoma in situ involving the urethra, prostatic ducts, and acini, and in some instances the ejaculatory ducts and seminal vesicles.
- Pagetoid spread is characteristic.
- Glandular differentiation is rare.
- Nuclei are pleomorphic with hyperchromasia, chromatin clumping, often angular nuclear borders, and single-to-multiple nucleoli; mitoses are frequent.
- Stromal invasion is associated with desmoplasia.

SPECIAL STAINS AND IMMUNOHISTOCHEMISTRY

- PSA and PAP immunostains are negative (the luminal surface of the cells may show some reactivity related to luminal secretions).
- High-molecular-weight cytokeratin is positive in up to 50% of high-grade transitional cell carcinomas.

DIFFERENTIAL DIAGNOSIS

- Prostate adenocarcinoma
- Prostatic intraepithelial neoplasia
- Basal cell hyperplasia
- Transitional cell metaplasia

References

Hardeman SW, Soloway MS. Transitional cell carcinoma of the prostate: Diagnosis, staging and management. World J Urol 6:170–174, 1988.

Seemayer TA, Knaack J, Thelmo WL, et al. Further observations on carcinoma in situ of the urinary bladder: Silent but extensive intraprostatic involvement. Cancer 36:514–520, 1975.

Wood DP Jr, Montie JE, Pontes JE, et al. Transitional cell carcinoma of the prostate in cystoprostatectomy specimens removed for bladder cancer. J Urol 141:346–349, 1989.

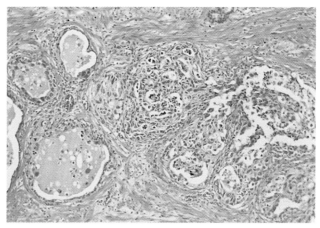

Figure 4–95. Transitional cell carcinoma. Transitional cell carcinoma in situ involving prostatic ducts and acini. Note the piling-up of the epithelial cells producing a cribriform-type appearance.

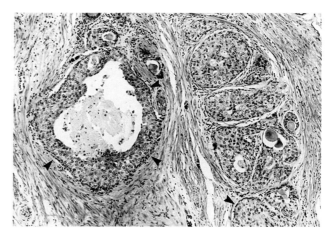

Figure 4–96. Transitional cell carcinoma. Transitional cell carcinoma in situ involving prostatic ducts. Residual concretions can be seen within the lumina and a residual layer of basal cells is evident even at this magnification *(arrowheads)*.

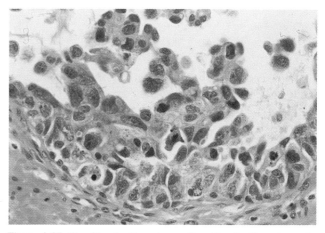

Figure 4–97. Transitional cell carcinoma. Transitional cell carcinoma in situ involving a prostatic duct highlighting the characteristic cytologic features. Note the marked nuclear pleomorphism and absence of single prominent nucleoli characteristic of ductal-type prostatic adenocarcinoma.

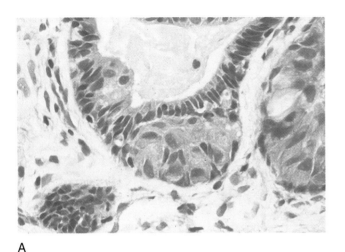

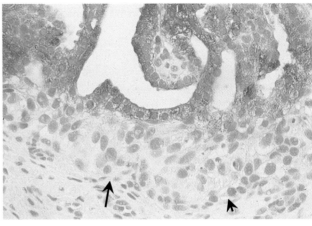

A

B

Figure 4–98. Transitional cell carcinoma. *A,* Transitional cell carcinoma in situ growing in a pagetoid fashion undermining the residual secretory cells. *B,* The secretory cells stain positively for prostate-specific antigen, but the transitional cell carcinoma cells are negative *(arrows).*

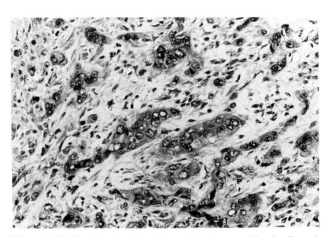

Figure 4–99. Transitional cell carcinoma. Invasive transitional cell carcinoma in the prostate gland. Note the striking stromal desmoplasia, a feature not usually seen with primary prostatic adenocarcinoma.

Adenoid Basal Cell Tumor, Basal Cell Carcinoma, Adenoid Cystic Carcinoma

CLINICAL

- No specific clinical features described.
- Have been reported over a wide age range.
- May present with obstructive symptoms or a mass.
- To date none of these lesions has been reported with invasion beyond the gland or with metastases.

GROSS

- No characteristic features

MICROSCOPIC

- These tumors have been viewed as a continuum by some authors, beginning with basal cell hyperplasia.
- Adenoid basal cell tumor is similar to basal cell hyperplasia but involves much more of the gland, producing a mass lesion.
- Adenoid basal cell tumor forms circumscribed nodules having typical basal cell hyperplasia-like areas admixed with adenoid cystic-like areas having basaloid cells surrounding spaces containing mucinous and eosinophilic material. The stroma is cellular and often loose or myxoid.
- Basal cell carcinoma has been diagnosed when similar lesions are associated with an infiltrative growth pattern and cytologic atypia (mitoses, enlarged nucleoli).

- Adenoid cystic carcinoma (adenoid cystic-like tumor) is diagnosed when features typical of adenoid cystic carcinoma elsewhere, including perineural invasion, are seen.

SPECIAL STAINS AND IMMUNOHISTOCHEMISTRY

- Mucinous material stains with acid and neutral mucin stains.
- PAS stain with and without diastase highlights the eosinophilic material.
- High-molecular-weight cytokeratin stains the basaloid cells (typically focal and weak).
- Secretory cells are PSA- and PAP-positive.
- S-100 protein and muscle-specific actin are negative.

DIFFERENTIAL DIAGNOSIS

- Basal cell hyperplasia

- Sclerosing adenosis
- Adenocarcinoma (cribriform type)

References

Cohen RJ, Goldberg RD, Verhaart MJ, et al. Adenoid cyst-like carcinoma of the prostate gland. Arch Pathol Lab Med 117:799–801, 1993.

Devaraj LT, Bostwick DG. Atypical basal cell hyperplasia of the prostate: Immunophenotypic profile and proposed classification of basal cell proliferations. Am J Surg Pathol 17:645–659, 1993.

Grignon DJ, Ro JY, Ordonez NG, et al. Basal cell hyperplasia, adenoid basal cell tumor, and adenoid cystic carcinoma of the prostate gland: An immunohistochemical study. Hum Pathol 19:1425–1433, 1988.

Ronnett BM, Epstein JI. A case showing sclerosing adenosis and an unusual form of basal cell hyperplasia of the prostate. Am J Surg Pathol 13:866–872, 1989.

Young RH, Frierson HF, Mills SE, et al. Adenoid cystic-like tumor of the prostate gland: A report of two cases and review of the literature on "adenoid cystic carcinoma" of the prostate. Am J Clin Pathol 89:49–56, 1988.

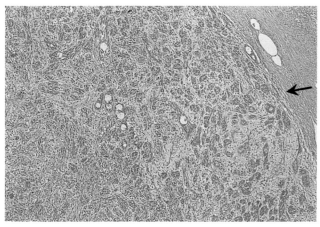

Figure 4–100. Adenoid basal cell tumor. Low-power photomicrograph showing the sharp demarcation of the lesion from the adjacent prostatic stroma *(arrow)*. The mixture of epithelial and stromal elements is readily apparent, even at this low magnification.

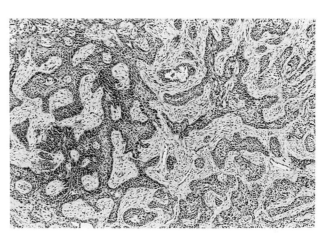

Figure 4–101. Adenoid basal cell tumor. In this focus the lesion consists of anastomosing islands of basaloid cells within a cellular stroma.

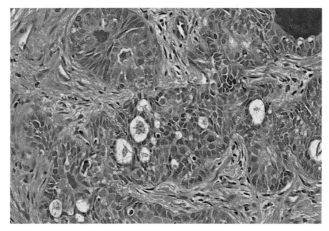

Figure 4–102. Adenoid basal cell tumor. Epithelial component showing basaloid cells with a focal cribriform architecture (periodic acid–Schiff stain).

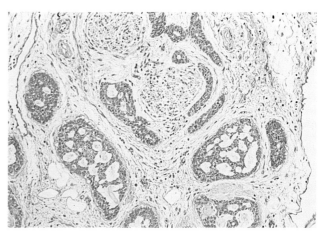

Figure 4–103. Adenoid cystic carcinoma. Prostatic tumor showing the characteristic histologic features of adenoid cystic carcinoma with cribriform architecture. Some spaces contain alcian blue–positive mucin, whereas others contain dense eosinophilic material.

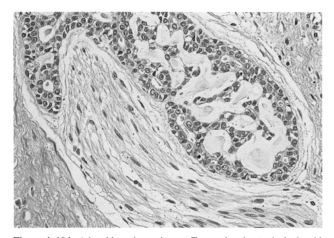

Figure 4–104. Adenoid cystic carcinoma. Tumor showing typical adenoid cystic carcinoma architecture with perineural invasion.

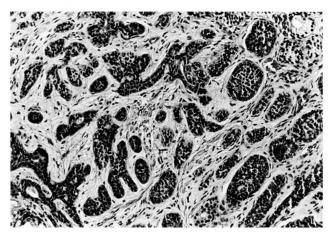

Figure 4–105. Basal cell carcinoma. Infiltrative tumor composed of basaloid cells with hyperchromatic nuclei and stromal desmoplasia.

Squamous and Adenosquamous Carcinoma

CLINICAL

- No specific features; presentation similar to other prostate cancers.
- PSA and PAP should not be elevated in pure tumors.
- Bone metastases are osteolytic.
- May be associated with *Schistosoma haematobium* infection.

GROSS

- No specific gross features

MICROSCOPIC

- May be pure or mixed with adenocarcinoma.
- Islands and cords of malignant cells with squamous differentiation.
- Criteria for diagnosis of pure squamous cell carcinoma include:
  - Unequivocal malignant growth.
  - Definite squamous features (keratin formation or intercellular bridges).
  - No glandular component.
  - No prior radiation or hormonal therapy.
  - Exclusion of primary origin elsewhere.
- Adenosquamous carcinoma is usually associated with prior radiation or hormonal therapy.

SPECIAL STAINS AND IMMUNOHISTOCHEMISTRY

- Reported cases of pure squamous cell carcinoma have been PSA-positive or -negative and PAP-negative.
- Adenosquamous carcinomas have PSA and PAP positivity in the glandular component.

DIFFERENTIAL DIAGNOSIS

- Squamous metaplasia
- Squamous carcinoma from elsewhere (especially bladder)
- Transitional cell carcinoma with squamous differentiation

References

Al Adani MS. Schistosomiasis, metaplasia and squamous cell carcinoma of the prostate: Histogenesis of the squamous cells determined by localization of specific markers. Neoplasma 32:613–622, 1991.

Gattuso P, Carson HJ, Candel A, et al. Adenosquamous carcinoma of the prostate. Hum Pathol 26:123–126, 1995.

Moskovitz N, Munichor M, Bolkier M, et al. Squamous cell carcinoma of the prostate. Urol Int 51:181–183, 1993.

Saito R, Davis BK, Ollipally EP. Adenosquamous carcinoma of the prostate. Hum Pathol 15:87–89, 1984.

Sarma DP, Weilbaecher TG, Moon TD. Squamous cell carcinoma of prostate. Urology 37:260–262, 1991.

Wernert N, Goebbels R, Bonkhoff H, et al. Squamous cell carcinoma of the prostate. Histopathology 17:339–344, 1990.

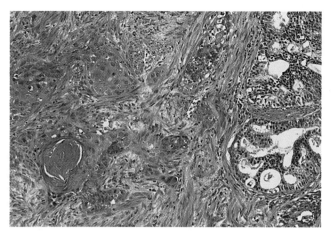

Figure 4–106. Adenosquamous carcinoma. Prostatic tumor showing a mixture of a squamous cell carcinoma *(left)* with a poorly differentiated adenocarcinoma *(right)*.

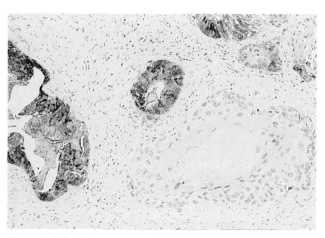

Figure 4–107. Adenosquamous carcinoma. Immunohistochemical stain for PSA showing positive reactivity in the glandular component and absence of staining in the squamous areas.

CHAPTER 5

Mesenchymal, Lymphoreticular, and Secondary Tumors

■ Mesenchymal Tumors

Stromal Nodule

CLINICAL

- Occurs in the setting of usual hyperplasia (BPH)

GROSS

- Usually microscopic

MICROSCOPIC

- Circumscribed proliferation of spindle-shaped cells without associated glandular elements.
- Cells arranged in fascicular or whorled pattern, often in a myxoid background.
- Individual cells are bland with no nuclear pleomorphism and absence of mitotic figures.
- Thick-walled blood vessels in background.
- Separation from leiomyoma somewhat arbitrary with the latter being encapsulated and greater than 1 cm in diameter.

SPECIAL STAINS AND IMMUNOHISTOCHEMISTRY

- Spindle cells are vimentin- and actin-positive.

DIFFERENTIAL DIAGNOSIS

- Leiomyoma
- Pseudosarcomatous fibromyxoid tumor
- Usual hyperplasia

Reference

Tetu B, Ro JY, Ayala AG, et al. Atypical spindle cell lesions of the prostate. Semin Diagn Pathol 5:284–293, 1988.

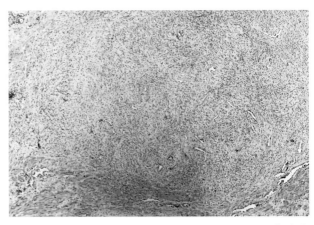

Figure 5–1. Stromal nodule. Circumscribed nodule composed of spindle-shaped cells with blood vessels scattered throughout.

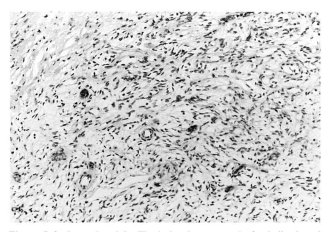

Figure 5–2. Stromal nodule. The lesion is composed of spindle-shaped cells in a loose myxoid background containing scattered small blood vessels.

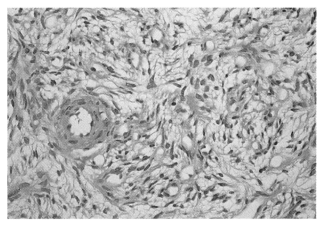

Figure 5–3. Stromal nodule. Spindle- and stellate-shaped cells in a loose myxoid background with scattered small blood vessels.

Leiomyoma

CLINICAL

• Wide age range but some cases reported under age 40

GROSS

• Whorled, bulging cut surface
• Usually over 1 cm

MICROSCOPIC

• Spindle cells in intersecting fascicles with a variably collagenized background
• Blunt-ended nuclei without significant nuclear pleomorphism or mitotic activity
• Encapsulated or sharply circumscribed without invasion into adjacent stroma or structures
• Absence of necrosis

SPECIAL STAINS AND IMMUNOHISTOCHEMISTRY

• Stains reflect the smooth muscle origin of the lesion— vimentin, muscle-specific actin, and desmin are all positive.

DIFFERENTIAL DIAGNOSIS

• Usual stromal nodule
• Pseudosarcomatous fibromyxoid tumor
• Leiomyosarcoma
• Other sarcomas
• Sarcomatoid carcinoma

References

Leonard A, Baert L, Van Praet F, et al. Solitary leiomyoma of the prostate. Br J Urol 60:184–187, 1988.
Regan JB, Barrett DM, Wold LE. Giant leiomyoma of the prostate. Arch Pathol Lab Med 111:381–383, 1987.

Pseudosarcomatous Fibromyxoid Tumor

CLINICAL

• Very rare lesion; may produce obstructive symptoms
• No prior history of operative procedure
• Important because may simulate sarcoma (mass lesion, spindle cells with atypia and mitoses, infiltrative growth)
• Cases reported to date not associated with recurrence or metastases

GROSS

• Nodular, fungating mass
• Average 4 to 5 cm in greatest dimension

MICROSCOPIC

• Ill-defined, infiltrative myxoid lesion with variable cellularity.
• Spindle cells have eosinophilic cytoplasm and may be elongate, plump, or stellate, with atypical cells present. The latter may be strap cell-like or tadpole-shaped.
• Nuclei are large and open with prominent nucleoli. Mitoses are present (<3 per 10 high-power field), but abnormal forms are not found.
• The background includes a granulation tissue-like vascular pattern and a prominent inflammatory infiltrate.

SPECIAL STAINS AND IMMUNOHISTOCHEMISTRY

- Spindle cells are vimentin- and smooth muscle actin (SMA)-positive, indicating fibroblastic or myofibroblastic differentiation.

DIFFERENTIAL DIAGNOSIS

- Stromal nodule, leiomyoma
- Postoperative spindle cell nodule

- Sarcoma
- Sarcomatoid carcinoma

References

Ro JY, El-Naggar A, Amin MB, et al. Pseudosarcomatous fibromyxoid tumor of the bladder and prostate: Immunohistochemical, ultrastructural, and DNA flow cytometric analysis of nine cases. Hum Pathol 24: 1203–1210, 1993.
Sahin AA, Ro JY, El-Naggar A, et al. Pseudosarcomatous fibromyxoid tumor of the prostate. Am J Clin Pathol 96:253–258, 1991.

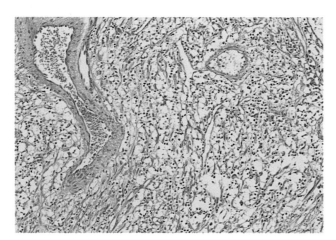

Figure 5–4. Pseudosarcomatous fibromyxoid tumor. Spindle- and stellate-shaped cells in a loose fibromyxoid background with scattered, variably sized blood vessels.

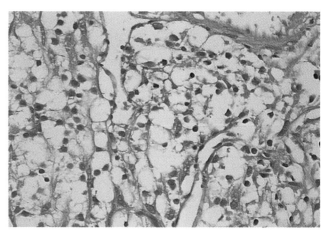

Figure 5–5. Pseudosarcomatous fibromyxoid tumor. Spindle- and stellate-shaped cells in loose fibromyxoid stroma with a sprinkling of inflammatory cells in the background.

Postoperative Spindle Cell Nodule

CLINICAL

- Develops in patients who have had prior surgery or instrumentation. The lesion itself is asymptomatic although it could possibly cause obstruction or hematuria.

GROSS

- Most are small (<1 cm), although lesions up to 4 cm have been described.

MICROSCOPIC

- Composed of intersecting fascicles of plump spindle cells having no nuclear pleomorphism.
- Generally uniformly cellular.
- Mitoses can be frequent (up to 25 per 10 high-power fields), but abnormal mitotic figures are absent.
- Background is edematous with scattered blood vessels and low-to-moderate numbers of inflammatory cells.

- Margins of the lesion are ill defined and it may have an infiltrative appearance.

SPECIAL STAINS AND IMMUNOHISTOCHEMISTRY

- Spindle cells are vimentin- and smooth muscle actin–positive. Desmin reactivity is variable.
- Cytokeratin positivity has been reported in some cases.

DIFFERENTIAL DIAGNOSIS

- Stromal nodule, leiomyoma
- Pseudosarcomatous fibromyxoid tumor
- Sarcoma
- Sarcomatoid carcinoma

References

Huang WL, Ro JY, Grignon DJ, et al. Postoperative spindle cell nodule of the prostate and bladder. J Urol 143:824–826, 1990.
Proppe KH, Scully RE, Rosai J. Postoperative spindle cell nodules of the genitourinary tract resembling sarcomas: A report of eight cases. Am J Surg Pathol 8:101–108, 1984.

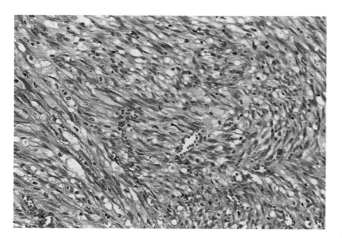

Figure 5–6. Postoperative spindle cell nodule. Cellular spindle cell lesion with poorly formed fascicles and congested small blood vessels.

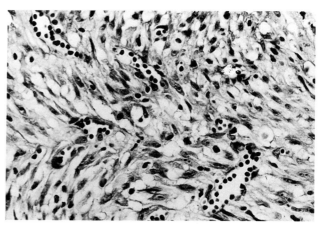

Figure 5–7. Postoperative spindle cell nodule. Cellular lesion composed of spindle-shaped cells without significant nuclear atypia. Mitotic figures may be frequent.

Phyllodes Tumor

CLINICAL

- Wide age range (23–78 years)
- Most often present with obstruction, but hematuria and dysuria have also been reported
- Most cured by resection, but local recurrences can develop

GROSS

- Gray-white, solid masses, sometimes with a spongy texture, usually between 4 and 25 cm, but examples up to 58 cm in diameter have been described

MICROSCOPIC

- Biphasic tumors with epithelial and stromal elements similar to those seen in phyllodes tumors of the breast.
- Epithelial cells are cuboidal to columnar with a double cell layer and are arranged in glands, cysts, or slitlike spaces.
- Stromal cells are spindle to stellate-shaped, arranged in a loose myxoid stroma with varying degrees of cellularity.
- Histologic evidence of malignancy, including pronounced hypercellularity, nuclear pleomorphism, and mitotic activity, have only rarely been reported, but are associated with a higher likelihood of recurrence.

SPECIAL STAINS AND IMMUNOHISTOCHEMISTRY

- Spindle cells are vimentin-positive, but smooth muscle actin and desmin are negative, indicating fibroblastic origin.
- Epithelial cells are prostate-specific antigen (PSA)- and prostatic acid phosphatase (PAP)-positive.

DIFFERENTIAL DIAGNOSIS

- Malignant phyllodes tumor
- Sarcoma
- Sarcomatoid carcinoma

References

Bostwick DG, Halling AC, Jones EC, et al. Prostatic phyllodes tumor: Proposed grading system based on clinicopathologic study of seven cases and review of the literature. In press.

Kevwitch MK, Walloch JL, Waters WB, et al. Prostatic cystic epithelial-stromal tumors: A report of 2 new cases. J Urol 149:860–864, 1993.

Maluf HM, King ME, DeLuca FR, et al. Giant multilocular prostatic cystadenoma: A distinctive lesion of the retroperitoneum in men. Am J Surg Pathol 15:131–135, 1991.

Young JF, Jensen PE, Wiley CA. Malignant phyllodes tumor of the prostate: A case report with immunohistochemical and ultrastructural findings. Arch Pathol Lab Med 116:296–299, 1992.

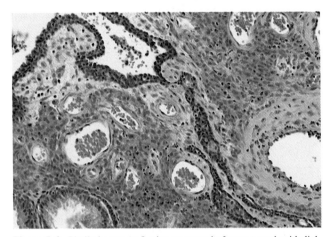

Figure 5–8. Phyllodes tumor. Lesion composed of compressed epithelial-lined structures with variable cellularity in the stroma.

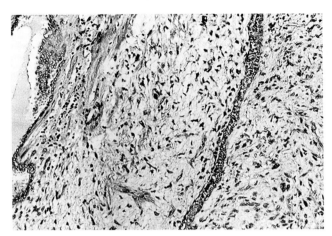

Figure 5–9. Phyllodes tumor. Mixture of compressed ductal structures with a loose spindle cell component. In this example the spindle cells have a stellate shape with a loose myxoid background.

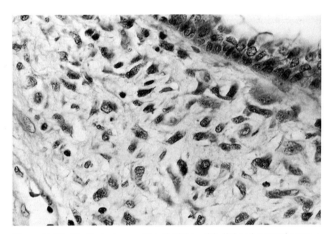

Figure 5–10. Phyllodes tumor. Detail of the epithelial and stromal components in a phyllodes tumor of the prostate. The stromal cells are spindle to stellate shaped without significant nuclear pleomorphism.

Atypical Smooth Muscle Lesions

CLINICAL

- Middle to older age group
- Obstructive symptoms
- No reports of recurrence or metastases in the few cases described

GROSS

- Nodular masses, variable size

MICROSCOPIC

- *Cellular leiomyoma* is made up of spindle cells without nuclear pleomorphism.
- *Symplastic leiomyoma* contains bizarre cells with large and frequently multiple nuclei having hyperchromasia. Nuclear chromatin is smudged, indicating degenerative change.
- In both, mitoses are absent or rare without abnormal forms.
- Necrosis is absent.

SPECIAL STAINS AND IMMUNOHISTOCHEMISTRY

- The cells react with smooth muscle markers (vimentin, SMA, desmin).

DIFFERENTIAL DIAGNOSIS

- Leiomyosarcoma
- Sarcomatoid carcinoma
- Stromal nodule with atypia

References

Persaud V, Douglas LL. Bizarre (atypical) leiomyoma of the prostate gland. West Indian Med J 60:184–187, 1982.
Tetu B, Ro JY, Ayala AG, et al. Atypical spindle cell lesions of the prostate. Semin Diagn Pathol 5:284–293, 1988.

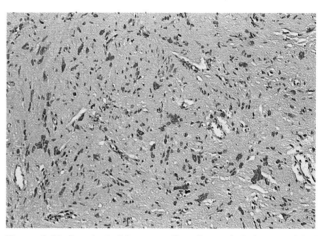

Figure 5–11. Symplastic leiomyoma. Smooth muscle lesion containing scattered atypical cells (see Figure 5–12).

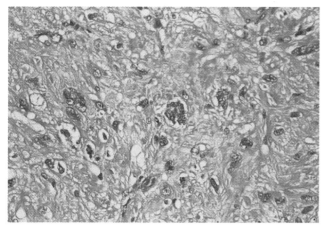

Figure 5–12. Symplastic leiomyoma. Detail of atypical cells in a symplastic leiomyoma. Despite the nuclear atypia, mitotic activity is absent.

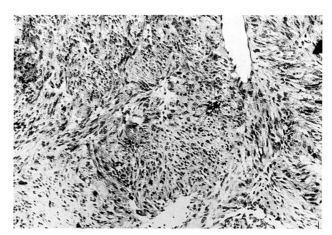

Figure 5–13. Cellular leiomyoma. Fascicles of spindle-shaped cells showing minimal nuclear atypia and no mitotic activity.

Leiomyosarcoma

CLINICAL

- Occurs in adults (fifth to eighth decades) with isolated cases in younger patients.
- Most common sarcoma in adults.
- Obstructive symptoms with enlarged prostate gland.
- Overall prognosis is poor with frequent recurrences and metastases.

GROSS

- Large, bulky gray-white masses with whorled or fleshy cut surface

MICROSCOPIC

- Interlacing fascicles of spindle cells with blunt-ended nuclei and eosinophilic cytoplasm.
- Nuclear atypia and mitoses are variable.
- Necrosis often present.
- No firm criteria exist to distinguish leiomyosarcoma from leiomyoma in the prostate. Features, which, if present, should lead to a diagnosis of malignancy include infiltrative growth pattern, frequent mitoses, and necrosis.

SPECIAL STAINS AND IMMUNOHISTOCHEMISTRY

- Tumor cells are vimentin-, SMA–, and desmin-positive.
- Cytokeratin is generally negative, although focal positivity can occur.

DIFFERENTIAL DIAGNOSIS

- Other sarcomas
- Sarcomatoid carcinoma
- Leiomyoma
- Pseudosarcomatous fibromyxoid tumor
- Postoperative spindle cell nodule

References

Meneses MF, Bostwick DG, Kleer E, et al. Leiomyosarcoma of the prostate (abstract). Mod Pathol 6:67A, 1993.
Witherow R, Molland E, Oliver T, et al. Leiomyosarcoma of prostate and superficial soft tissue. Urology 15:513, 1980.

Rhabdomyosarcoma

CLINICAL

- The most common sarcoma of the prostate.
- Majority under 20 years of age; rare cases reported in adults.
- The genitourinary tract accounts for 21% of childhood rhabdomyosarcomas.
- Present with pelvic mass.
- With current combined therapy regimens, overall 3-year survival is over 70%.

GROSS

- Usually large and extensive at diagnosis
- Soft, gray-white, grossly circumscribed, but histologically infiltrative

MICROSCOPIC

- Embryonal type most common followed by alveolar; pleomorphic type is rare.
- Botryoid pattern can be seen if tumor extends into urethra or bladder.

- Sheets of immature round-to-spindled cells in a loose, myxoid stroma.
- Occasional cells have intensely eosinophilic cytoplasm.
- Strap cells or rhabdomyoblasts, with cross striations, are diagnostic when present.
- Ultrastructural examination may reveal cells containing sarcomeres and glycogen.

SPECIAL STAINS AND IMMUNOHISTOCHEMISTRY

- Cells are vimentin-, muscle-specific actin–, desmin-, and variably myoglobin-positive.
- PAS with and without diastase digestion demonstrates glycogen.
- Cytokeratin, neuron-specific enolase (NSE), and leukocyte common antigen (LCA) are negative.

DIFFERENTIAL DIAGNOSIS

- Lymphoma/leukemia
- Neuroblastoma
- Peripheral neuroectodermal tumor
- Wilms' tumor
- Other small, blue, round cell tumors

References

Asmar L, Gehan EA, Newton WA, et al. Agreement among and within groups of pathologists in the classification of rhabdomyosarcoma and related childhood sarcomas: Report of an international study of four pathology classifications. Cancer 74:2579–2588, 1994.
Loughlin KR, Retik AB, Weinstein HJ, et al. Genitourinary rhabdomyosarcoma in children. Cancer 63:1600–1606, 1989.
Raney RB Jr, Gehan EA, Hays DM, et al. Primary chemotherapy with or without radiation therapy and/or surgery for children with localized sarcoma of the bladder, prostate, vagina, uterus, and cervix: A comparison of the results in Intergroup Rhabdomyosarcoma Studies I and II. Cancer 66:2072–2081, 1990.

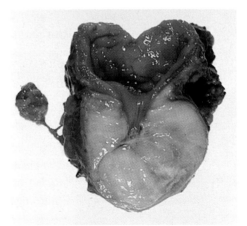

Figure 5–14. Rhabdomyosarcoma. The prostate gland is replaced by a bulging, soft, fleshy, gray-white mass typical of rhabdomyosarcoma in a child.

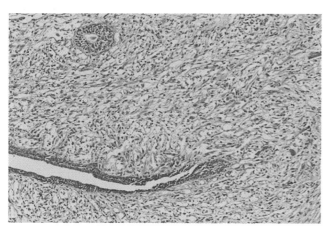

Figure 5–15. Rhabdomyosarcoma. Prostatic rhabdomyosarcoma in a child. This tumor is composed of spindle cells in a loose background.

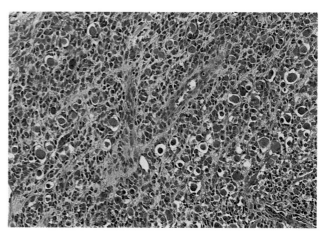

Figure 5–16. Rhabdomyosarcoma. Embryonal rhabdomyosarcoma of the prostate in a child. This tumor is composed of small, blue, round cells with numerous rhabdomyoblasts.

Other Sarcomas

CLINICAL

- Isolated cases of other types of sarcoma reported in the prostate have no specific clinical features.

GROSS

- Most are large, bulky tumors.

MICROSCOPIC

- Histologic features of each type of sarcoma are the same as elsewhere.
- Types reported in the prostate include fibrosarcoma, malignant fibrous histiocytoma, osteosarcoma, chondrosarcoma, angiosarcoma, neurofibrosarcoma, liposarcoma, and unclassified sarcomas.

SPECIAL STAINS AND IMMUNOHISTOCHEMISTRY

- Immunohistochemical staining should correspond to that expected for the given sarcoma type.

DIFFERENTIAL DIAGNOSIS

- Sarcomatoid carcinoma
- Pseudosarcomatous fibromyxoid tumor
- Postoperative spindle cell nodule

References

Chin W, Fay R, Ortega P. Malignant fibrous histiocytoma of prostate gland. Urology 27:363–365, 1986.

Smith DM, Manivel C, Kapps D, et al. Angiosarcoma of the prostate: Report of 2 cases and review of the literature. J Urol 135:382–384, 1986.

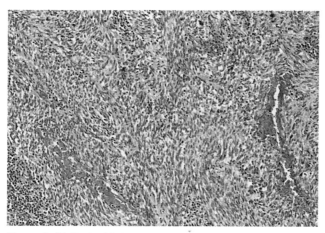

Figure 5–17. Unclassified sarcoma. Unclassified high-grade sarcoma involving the prostate gland.

■ Lymphoreticular and Hematologic Tumors

Lymphoma

CLINICAL

- Wide age range, most commonly older (mean 61 years).
- Secondary involvement more common than primary.
- Criteria for diagnosis of primary lymphoma:
  - Symptoms related to prostate involvement.
  - Lymphoma mainly involves prostate gland.
  - No involvement of liver, spleen, lymph nodes, or peripheral blood within 1 month of diagnosis.
- Systemic symptoms are infrequent.
- Prognosis is poor with most patients dying within 2 years.

GROSS

- Diffuse enlargement of gland

MICROSCOPIC

- Diffuse sheets or patchy infiltration of stroma by neoplastic lymphoid cells with sparing of ducts and acini.
- Infiltration of epithelium is uncommon.
- Extension into surrounding tissue often present.
- Most frequent type is diffuse non-Hodgkin's lymphoma (small cleaved, large cell, or mixed, and of B-cell origin).
- Hodgkin's disease reported but extremely rare.

SPECIAL STAINS AND IMMUNOHISTOCHEMISTRY

- Non-Hodgkin's lymphoma is LCA-positive.
- Other lymphoid markers are as expected for the type.

DIFFERENTIAL DIAGNOSIS

- Chronic prostatitis
- Granulomatous prostatitis
- Leukemia
- Small cell carcinoma
- Rhabdomyosarcoma

References

Amin MB, Osborne B, Discigel C, et al. Malignant lymphoma involving the prostate: Report of 52 cases (abstract). Mod Pathol 6:54A, 1993.

Banerjee SS, Harris M. Angiotropic lymphoma presenting in the prostate. Histopathology 12:667–683, 1988.

Bostwick DG, Mann RB. Malignant lymphomas involving the prostate: A study of 13 cases. Cancer 56:2932–2938, 1985.

Fell P, O'Connor M, Smith JM. Primary lymphoma of prostate presenting as bladder outlet obstruction. Urology 29:555–559, 1987.

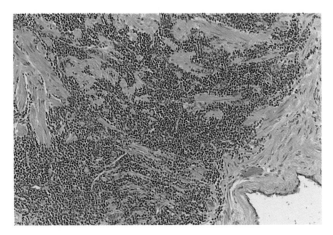

Figure 5–18. Malignant lymphoma. Involvement of the prostate gland by poorly differentiated lymphocytic lymphoma. The neoplastic cells permeate the stroma diffusely, sparing the epithelial structures.

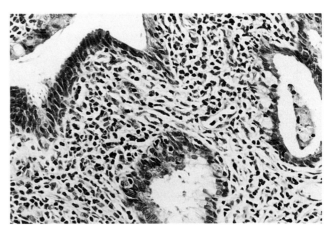

Figure 5–19. Malignant lymphoma. Poorly differentiated lymphocytic lymphoma infiltrating prostatic stroma and sparing the epithelial elements.

Leukemia

CLINICAL

- At autopsy up to 20% of patients with leukemia have prostatic involvement.
- Less than 1% have symptoms attributable to the infiltration.

GROSS

- Usually no gross abnormality

MICROSCOPIC

- Chronic lymphocytic leukemia (CLL) is most frequent.
- There is diffuse or multifocal stromal permeation.

SPECIAL STAINS AND IMMUNOHISTOCHEMISTRY

- CLL is LCA-positive.

DIFFERENTIAL DIAGNOSIS

- Chronic prostatitis
- Malignant lymphoma
- Small cell carcinoma

References

Cachia PG, McIntyre MA, Dewar AE, et al. Prostatic infiltration in chronic lymphatic leukemia. J Clin Pathol 40:342–345, 1987.
Thalhammer F, Gisslinger H, Chott A, et al. Granulocytic sarcoma of the prostate as the first manifestation of a late relapse of acute myelogenous leukemia. Ann Hematol 68:97–99, 1994.

Multiple Myeloma

CLINICAL

- Secondary involvement of the prostate is very rare, with most cases being incidental findings at autopsy.

GROSS

- No specific features

MICROSCOPIC

- Involvement by neoplastic plasma cells

SPECIAL STAINS AND IMMUNOHISTOCHEMISTRY

- IgD and IgA myelomas described
- Monoclonal light chain expression

DIFFERENTIAL DIAGNOSIS

- Chronic prostatitis
- Plasmacytoid lymphoma
- Plasmacytoma

Reference

Yasuda N, Ohmori S-I, Usui T. IgD myelomas involving the prostate. Am J Hematol 47:65–66, 1994.

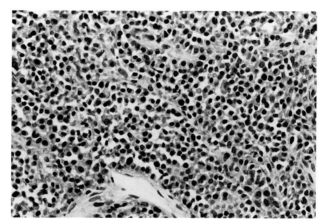

Figure 5–20. Multiple myeloma. Involvement of the prostate gland by sheets of malignant plasma cells in a patient with multiple myeloma.

■ Secondary Tumors

CLINICAL

- Excluding lymphoma and leukemia, contiguous spread from adjacent organs is most common, especially bladder and colon.
- Metastases to gland uncommon at autopsy and rarely symptomatic.

- Most frequent origin of metastases is lung followed by melanoma, gastrointestinal tract, and kidney.

GROSS

- No characteristic features.
- Metastatic melanoma may have black discoloration.

MICROSCOPIC

• Depends on specific tumor type

SPECIAL STAINS AND IMMUNOHISTOCHEMISTRY

• As appropriate for tumor type

DIFFERENTIAL DIAGNOSIS

• For colon cancer: cribriform, endometrioid, and mucinous types of prostate carcinoma; high-grade prostatic intra-epithelial neoplasia

References

Johnson DE, Chalbaud R, Ayala AG. Secondary tumors of the prostate. J Urol 112:507–508, 1974.

Simon A, Addonizio JC, Stahl RE. Prostatic invasion of rectal carcinoma: Does transurethral surgery alter prognosis? Urology 29:71–72, 1987.

Zein TA, Huben R, Lane W, et al. Secondary tumors of the prostate. J Urol 133:615–616, 1985.

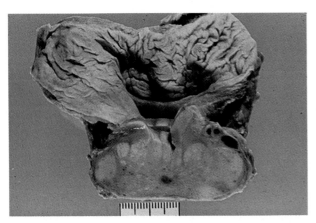

Figure 5–21. Metastatic carcinoma. Example of prostate gland involved by metastatic adenocarcinoma of pancreatic origin. Note the multiple nodules throughout the peripheral and transition zones of the gland.

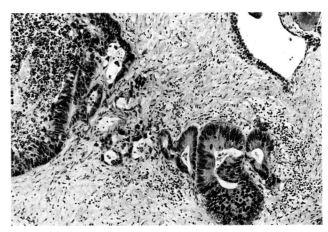

Figure 5–22. Metastatic carcinoma. Involvement of the prostate gland by direct extension of a rectal adenocarcinoma. This tumor must be differentiated from the ductal (endometrioid) type of prostate carcinoma.

CHAPTER 6

Seminal Vesicles

■ Normal Anatomy and Histology

- The seminal vesicles are paired organs situated proximal to the prostate gland and posterior to the base of the bladder.
- The proximal portion of each seminal vesicle joins the vas deferens to form the ejaculatory duct.
- The mucosal surface is highly convoluted, resulting in a papillary architecture with small acinar structures in the underlying stroma.
- The lining is two cell layers thick with an inner layer of tall columnar epithelium and outer layer of flattened basal cells; the latter stain positively with high-molecular-weight cytokeratin antibodies.

- The columnar cells characteristically contain abundant lipofuscin pigment which accumulates with age.
- The nuclei of the columnar cells often are large and pleomorphic with hyperchromasia ("monster nuclei"). Nuclear pseudoinclusions are seen and mitoses are absent.
- The lumen is surrounded by a thick muscular wall composed of compact smooth muscle fibers.

Reference

Kuo T, Gomez LG. Monstrous epithelial cells in human epididymis and seminal vesicles: A pseudomalignant change. Am J Surg Pathol 5: 483–490, 1981.

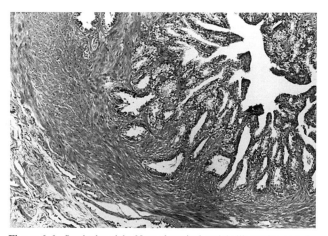

Figure 6–1. Seminal vesicle. Normal seminal vesicle illustrating complex mucosal surface with formation of small acinar structures in a dense smooth muscle wall (see also Figure 1–18).

■ Seminal Vesiculitis

CLINICAL

- Primary seminal vesiculitis is rare and is usually secondary to prostatitis.
- Pathogenic organisms include gonococci, *Escherichia coli*, and other coliforms.
- Acute and chronic forms occur.

GROSS

- No specific findings

MICROSCOPIC

- In acute cases, neutrophils are present in the lumen with involvement of the mucosal surface.
- In chronic cases, lymphocytes and plasma cells infiltrate the wall.

SPECIAL STAINS AND IMMUNOHISTOCHEMISTRY

- None

DIFFERENTIAL DIAGNOSIS

- None

■ Localized Amyloidosis

CLINICAL

- Primary localized amyloidosis is common (21% of men over 75 years of age).
- Rarely symptomatic.

GROSS

- Wall may appear normal or thickened with reduced or absent lumina.

MICROSCOPIC

- Deposits tend to be nodular and subepithelial. Involvement of vessel walls is not seen in the localized form.
- The nature of the eosinophilic material is confirmed by positive staining and apple-green birefringence with Congo red staining.

SPECIAL STAINS AND IMMUNOHISTOCHEMISTRY

- Congo red

DIFFERENTIAL DIAGNOSIS

- Systemic amyloidosis

Reference

Pitkanen P, Westermark P, Cornwell GG III, et al. Amyloid of the seminal vesicles: A distinctive and common localized form of senile amyloidosis. Am J Pathol 110:64–69, 1983.

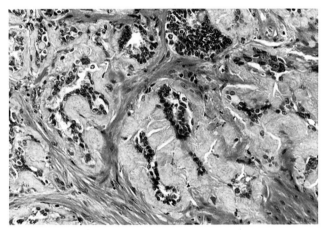

Figure 6–2. Localized amyloidosis. The seminal vesicle is distorted by the deposition of fine fibrillar eosinophilic material in a subepithelial location.

■ Cysts

CLINICAL

- Majority are acquired but congenital forms do occur.
- Congenital cysts are due to developmental abnormalities of the mesonephric duct and are often associated with unilateral renal agenesis.
- Acquired cysts are due to obstruction and are most often associated with chronic prostatitis.
- When symptomatic, can result in hematuria and painful ejaculation.

GROSS

- Most are single and unilateral (both types).
- Variable size; may be very large ("hydrops").

MICROSCOPIC

• Lined by flattened-to-cuboidal epithelium having characteristics of seminal vesicle epithelium—lipofuscin pigment and large hyperchromatic nuclei.

SPECIAL STAINS AND IMMUNOHISTOCHEMISTRY

• None

DIFFERENTIAL DIAGNOSIS

• Cystadenoma

References

Ejeckham GC, Govatsos S, Lewis AS. Cyst of seminal vesicle associated with ipsilateral renal agenesis. Urology 24:372–374, 1984.
Steers WD, Corriere JD. Case profile: Seminal vesicle cyst. Urology 27:177–178, 1986.

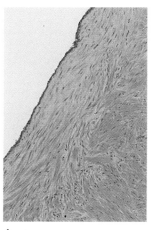
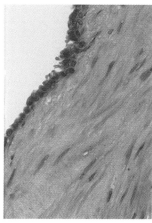

A   B

Figure 6–3. Seminal vesicle cyst. The cyst is lined by a flattened epithelium with the wall being made up of fibromuscular tissue. Note the atypical, hyperchromatic nuclei; at high magnification lipofuscin pigment can be identified (*A*, low power; *B*, high power).

■ Cystadenoma

CLINICAL

• Rare neoplasms with only a few reported cases
• Usually asymptomatic

GROSS

• Unilateral
• Variable size, up to 10 cm in diameter
• Multilocular with septa of varying thickness

MICROSCOPIC

• Cysts lined by a single layer of columnar cells.
• Lipofuscin pigment may be found.
• No significant pleomorphism or mitoses.
• Loose fibrous stroma with scattered chronic inflammatory cells.

SPECIAL STAINS AND IMMUNOHISTOCHEMISTRY

• PSA and PAP to exclude prostatic origin

DIFFERENTIAL DIAGNOSIS

• Seminal vesicle cyst
• Adenocarcinoma (primary or secondary)

Reference

Lundhus E. Bundgaard N, Sorensen FB. Cystadenoma of the seminal vesicle. Scand J Urol Nephrol 18:341–342, 1984.

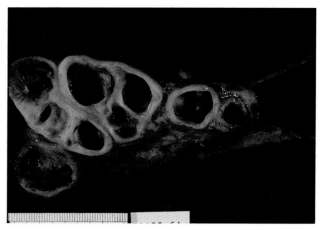

Figure 6–4. Seminal vesicle cystadenoma. Gross specimen demonstrating multiloculated cystic mass. (Photograph courtesy of Dr. David Bostwick, Rochester, MN.)

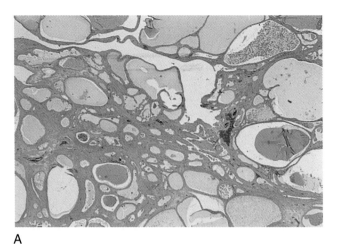
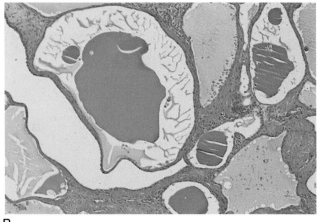

A   B

Figure 6–5. Seminal vesicle cystadenoma. The lesion is composed of variably sized cysts with intervening fibrous stroma (*A*, low power; *B*, high power). (Photomicrograph courtesy of Dr. David Bostwick, Rochester, MN.)

■ Primary Adenocarcinoma

CLINICAL

- Very rare tumors with most reported cases likely representing prostatic carcinoma involving the seminal vesicles.
- Recommended minimal criteria for the diagnosis include:
  - Tumor epicenter should be localized to seminal vesicle region, superior to the prostate gland.
  - There should be no other primary tumor (particularly of bladder, anorectal, or prostate origin).
  - Histologically, the tumor should have papillary or anaplastic features.
  - The tumor should be PSA- and PAP-negative.
  - An in situ component is present in adjacent seminal vesicle epithelium.
- Wide age range reported (24–90 years; mean 62 years).
- Present with bladder outlet obstruction, hematospermia, mass.
- Prognosis is poor.

GROSS

- Solid, gray-white, with tumor epicenter in region of seminal vesicles

MICROSCOPIC

- Variety of architectural patterns with papillary most frequent
- High-grade cytology, frequently anaplastic
- Mucin production always present

SPECIAL STAINS AND IMMUNOHISTOCHEMISTRY

- Mucin stains (alcian blue, mucicarmine)
- PSA and PAP: uniformly negative
- Carcinoembryonic antigen (CEA): positive in most

DIFFERENTIAL DIAGNOSIS

- Cystadenoma
- Secondary carcinoma

References

Benson RC Jr, Clark WR, Farrow GM. Carcinoma of the seminal vesicle. J Urol 132:483–485, 1984.

Okada Y, Tanaka H, Takeuchi H, et al. Papillary adenocarcinoma in a seminal vesicle cyst associated with ipsilateral renal agenesis: A case report. J Urol 148:1543–1545, 1992.

Tanaka T, Takeuchi T, Oguchi K, et al. Primary adenocarcinoma of the seminal vesicle. Hum Pathol 18:200–202, 1987.

■ Other Neoplasms

- A wide range of other neoplasms originating in the seminal vesicles have been described in isolated case reports.

References

Kinas H, Kuhn MJ. Mesonephric hamartoma of the seminal vesicle: A rare cause of retrovesical mass. N Y State J Med 87:48, 1987.

Laurila P, Leivo I, Makisalo H, et al. Müllerian adenocarcinoma-like tumor of the seminal vesicle: A case report with immunohistochemical and ultrastructural observations. Arch Pathol Lab Med 116:1072–1076, 1992.

Mazur MT, Myers JL, Maddox WA. Cystic epithelial-stromal tumor of the seminal vesicle. Am J Surg Pathol 11:210–217, 1987.

Schned AR, Ledbetter JS, Selikowitz SM. Primary leiomyosarcoma of the seminal vesicle. Cancer 57:2202–2206, 1986.

Secondary Neoplasms

CLINICAL

- Secondary involvement of the seminal vesicle by other tumors much more common than primary neoplasms.
- Most frequent tumors involving the seminal vesicles are prostate adenocarcinoma and urothelial carcinoma of the bladder.
- Presentation is typical of the primary site.

GROSS

- Tumor epicenter is in primary organ.
- In many cases involvement is histologic.

MICROSCOPIC

- Histologic features are typical of the primary tumor.
- Urothelial carcinoma can involve the seminal vesicle by in situ pagetoid spread.

SPECIAL STAINS AND IMMUNOHISTOCHEMISTRY

- Prostate carcinomas are PSA- and PAP-positive.

DIFFERENTIAL DIAGNOSIS

- Primary adenocarcinoma

Reference

Ro JY, Ayala AG, el-Naggar A, et al. Seminal vesicle involvement by in situ and invasive transitional cell carcinoma of the bladder. Am J Surg Pathol 12:951–958, 1987.

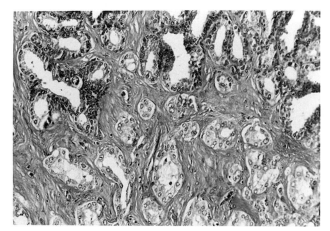

Figure 6–6. Secondary prostate carcinoma. The wall of the seminal vesicle is infiltrated by prostatic adenocarcinoma; note the differences in cytologic features between the seminal vesicle epithelium and that of the carcinoma (see also Figures 2–30 and 2–31).

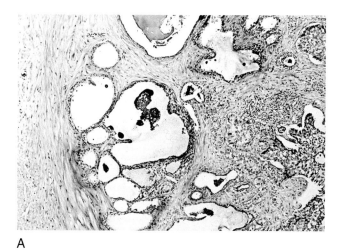

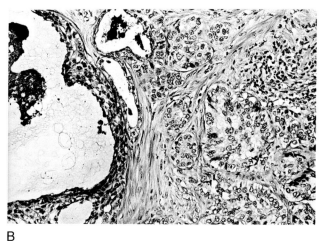

A   B

Figure 6–7. Urothelial carcinoma. Involvement of the seminal vesicle epithelium by urothelial carcinoma spreading in a pagetoid fashion (A, low power; B, high power).

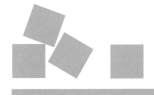

THE TESTIS

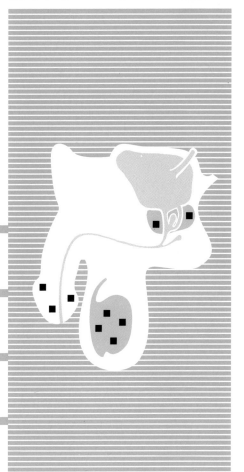

CHAPTER 7

Normal Anatomy and Histology of the Testis

- Paired ovoid organ, average weight 15 to 19 g and dimensions $4 \times 3 \times 2$ cm.
- Supporting frameworks of the testis:
  - Capsule.
  - Mediastinum.
  - Fibrous septa.
- The capsule is composed of three layers: tunica vaginalis (mesothelia-lined), tunica albuginea (layer of collagen fibers), and tunica vasculosa (loose vascular connective tissue).
- The mediastinum contains blood vessels, lymphatics, and the intratesticular portion of the rete testis.
- The fibrous septa divide the testis into approximately 250 lobules.
- Each lobule contains up to four seminiferous tubules (average diameter of tubule, 180 μm).
- The seminiferous tubules are composed of Sertoli and germ cells in varying stages of differentiation.
- Germ cells outnumber Sertoli cells and primary spermatocytes are the most preponderant type of germ cell.
- Sertoli cells are roughly triangular, columnar, or elongated cells oriented with their base to the tubular basement membrane. The cell outline is irregular and indistinct, and the cytoplasm is clear, pale, or faintly eosinophilic. The nuclei are irregularly shaped and have vesicular chromatin and a prominent nucleolus. Sertoli cells constitute 10% to 15% of the cellular components of seminiferous tubules.
- The germ cells mature from base to center of the lumen. Based on the level of maturation the germ cells may be classified as:
  - Spermatogonia: these are situated along the basement membrane and have round, dense nuclei with nucleoli.
  - Primary spermatocytes: larger than spermatogonia; located more centrally than spermatogonia and have a nucleus with beaded cytoplasm; largest cell type.
  - Secondary spermatocytes: smaller than primary spermatocytes, fewer in number, fine granular chromatin, no nucleoli.
  - Spermatids: small cells with darkly stained chromatin and slight depression on the surface of the nucleus; cells

are found toward the lumen; approximately half of the germ cells are in this stage.
  - Spermatozoa: elongated eccentric nucleus with long cytoplasmic tail.
- The interstitium is divided into intertubular and peritubular regions. Peritubular interstitium contains a basement membrane and a thin lamina propria which envelops the tubules. Intertubular interstitium is made up of the remainder of mesenchymal cells between tubules.
- Leydig cells are found singly, or in clusters of various size within the interstitium. The cytoplasm is abundant and eosinophilic. The nucleus of Leydig cells is oval to round with a vesicular chromatin containing one or two eccentrically located nucleoli.
- Leydig cells contain lipofuscin pigment and Reinke crystalloids. They are present only in the postpubertal testis.
- Ectopic Leydig cells may be seen in the tunica albuginea, epididymis, spermatic cord, and mediastinum testis. They are located in intimate association with nerve fibers and vessels. Therefore, these ectopic Leydig cells may be confused with metastatic carcinoma cells, particularly with prostate carcinoma.
- The blood supply is derived from the testicular artery, which originates from the abdominal aorta.
- The right spermatic vein drains into the inferior vena cava and the left drains into the renal vein.
- Lymphatic spaces are found in the interstitium adjacent to Leydig cell clusters. Lymphatic channels drain into the septa and then to either the capsule or mediastinum testis. They anastomose with lymphatic channels from the epididymis and enter the spermatic cord.
- Rete testis is divided into three compartments: tubular rete, mediastinal rete, and extratesticular rete.
- Rete epithelium is of low cuboidal type with surface microvilli.
- Efferent ductules emerge from the rete testis to form lobules of epididymis.
- Epididymis is longitudinally oriented along the lateral posterior aspect of the testis.
- Epididymal ducts are lined by tall columnar chief cells

with microvilli (stereocilia), clear cells, and basal cells. The chief cells contain lipid and lipofuscin. Epididymal epithelial cells have intranuclear inclusions (these inclusions can be seen in vas deferens and less commonly in the seminal vesicle). Coarsely granular eosinophilic cytoplasmic change of the epididymal cells has been described as Paneth cell-like change. Cells with monster nuclei can be seen. Cribriform hyperplasia can be seen as a normal variant.

References

Mai KT. Cytoplasmic eosinophilic granular change of the ductuli efferentes: A histological, immunohistochemical, and electron microscopic study. J Urol Pathol 2:273–282, 1994.

Schned AR, Memoli VA. Coarse granular cytoplasmic change of the epididymis: An immunohistochemical and ultrastructural study. J Urol Pathol 2:213–222, 1994.

Sharp SC, Batt MA, Lennington WJ. Epididymal cribriform hyperplasia. A variant of normal epididymal histology. Arch Pathol Lab Med 118:1020–1022, 1994.

Trainer TD. Histology of the normal testis. Am J Surg Pathol 11:797–809, 1987.

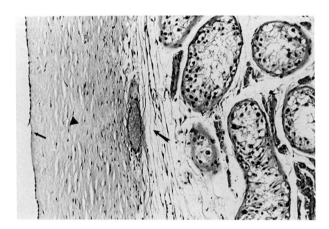

Figure 7–1. Normal testis. This illustration shows seminiferous tubules and the capsule. The capsule is composed of the tunica vaginalis *(thin arrow),* tunica albuginea *(arrowhead),* and tunica vasculosa *(large arrow).* The tunica vaginalis is lined by flattened mesothelial cells.

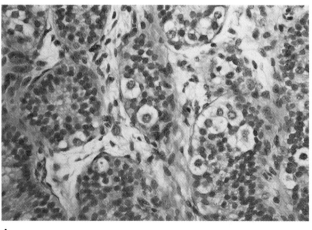

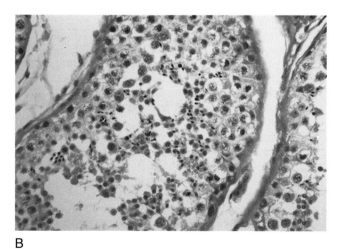

A   B

Figure 7–2. Normal testis. *A,* Infantile testis showing a few scattered germ cells and primitive Sertoli cells. *B,* Adult testis showing spermatogenesis with varying stages of differentiation of germ cells.

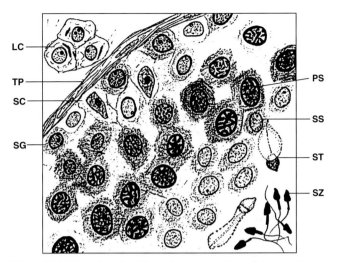

Figure 7–3. Normal testis. Schematic representation of the constituent cells of the seminiferous tubule and the interstitium. *LC,* Leydig cell; *TP,* tunica propria; *SC,* Sertoli cell; *SG,* spermatogonia; *PS,* primary spermatocyte; *SS,* secondary spermatocyte; *ST,* spermatid; *SZ,* spermatozoa. (Diagram created by Dr. A. Savera, Senior Resident, Department of Pathology, Henry Ford Hospital, Detroit.)

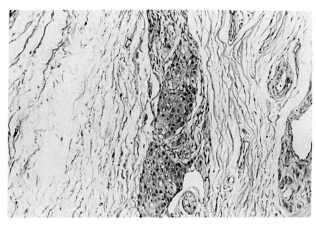

Figure 7–4. Ectopic Leydig cells. This illustration shows clusters of Leydig cells intimately associated with a nerve trunk in the spermatic cord.

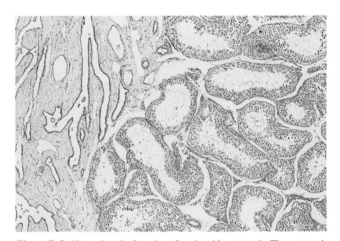

Figure 7–5. Normal testis. Junction of testis with rete testis. The rete testis is lined by a single layer of low cuboidal epithelial cells.

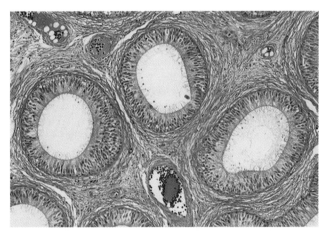

Figure 7–6. Normal epididymis. Epididymal ducts are lined by tall columnar chief cells with microvilli, clear cells, and basal cells.

CHAPTER 8

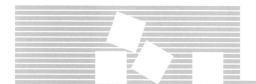

Congenital Abnormalities

■ Cryptorchidism

CLINICAL

- Prevalence of 0.03% to 0.4% among adult males.
- Mostly unilateral, with a slight predilection for the right testis; testis may be intraabdominal (10%), inguinal (42%), or upper scrotal (48%). The testis may be found in ectopic sites (off normal pathway of descent). The five major sites of testicular ectopia are the perineum, the femoral canal, the superficial inguinal pouch, the suprapubic area, and the opposite scrotal compartment.
- Complications: torsion, infarction, infertility, and germ cell neoplasms.
- Risk of developing a germ cell malignancy in a cryptorchid testis is 35-fold that of the normal adult population, and estimated at 5% to 10%.
- Seminoma, embryonal carcinoma, and mixed germ cell tumors (MGCTs) frequently arise in cryptorchid testis, but spermatocytic seminoma has not been reported.

GROSS

- Atrophy, characterized by diminished size and firm consistency.
- Surgically excised specimens should be closely examined for scars or infarcts which may be sites of previous tumors (now regressed). Minute nodules may represent Pick's adenoma (see Microscopic section).

MICROSCOPIC

- Prepubertal: diminished tubular diameter, Leydig cell hypoplasia, reduced germ cells. Tunica propria thickening occurs in the first year of life. Miscellaneous changes: microcalcifications in tubules, increased interstitium
- Postpubertal: tunica propria thickening, reduced tubular diameter, tubular sclerosis, Leydig cell hyperplasia, interstitial fibrosis
- Intratubular germ cell neoplasia (ITGCN): rare in prepubertal, up to 8% in postpubertal testis. Morphologic features described in Chapter 10
- Sertoli cell adenoma (Pick's adenoma) characterized by congeries of complex tubular structures lined by immature Sertoli cells

SPECIAL STAINS AND IMMUNOHISTOCHEMISTRY

- Stains to confirm ITGCN:
  - PAS with and without diastase
  - Placental alkaline phosphatase (PLAP)
  - NSE
  - Monoclonal antibody M2A and 43-9F
- All stains positive in cells of ITGCN

DIFFERENTIAL DIAGNOSIS

- Other causes of atrophy of the testes should be excluded—clinical information and correlation essential
  - Klinefelter's syndrome
  - Obstruction to outflow of semen
  - Administration of estrogen, most commonly for the treatment of prostatic carcinoma
  - Hypopituitarism
  - Aging
  - Malnutrition and cachexia
  - Inflammatory diseases such as mumps orchitis
  - Radiation
  - Alcoholic cirrhosis

References

Batata MA, Chu FCH, Hilaris BS, et al. Testicular cancer in cryptorchids. Cancer 49:1023–1030, 1982.

Muller J, Skakkebaek NE. Abnormal germ cells in maldescended testes: A study of cell density, nuclear size and deoxyribonucleic acid content in testicular biopsies from 50 boys. J Urol 131:730–733, 1984.

Muller J, Skakkebaek NE, Nielsen OH, et al. Cryptorchidism and testis cancer. Atypical infantile germ cells followed by carcinoma in situ and invasive carcinoma in adulthood. Cancer 54:629–634, 1984.

Nistal M, Paniagua R, Diez-Pardo JA. Histologic classification of undescended testes. Hum Pathol 11:666–674, 1980.

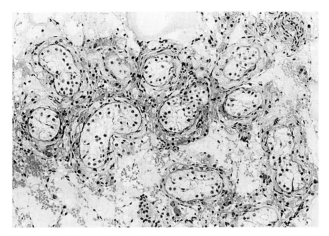

Figure 8–1. Cryptorchidism. Postpubertal testis shows reduced tubular diameter, tubular sclerosis, and Leydig cell hyperplasia.

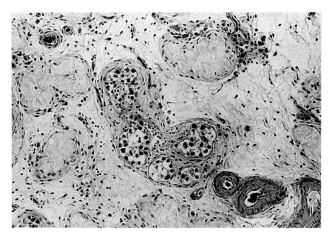

Figure 8–2. Cryptorchidism. Intratubular germ cell neoplasia may be associated with the cryptorchid testis seen in this illustration.

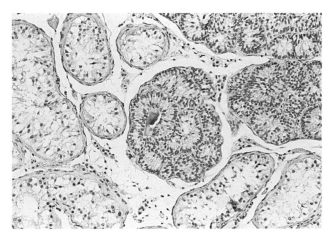

Figure 8–3. Pick's adenoma. In the center of the picture and toward one corner *(right)* is a conglomerate of tubules lined by basally located hyperchromatic Sertoli cells that are perpendicularly oriented in relation to the basement membrane.

■ Klinefelter's Syndrome

CLINICAL

- Prevalence: 0.2% of male population.
- Male hypogonadism characterized by gynecomastia, eunuchoid habitus, absent spermatogenesis, increased follicle-stimulating hormone secretion, and apparently normal Leydig cell function.
- Abnormal karyotype, most commonly 47, XXY.
- Responsible for about 3% of cases of infertility in males.

- Increased incidence of mediastinal germ cell tumors, but not of retroperitoneal or testicular germ cell tumors. Breast cancer occurs in patients with Klinefelter's syndrome with the same frequency as in adult females.
- Cases of Leydig cell tumor, epidermoid cyst, and germ cell tumor of the testis have been reported to be associated with Klinefelter's syndrome.

GROSS

- Small testes

MICROSCOPIC

- Prepubertal:
  - At birth: normal or reduced germ cells
  - Childhood: variable reduction of germ cells; some may only contain Sertoli cells
- Postpubertal:
  - Reduced or absent spermatogenesis
  - Tubular sclerosis with diminished or absent elastic fibers
- Leydig cell hyperplasia

SPECIAL STAINS AND IMMUNOHISTOCHEMISTRY

- None

DIFFERENTIAL DIAGNOSIS

- Cryptorchidism

References

Dexeus FH, Logothetis CJ, Chong C, et al. Genetic abnormalities in men with germ cell tumors. J Urol 140:80–84, 1988.

Gordon DL, Krmpotic E, Thomas W, et al. Pathologic testicular findings in Klinefelter's syndrome. 47,XXY vs 46,XY/47,XXY. Arch Intern Med 130:726–729, 1972.

Hasle H, Mellemgaard A, Nielsen J, et al. Cancer incidence in men with Klinefelter syndrome. Br J Cancer 71:416–420, 1995.

Regadera J, Codesai J, Paniagua R, et al. Immunohistochemical and quantitative study of interstitial and intratubular Leydig cells in normal men, cryptorchidism, and Klinefelter's syndrome. J Pathol 164:299–306, 1991.

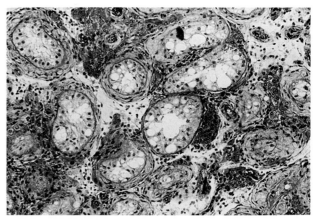

Figure 8–4. Klinefelter's syndrome. This illustration shows tubular sclerosis, absent spermatogenesis with Sertoli cells only, and Leydig cell hyperplasia.

■ Splenic-Gonadal Fusion

CLINICAL

- Rare.
- Usually involves left testis.
- A discrete mass, usually small.
- Mass is almost always fused to the upper pole of the testis or to the head of the epididymis.
- Testis may be atrophic or may show hypoplasia.

GROSS

- Reddish-brown nodule resembling splenic tissue separated from testicular tissue by band of fibrous tissue

MICROSCOPIC

- Histologically normal splenic tissue separated from testicular tissue by band of fibrous tissue

SPECIAL STAINS AND IMMUNOHISTOCHEMISTRY

- None

DIFFERENTIAL DIAGNOSIS

- Mature teratoma

References

Andrews RW, Copeland DD, Fried FA. Splenogonadal fusion. J Urol 133:1052–1053, 1985.

Ceccacci L, Tosi S. Splenic-gonadal fusion: Case report and review of the literature. J Urol 126:558–559, 1981.

Knorr PA, Borden TA. Splenogonadal fusion. Urology 44:136–138, 1994.

Mendez R, Morrow JW. Ectopic spleen simulating testicular tumor. J Urol 102:598–601, 1969.

Putschar WGJ, Manion WC. Splenic gonadal fusion. Am J Pathol 32:15–33, 1956.

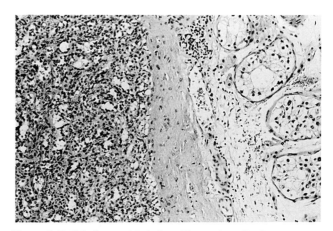

Figure 8–5. Splenic-gonadal fusion. The tunica albuginea separates splenic tissue *(left side)* from the seminiferous tubules *(right side)*.

■ Adrenal Rests

CLINICAL

- Ectopic adrenocortical tissue in the spermatic cord, rete testis, epididymis, and tunica albuginea
- Found in approximately 10% of infants

GROSS

- Small yellow nodules (usually <1 cm in diameter).
- Usually forms an encapsulated nodule.
- Cut section may show zones of normal adrenal gland.

MICROSCOPIC

- Solid sheets and nests of polygonal cells
- Abundant cytoplasm
- Bland cytology
- Absent adrenal medullary tissue

SPECIAL STAINS AND IMMUNOHISTOCHEMISTRY

- None

DIFFERENTIAL DIAGNOSIS

- Leydig cell hyperplasia involving cord
- Leydig cell tumor
- Tumor of adrenogenital syndrome
- Nelson's syndrome

References

Dahl EV, Bahn RC. Aberrant adrenal cortical tissue near the testis in human infants. Am J Pathol 40:587–598, 1962.
Habuchi T, Mizutani Y, Miyakawa M. Ectopic aberrant adrenals with epididymal abnormality. Urology 39:251–253, 1992.
Mares AJ, Shkolnik A, Sacks M, et al. Aberrant (ectopic) adrenocortical tissue along the spermatic cord. J Pediatr Surg 15:289–292, 1980.
Nelson AA. Accessory adrenal cortical tissue. Arch Pathol 27:955–965, 1939.

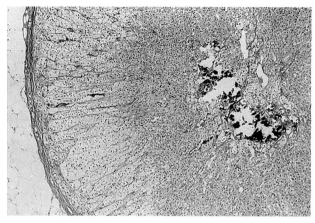

Figure 8–6. Adrenal rest. Histologically, this lesion resembles normal adrenal cortex.

■ Testicular Feminization Syndrome (Androgen-Insensitivity Syndrome)

CLINICAL

- A rare inherited form of male pseudohermaphroditism.
- Associated with undescended testis (intraabdominal or inguinal).
- Pelvic mass may be a presenting symptom.
- Male karyotype (XY) and negative sex chromatin.
- Increased risk of undergoing malignant germ cell tumor transformation of the undescended gonad; germ cell tumors increase in incidence with age. All types of germ cell tumors have been reported.

GROSS

- Tan-to-brown parenchyma with multiple, pale-tan nodules

MICROSCOPIC

- Three characteristic features:
  - Small-sized seminiferous tubules with mostly immature Sertoli cells.
  - Leydig cell hyperplasia.
  - Ovarian-like stroma.
- Other features:
  - Spermatogonia and spermatocytes are usually sparse in seminiferous tubules.
  - Sertoli cell adenoma: increased number of seminiferous tubules, Sertoli cell immaturity, and reduced number of Leydig cells relative to surrounding testis parenchyma.

SPECIAL STAINS AND IMMUNOHISTOCHEMISTRY

- None

DIFFERENTIAL DIAGNOSIS

• Leydig cell hyperplasia
• Sertoli cell tumor

References

Collins GM, Kim DU, Logrono R, et al. Pure seminoma arising in androgen insensitivity syndrome (testicular feminization syndrome): A case report and review of the literature. Mod Pathol 6:89–93, 1993.

Ramaswamy G, Jagadha V, Tchertkoff V. A testicular tumor resembling the sex cord with annular tubules in a case of the androgen insensitivity syndrome. Cancer 55:1607–1611, 1985.

Rutgers JL, Scully RE. Pathology of the testis in intersex syndromes. Semin Diagn Pathol 4:275–291, 1987.

■ Other Abnormalities

• Anorchidism (absent testes)
• Monorchidism (absent one testis): 1 in 5,000 males; bilatral anorchidism: 1 in 20,000 males
• Polyorchidism (more than two testes)

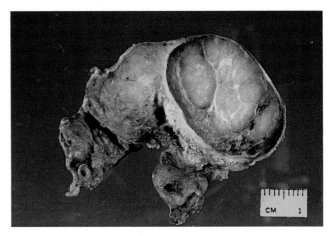

Figure 8–7. Testicular feminization syndrome. Tan-to-brown parenchyma with multiple firm nodules. (Courtesy of Dr. M.E. Kirk, London, Ontario, Canada.)

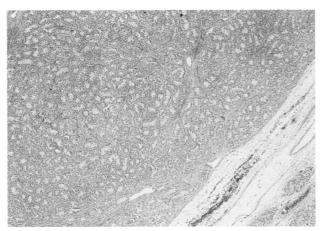

Figure 8–8. Testicular feminization syndrome. Small-sized seminiferous tubules contain mostly immature Sertoli cells.

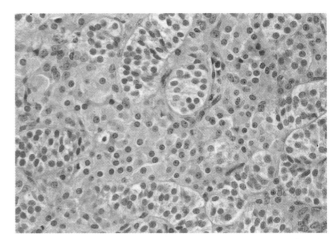

Figure 8–9. Testicular feminization syndrome. A few seminiferous tubules with Sertoli cells and Leydig cell hyperplasia. Other features include areas of ovarian-like stroma (not shown here).

CHAPTER 9

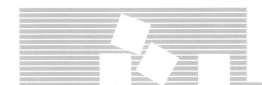

Inflammatory Diseases

■ Acute Orchitis

CLINICAL

- Frequently with concurrent involvement of ipsilateral epididymis.
- Most cases have an underlying gram-negative bacterial infection, frequently associated with urinary tract infection. Gram-positive organisms (staphylococci and streptococci) may also be causative agents.

GROSS

- Variable: hyperemia, microabscesses, or discrete abscess formation with massive destruction of parenchyma

MICROSCOPIC

- Acute inflammation, including abscess formation composed of many neutrophils predominantly in seminiferous tubules; interstitium is also affected.

SPECIAL STAINS AND IMMUNOHISTOCHEMISTRY

- Gram stain: may be positive

DIFFERENTIAL DIAGNOSIS

- Malignant lymphoma
- Mumps orchitis
- Idiopathic granulomatous orchitis

References

de la Maza LM, Peterson EM. Genital infections. Med Clin North Am 67:1059–1073, 1983.
Mikuz G, Damjanov I. Inflammation of the testis, epididymis, peritesticular membranes, and scrotum. Pathol Annu 17(1):101–128, 1982.

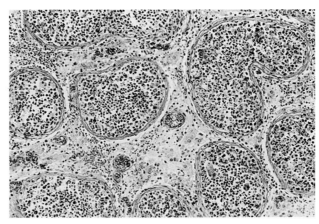

Figure 9–1. Acute orchitis. The seminiferous tubules are largely destroyed by acute inflammatory cells. The stroma is edematous.

■ Chronic Orchitis

CLINICAL

- Failure of resolution of the acute orchitis leads to chronic orchitis.

GROSS

- Fibrotic gray-white parenchyma, which may be adherent to adjacent tissues

MICROSCOPIC

- Chronic inflammatory cells, lymphocytes, and plasma cells, predominantly in interstitium
- Granulation tissue
- Fibrosis

SPECIAL STAINS AND IMMUNOHISTOCHEMISTRY

- Gram stain: usually negative
- Acid-fast bacillus (AFB): negative
- Gomori's methenamine silver stain (GMS): negative

DIFFERENTIAL DIAGNOSIS

- Malignant lymphoma
- Seminoma
- Mumps orchitis

References

de la Maza LM, Peterson EM. Genital infections. Med Clin North Am 67:1059–1073, 1983.

Mikuz G, Damjanov I. Inflammation of the testis, epididymis, peritesticular membranes, and scrotum. Pathol Annu 17(1):101–128, 1982.

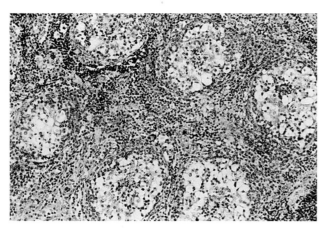

Figure 9–2. Chronic orchitis. The interstitial tissue is expanded by a heavy chronic inflammatory infiltrate. Note some residual spermatogenesis in the tubules.

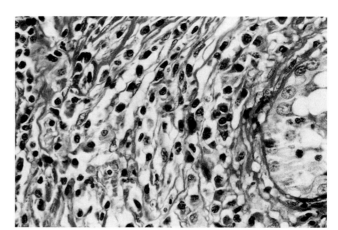

Figure 9–3. Chronic orchitis. This high-power view shows plasma cells and lymphocytes embedded in a reticulated stroma. A portion of a seminiferous tubule is also present.

■ Mumps Orchitis

CLINICAL

- Most common viral orchitis.
- Mumps orchitis is caused by paramyxovirus species.
- Complicates 20% of mumps occurring in adults; uncommon in prepubertal patients.
- Testicular swelling and pain with or without evidence of systemic involvement (1 week after onset of parotid gland swelling).
- Most commonly unilateral; bilateral in 25%.
- Epididymal involvement is high (85%).
- Subsequent sterility is rare (<2%).
- Little evidence to verify a significant risk of future testicular tumor developing after mumps orchitis
- Other viral orchitides caused by coxsackievirus, infectious mononucleosis (Epstein-Barr) virus, adenovirus, arbovirus, influenza virus, echovirus, etc., have been reported.

GROSS

- Early stage: enlarged testis with edema and congestion
- Late stage: atrophy

MICROSCOPIC

- Characterized by focal nature of inflammation.
- Interstitial edema.
- Vascular congestion surrounded by cuffs of lymphocytes.
- Focal interstitial hemorrhage and exudation of fibrin and leukocytes.
- Primarily lymphocytes and plasma cells in the interstitium and seminiferous tubules; neutrophils and macrophages can be present in severely affected gonads.
- Degeneration of germ cells is a frequent finding, but Sertoli and Leydig cells show little evidence of degeneration.
- Interstitial deposition of collagen with concentric peritubular fibrosis.
- Tubular atrophy—late stage.

SPECIAL STAINS AND IMMUNOHISTOCHEMISTRY

- Gram stain: negative
- GMS: negative
- AFB: negative

DIFFERENTIAL DIAGNOSIS

- Acute orchitis
- Chronic orchitis
- Malignant lymphoma
- Leukemia

References

Beard CM, Benson RC, Kelalis PP, et al. The incidence and outcome of mumps orchitis in Rochester, Minnesota, 1935 to 1974. Mayo Clin Proc 52:3–10, 1977.
Manson AL. Mumps orchitis. Urology 36:355–358, 1990.
Werner CA. Mumps orchitis and testicular atrophy. Ann Intern Med 32: 1066–1086, 1950.

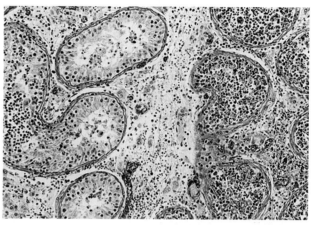

Figure 9–4. Mumps orchitis. This testicular biopsy shows the focal and patchy nature of inflammation. Some seminiferous tubules *(right half)* are heavily inflamed, but the others are mildly involved. The interstitium is edematous and contains a few inflammatory cells.

■ Nonspecific (Idiopathic) Granulomatous Orchitis

CLINICAL

- Well-defined clinicopathologic entity of unknown cause.
- Usually presents with a unilateral testicular enlargement (most common); may be accompanied by pain, tenderness, a dragging sensation, or heaviness. Rare cases have been bilateral.
- Middle-aged men.
- Trauma, infection, extravasated sperm, autoimmune disease have been postulated as possible pathogenic mechanism.

GROSS

- Moderately enlarged and indurated testis, with a thickened tunica.
- Cut surface: homogeneous, gray-white-to-tan areas of induration obscuring testicular architecture; the gross appearance may resemble that of lymphoreticular neoplasms, seminoma, and malacoplakia.
- Epididymis and tunics may be simultaneously involved.

MICROSCOPIC

- No distinct granulomas, but intratubular aggregation of epithelioid histiocytes and plasma cells impart a granulomatous appearance.
  - Early stage: predominantly intratubular, with destruction of germ cells and to a lesser extent of Sertoli cells. Interstitium is also involved.
  - Later stage: tubular destruction with extensive fibrosis. Lymphocytes, plasma cells, and histiocytes with occasional multinucleated giant cells replace entire tubules.

SPECIAL STAINS AND IMMUNOHISTOCHEMISTRY

- Gram stain: negative
- AFB: negative
- GMS: negative

DIFFERENTIAL DIAGNOSIS

- Malignant lymphoma
- Tuberculosis
- Sperm granuloma

- Malacoplakia
- Seminoma with extensive granulomatous change

References

Elicker ER, Evans AT. Granulomatous orchitis. J Urol 113:199–200, 1975.

Kahn RI, McAninch JW. Granulomatous disease of the testis. J Urol 123:868–871, 1980.

Perimenis P, Athanasopoulos A, Venetsanou-Petrochilou C, et al. Idiopathic granulomatous orchitis. Eur Urol 19:118–120, 1991.

Sporer A, Seebode JJ. Granulomatous orchitis. Urology 19:319–321, 1982.

Wegner HE, Loy V, Dieckmann KP. Granulomatous orchitis: An analysis of clinical presentation, pathological anatomic features and possible etiologic factors. Eur Urol 26:56–60, 1994.

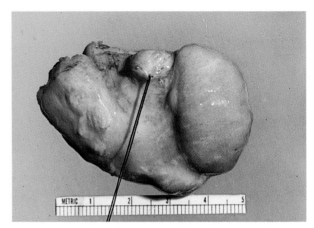

Figure 9–5. Idiopathic granulomatous orchitis. This gross illustration shows a bivalved testis exhibiting a bulging edematous parenchyma including some ill-defined prominent nodules.

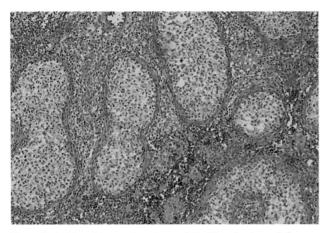

Figure 9–6. Idiopathic granulomatous orchitis. There is a heavy inflammatory infiltrate in both the tubules and stroma. Note also the increased vascularity.

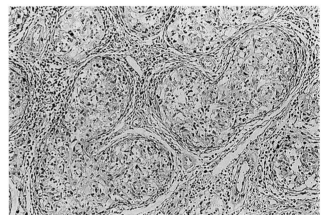

Figure 9–7. Idiopathic granulomatous orchitis. The seminiferous tubules are mildly to moderately enlarged by a histiocytic-granulomatous inflammatory reaction that has replaced the normal germinative epithelium. Some mild round cell inflammatory infiltrate is also seen in the stroma.

■ Syphilis

CLINICAL

- Testis may be involved in congenital syphilis and in the tertiary stage of acquired syphilis.
- Presents as bilateral, painless testicular enlargement.
- Gummas in tertiary syphilis.

GROSS

- Enlarged, nodular, firm testis
- Gumma: a circumscribed zone of necrosis surrounded by a fibrous capsule

MICROSCOPIC

- Interstitial mononuclear inflammation composed predominantly of plasma cells with occasional lymphocytes
- Endothelial cell proliferation with endarteritis
- Fibrosis may be extensive
- Gumma: sharply circumscribed granuloma with central necrosis lying adjacent to testicular tissue

SPECIAL STAINS AND IMMUNOHISTOCHEMISTRY

- Warthin-Starry stain may demonstrate spirochetes in gummatous stage.

DIFFERENTIAL DIAGNOSIS

• Granulomatous orchitis
• Tuberculosis

References

Nistal M, Paniagua R. Inflammatory diseases of the epididymis and testis. In Nistal M, Paniagua R (eds). *Testicular and Epididymal Pathology.* New York, Thieme-Stratton, 1984, pp 268–269.
Persaud V, Rao A. Gumma of the testis. Br J Urol 49:142, 1977.

■ Tuberculosis

CLINICAL

• One third of cases of genitourinary tuberculosis are caused by *Mycobacterium tuberculosis.*
• The epididymis is the primary site of disease; the testis is usually affected only in the late stages of disease.
• Bilateral involvement (30%).
• Formation of abscess or sinus tract (50%).
• Atypical mycobacteria, including *M. kansasii* and *M. avium–intracellulare* may also involve testis and epididymis.
• Cases of epididymo-orchitis have been reported as a late manifestation of intravesical bacille Calmette-Guérin (BCG) therapy.

GROSS

• Nodule(s) with central caseation necrosis; confluent nodules produce mass with caseation necrosis

MICROSCOPIC

• Multiple confluent granulomas with central caseation necrosis

• Epithelioid cell clusters with peripheral rim of lymphocytes
• Langhans' giant cells
• Fibrosis or fibroblastic response

SPECIAL STAINS AND IMMUNOHISTOCHEMISTRY

• AFB: positive
• GMS: negative

DIFFERENTIAL DIAGNOSIS

• Granulomatous orchitis
• Syphilis
• Malacoplakia
• Seminoma with extensive granulomatous inflammation

References

Christensen WI. Genitourinary tuberculosis. A review of 102 cases. Medicine (Baltimore) 53:377–390, 1974.
Cos LR, Cockett ATK. Genitourinary tuberculosis revisited. Urology 20:111–117, 1982.
Jocobs SC. Spermatic cord tuberculoma. Urology 9:566–567, 1977.
Riehle RA Jr, Jayaraman K. Tuberculosis of testis. Urology 20:43–46, 1982.
Stein AL, Miller DB. Tuberculous epididymo-orchitis: A case report. J Urol 129:613, 1983.
Truelson T, Wishnow KI, Johnson DE. Epididymo-orchitis developing as a late manifestation of intravesical bacillus Calmette-Guérin therapy and masquerading as a primary testicular malignancy: A report of 2 cases. J Urol 148:1534–1535, 1992.
Wechsler H, Westfall M, Lattimer JK. The earliest signs and symptoms in 127 male patients with genitourinary tuberculosis. J Urol 83:801–803, 1960.
Wolf JS, McAninch JW. Tuberculous epididymo-orchitis: Diagnosed by fine needle aspiration. J Urol 145:836–838, 1991.

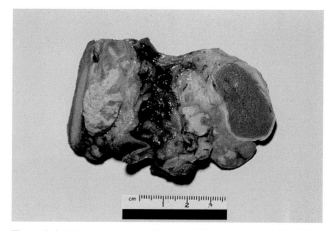

Figure 9–8. Tuberculosis, gross. There are ill-defined necrotizing lesions involving testis and epididymis. (Courtesy of Dr. S. Fligiel, Detroit.)

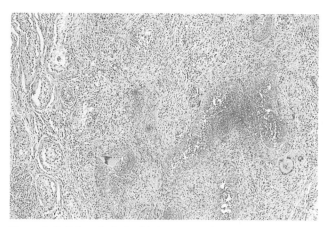

Figure 9–9. Tuberculosis. In this low-power view there are necrotizing granulomas with central caseous necrosis, and epithelioid histiocytes, lymphocytes, and plasma cells at the periphery.

■ Fungal Infections

CLINICAL

- Usually occur as part of systemic illness; may rarely present as a de novo testicular lesion.
- Organisms include *Blastomyces, Cryptococcus, Candida, Coccidioides, Histoplasma, Aspergillus,* etc.

GROSS

- Discrete circumscribed zone or confluent parenchymal destruction

MICROSCOPIC

- Mixed inflammatory infiltrate: neutrophils, lymphocytes, plasma cells, histiocytes.
- Granulomatous inflammation with or without necrosis.
- Fungal organisms may or may not be apparent on H&E sections.

SPECIAL STAINS AND IMMUNOHISTOCHEMISTRY

- GMS or Grocott: positive, showing distinctive morphology

DIFFERENTIAL DIAGNOSIS

- Granulomatous orchitis
- Malacoplakia
- Seminoma with extensive granulomatous inflammation
- Tuberculosis
- Syphilis

References

James CL, Lomax-Smith JD. Cryptococcal epididymo-orchitis complicating steroid therapy for relapsing polychondritis. Pathology 23:256–258, 1991.

Monroe M. Granulomatous orchitis due to *Histoplasma capsulatum* masquerading as a sperm granuloma. J Clin Pathol 4:927–929, 1974.

CHAPTER 10

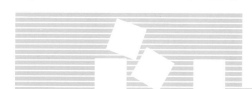

Germ Cell Tumors of the Testis

■ **Gross Examination**

- Measure and weigh the testicle and spermatic cord.
- Take a section of the spermatic cord margin before opening the testis (to avoid contamination of surgical margin by tumor) (see Fig. 10–43).
- Bivalve the testis completely, including the tumor.
- Cut epididymis longitudinally throughout its length; examine for tumor extension.
- Cut spermatic cord at several levels; examine for gross tumor.
- Sections to be submitted:
  - Spermatic cord margin.
  - Spermatic cord, random sections (two to three sections).
  - Tumor (at least one section per centimeter of tumor).
  - Sample hemorrhagic and necrotic areas of tumor and areas that have different gross appearance.
  - Two to three sections of uninvolved testis.
  - Rete testis and epididymis.

■ **Information to Be Included in Surgical Pathology Report**

- Specify tumor type: seminoma, nonseminomatous germ cell tumor (NSGCT), sex cord–stromal tumor, others.
- If NSGCT, indicate the different components with their relative amounts expressed as a percentage.
- Presence of vascular or lymphatic invasion: specify location in relation to the tumor.
- Spermatic cord: if involved by tumor, indicate the status of cord margin.
- Epididymis.
- Involvement of tunica, if present.
- Uninvolved testis: presence of intratubular germ cell neoplasia, features of cryptorchidism, prior therapy effect, etc.

■ **Classification of Testicular Tumors**

Germ cell tumors
    Intratubular germ cell neoplasia (ITGCN)
    Seminoma
        Classic seminoma
        Tubular seminoma
      Spermatocytic seminoma
    Nonseminomatous germ cell tumors
        Embryonal carcinoma (EC)
        Yolk sac tumor (YST; endodermal sinus tumor [EST]
        Teratoma, mature and immature
        Choriocarcinoma
        Mixed germ cell tumor (MGCT)
        Polyembryoma
        Diffuse embryoma
    Others
        Carcinoid tumor
Sex cord–stromal tumors
    Leydig cell tumor
    Sertoli cell tumor
        Large cell calcifying Sertoli cell tumor
        Sclerosing Sertoli cell tumor
    Granulosa cell tumor (GCT)
        Juvenile GCT
        Adult GCT
    Tumor of adrenogenital syndrome
    Mixed and unclassified sex cord–stromal tumor
Germ cell and sex cord–stromal tumors
    Gonadoblastoma
    Unclassified germ cell and sex cord–stromal tumor
Lymphoreticular neoplasms
    Malignant lymphoma
    Leukemia
    Plasmacytoma
Metastatic tumors
Tumorous conditions
    Epidermoid cyst
    Malacoplakia
    Sclerosing lipogranuloma
    Sperm granuloma
    Vasitis nodosa
    Fibrous pseudotumor
Tumors of rete testis
    Adenomatous hyperplasia
    Adenocarcinoma of rete testis

Tumors of tunica and mesothelium
    Mesothelioma
    Tumors of Müllerian origin
Tumors of paratesticular region
    Adenomatoid tumor
    Papillary cystadenoma
    Melanotic neuroectodermal tumor
    Paratesticular sarcoma

■ Staging of Germ Cell Tumors (TNM)

AMERICAN JOINT COMMITTEE ON CANCER (AJCC) STAGING SYSTEM (1992)

Primary Tumor (T)

pTX   Primary tumor cannot be assessed (if no radical orchiectomy has been performed, TX is used).

pT0   No evidence of primary tumor (e.g., histologic scar in testis).

pTis   Intratubular tumor; preinvasive cancer.

pT1   Tumor limited to the testis, including the rete testis.

pT2   Tumor invades beyond the tunica albuginea or into the epididymis.

pT3   Tumor invades the spermatic cord.

pT4   Tumor invades the scrotum.

Regional Lymph Nodes (N)

NX   Regional lymph nodes cannot be assessed.

N0   No regional lymph node metastasis.

N1   Metastasis in a single lymph node, 2 cm or less in greatest dimension.

N2   Metastasis in a single lymph node, more than 2 cm but not more than 5 cm in greatest dimension; or multiple lymph nodes, none more than 5 cm in greatest dimension.

N3   Metastasis in a lymph node more than 5 cm in greatest dimension.

Distant Metastasis (M)

MX   Presence of distant metastasis cannot be assessed.

M0   No distant metastasis.

M1   Distant metastasis.

Stage Grouping

Stage	0	pTis	N0	M0
Stage	I	Any pT	N0	M0
Stage	II	Any pT	N1	M0
		Any pT	N2	M0
		Any pT	N3	M0
Stage	III	Any pT	Any N	M1

M.D. ANDERSON CANCER CENTER (MDACC) STAGING SYSTEM FOR SEMINOMA

Stage	I	Tumor confined to the testis
Stage	II	Nodal metastases, but limited to the infradiaphragmatic lymph nodes
	IIA	Mass less than 10 cm
	IIB	Mass 10 cm or larger
Stage	III	Nodal metastases above diaphragm or visceral metastases

MDACC STAGING SYSTEM FOR NONSEMINOMATOUS GERM CELL TUMOR

Stage	I	Tumor confined to the testis
Stage	II	Nodal metastasis limited to the infradiaphragmatic lymph nodes
	IIA	Rising levels of serum biomarkers (alpha-fetoprotein, human chorionic gonadotropin)
	IIB	Metastases less than 2 cm
	IIC	Metastases 2 to less than 5 cm
	IID	Metastases 5 cm or greater, but less than 10 cm
Stage	III	Metastases 10 cm or greater or lymph node metastases above the diaphragm or visceral metastases

Other staging systems include International Union Against Cancer (UICC) TNM, Boden/Gibb, Memorial Sloan-Kettering Cancer Center, Royal Marsden, Skinner, and Massachusetts General Hospital staging system.

■ Germ Cell Tumors

Intratubular Germ Cell Neoplasia (ITGCN)

CLASSIFICATION OF ITGCN

Unclassified (undifferentiated)
Differentiated types
    Intratubular seminoma
    Intratubular embryonal carcinoma
    Intratubular yolk sac tumor (YST)
    Intratubular teratoma
    Intratubular choriocarcinoma

CLINICAL

- Precursor lesion of invasive germ cell tumors seen in virtually all cases of germ cell tumors.
- Also seen in 0.5% to 1.0% of infertile patients with severe oligospermia, in 2% to 8% of those with cryptorchidism, and in 5% of those with a history of testicular cancer; increased risk in patients with gonadal dysgenesis and androgen-insensitivity syndrome.
- Fifteen percent to 20% risk for development of a tumor in the remaining or contralateral testis in patients with a history of undescended testis and testicular carcinoma.
- Fifty percent of patients with ITGCN progress to invasive carcinoma within 5 years. In some cases, development of the invasive tumor may take longer.
- Most patients with ITGCN develop seminoma, although NSGCTs can also occur.
- ITGCN has not been noted in spermatocytic seminoma, indicating lack of its role in development of this tumor.
- The role of ITGCN in the development of pediatric germ cell tumors (YST, teratoma, NSGCT) is not clear and is currently a controversial issue.

GROSS

- No demonstrable testicular mass
- Testis usually smaller than normal (especially cryptorchid testis)

MICROSCOPIC

- Seminiferous tubules with decreased diameter and thickened tubular wall and decreased or absent spermatogenesis.
- Early stage: large atypical cells with enlarged central nuclei and abundant clear to faintly eosinophilic cytoplasm (containing lipid and glycogen) at the periphery of tubules, often forming a distinct rim around the tubules (morphologically the cells of ITGCN are identical to those of seminoma); large nuclei with evenly distributed chromatin pattern and large, prominent, irregular nucleoli. Mitotic figures, including abnormal forms, may be seen. The center of the seminiferous tubules may contain maturing germ cells and even spermatozoa. Rete testis can be involved by ITGCN ("pagetoid spread").
- Later stage: extensive replacement of the normal tubular components by atypical cells.
- Intratubular microcalcifications are more frequently seen in ITGCN specimens than in control samples.
- Pagetoid spread of ITGCN into rete testis is frequently seen in testis with invasive germ cell tumors (more common in NSGCTs than in seminomas).
- No extratubular extension.
- Intratubular seminoma and intratubular embryonal carcinoma can be seen; rarely intratubular YST, intratubular choriocarcinoma, and intratubular teratoma. This terminology of intratubular seminoma or embryonal carcinoma is reserved for complete packing of seminiferous tubules by neoplastic cells that are readily characterizable as a distinct germ cell tumor type. Alternative terms are seminoma in situ, embryonal carcinoma in situ, etc.

SPECIAL STAINS AND IMMUNOHISTOCHEMISTRY

- PAS with and without diastase: positive for glycogen in cytoplasm
- Cytokeratin: negative; may be focally positive
- PLAP: positive, highly sensitive
- Alpha-fetoprotein (AFP) and human chorionic gonadotropin (HCG): negative
- Monoclonal 43–9F and M2A: positive
- NSE: positive
- Ferritin: positive

DIFFERENTIAL DIAGNOSIS

- Normal spermatogenic cells

References

Burke AP, Mostofi FK. Intratubular malignant germ cells in testicular biopsies: Clinical course and identification by staining for placental alkaline phosphatase. Mod Pathol 1:475–479, 1988.

Coffin CM, Ewing S, Dehner LP. Frequency of intratubular germ cell neoplasia with invasive testicular germ cell tumors: Histologic and immunohistochemical features. Arch Pathol Lab Med 109:555–559, 1985.

Gondos B, Migliozzi JA. Intratubular germ cell neoplasia. Semin Diagn Pathol 4:292–303, 1987.

Jacobsen GK, Henriksen OB, Der Maase HV. Carcinoma in situ of testicular tissue adjacent to malignant germ cell tumors: A study of 105 cases. Cancer 47:2660–2662, 1981.

Kang JL, Rajpert-de Meyts E, Giwercman A, et al. The association of testicular carcinoma in situ with intratubular microcalcifications. J Urol Pathol 2:235–242, 1994.

Nistal M, Codesai J, Paniagua R. Carcinoma in situ of the testis in infertile men. A histological, immunocytochemical, and cytophotometric study of DNA content. J Pathol 159:205–210, 1989.

Perry A, Wiley EL, Albores-Saavedra J. Pagetoid spread of intratubular germ cell neoplasia into rete testis: A morphologic and histochemical study of 100 orchiectomy specimens with invasive germ cell tumors. Hum Pathol 25:235–239, 1994.

Scully RE. Testis. In Hedson DE, Albores-Saavedra J (eds). *The Pathology of Incipient Neoplasia.* Philadelphia, WB Saunders, 1986, pp 329–343.

Skakkebaek NE. Carcinoma-in-situ of the testis: Frequency and relationship to invasive germ cell tumours in infertile men. Histopathology 2:157–170, 1978.

Skakkebaek NE, Berthelsen JG, Muller J. Carcinoma-in-situ of the undescended testis. Urol Clin North Am 9:377–385, 1982.

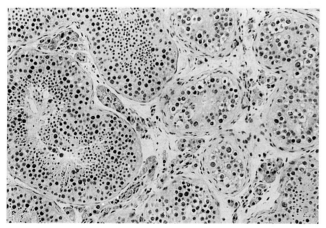

Figure 10–1. Intratubular germ cell neoplasia (ITGCN). The smaller tubules exhibit the presence of large cells with abundant clear cytoplasm and a centrally placed nucleus; these cells are seen at the periphery of the tubule in contact with the basement membrane. The larger seminiferous tubules display active spermatogenesis.

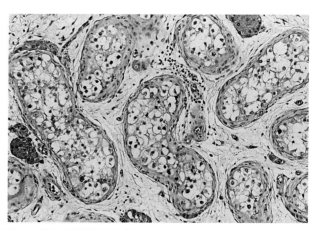

Figure 10–2. ITGCN. All of the tubules show the prominent large cytoplasmic cells, not only at the periphery of the tubule but also within the entire width of the tubule.

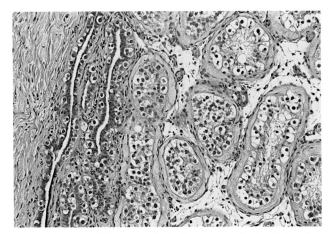

Figure 10–3. ITGCN. Large atypical cells are present in the tubules. Note pagetoid spread of these cells into the adjacent rete testis.

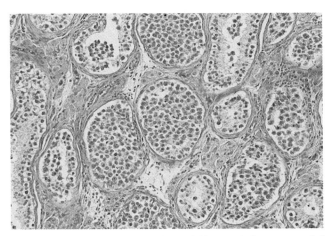

Figure 10–4. Seminoma in situ. The seminiferous tubules are expanded and completely replaced by proliferation of seminomatous cells.

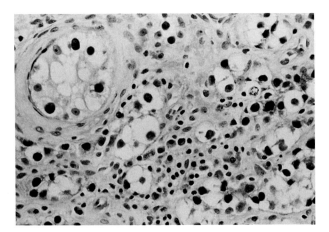

Figure 10–5. ITGCN with microinvasion. This example shows a tubule with ITGCN and few isolated single cells of invasive seminoma in the stroma accompanied by some lymphocytic infiltration.

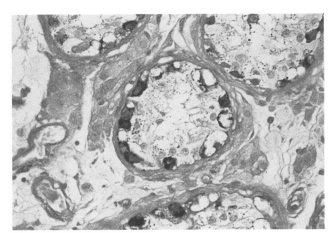

Figure 10–6. ITGCN. The high content of cytoplasmic glycogen in the cells of ITGCN is reflected by the strong PAS-positive reaction which disappears after diastase digestion.

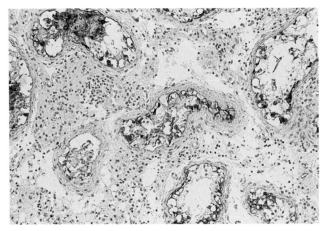

Figure 10–7. ITGCN. Placental alkaline phosphatase (PLAP) immunoreactivity of the neoplastic cells. Normal spermatogenic cells are negative for PLAP.

Classic Seminoma

CLINICAL

- Accounts for 40% to 50% of testicular germ cell tumors (the most common testicular tumor).
- Most frequent germ cell tumor in patients with bilateral germ cell tumors (2%) except for spermatocytic seminoma (4%–10%).
- Occurs in undescended testis in 5% to 8%.
- Most common in 35- to 45-year-olds, relatively uncommon in men over 50 years of age, and rare in children.
- More than 70% present with testicular enlargement with or without pain.
- Presentation with symptoms of metastases (10%).
- Asymptomatic (4%).
- Gynecomastia or exophthalmos can rarely be presenting symptoms (usually due to HCG production).
- Good prognosis with therapy.
- Elevated serum PLAP (40%) and HCG (10%).
- Presence of elevated serum HCG does not change classification and has no known clinical significance. Presence of elevated serum AFP, however, indicates an NSGCT even though histologic examinations disclose only seminomatous component.
- Anaplastic seminoma: defined as seminoma with three or more mitoses per high-power field in most fields and pleomorphism of tumor cells. Accounts for 5% to 15% of seminomas. Controversial survival data: some claim it has worse prognosis than classic seminoma, but most authors do not agree. Most believe that this is not a separate entity.

GROSS

- Well-demarcated, homogeneous, soft mass
- White-gray to tan, coarsely lobulated, bulging
- Hemorrhage and necrosis uncommon except for large tumors
- Usually confined to testis; extension to the spermatic cord or epididymis in 5% to 8%

MICROSCOPIC

- Diffuse proliferation of large, uniform tumor cells arranged in a lobular pattern.
- Sheets, nests, cords of tumor cells.
- Regularity of the supporting fibrovascular stroma containing variable amount of lymphocytes.
- Papillary, cribriform, cystic, tubular, and acinar patterns (tubular seminoma) are extremely rare and extensive tubulopapillary or acinar arrangement should arouse suspicion of NSGCT component; in most cases, tubular or papillary structures are artifacts.
- Edema with proteinaceous fluid and microcystic appearance; usually focal.
- Seminiferous tubules may be entrapped within tumor (usually at periphery).

- Discrete or diffuse granulomatous reaction with or without Langhans' giant cells (30%–50%); granulomas may be seen in seminiferous tubules.
- Stromal sclerosis and artifactual distortion are frequently seen.
- Calcification and, rarely, ossification may be seen.
- The tumor cells are relatively large, uniform cells with a large, polygonal or round central nucleus surrounded by clear or eosinophilic cytoplasm.
- The tumor cells are evenly spaced without nuclear overlapping. The cell border is characteristically distinct.
- Mitotic figures are common, especially in so-called anaplastic seminoma.
- The nucleus is traversed by thin bands of chromatin, which is finely granular and uniform and contains one or two prominent nucleoli.
- Scattered syncytiotrophoblasts in 10% to 20% (may be associated with microscopic "blood lakes"); choriocarcinoma component with seminoma without other germ cell components is nonexistent or extremely rare.
- Pagetoid spread of seminoma cells to rete testis may occur.

SPECIAL STAINS AND IMMUNOHISTOCHEMISTRY

- PAS with and without diastase: positive for glycogen in the cytoplasm of the tumor cells
- Cytokeratin: negative; may be positive in scattered cells (mainly cytokeratin 8 and 18); diffuse and intense staining usually rules out seminoma
- Vimentin: may be positive
- HCG: positive in syncytiotrophoblast
- PLAP: usually diffusely positive
- NSE: usually positive
- Ki-1: negative

DIFFERENTIAL DIAGNOSIS

- Malignant lymphoma (Table 10–1)
- Granulomatous orchitis
- Embryonal carcinoma (Table 10–2)
- Yolk sac tumor (YST): usually in children (Table 10–3)
- Spermatocytic seminoma

References

Babaian RJ, Zagars GK. Testicular seminoma: The M.D. Anderson experience. An analysis of pathological and patient characteristics and treatment recommendations. J Urol 139:311–314, 1988.

Bell DA, Flotte TJ, Bhan AK. Immunohistochemical characterization of seminoma and its inflammatory cell infiltrate. Hum Pathol 18:511–520, 1987.

Cockburn AG, Vugrin D, Batata M, et al. Poorly differentiated (anaplastic) seminoma of the testis. Cancer 53:1991–1994, 1984.

Eglen DE, Ulbright TM. The differential diagnosis of yolk sac tumor and seminoma. Usefulness of cytokeratin, alpha-fetoprotein, and alpha-1-antitrypsin immunoperoxidase reactions. Am J Clin Pathol 88:328–332, 1987.

Johnson DE, Gomez JJ, Ayala AG. Anaplastic seminoma. J Urol 114:80–82, 1975.

Table 10–1

DIFFERENTIAL FEATURES BETWEEN
SEMINOMA AND LYMPHOMA

	Seminoma	Lymphoma
Age (yr)	35–45	>60
Bilaterality	2%	20%
Spermatic cord involvement	5%–8%	50%
Growth pattern	Diffuse	Interstitial
Lobular arrangement	Present	Absent
Fibrovascular septa	Present	Absent
Granulomas	Present	Absent
Tumor cells	Polygonal/round	Oval/round
Tumor cell nucleus	Uniform	Pleomorphic
Nuclear chromatin	Fine	Coarse
Tumor cell spacing	Evenly spaced	Overlapping
Cell boundary	Distinct	Variable
PLAP	+	−
LCA	−	+
Glycogen	+	±
ITGCN	Present	Absent

PLAP, placental alkaline phosphatase; LCA, leukocyte common antigen;
ITGCN, intratubular germ cell neoplasia.

Table 10–2

DIFFERENTIAL FEATURES BETWEEN
SEMINOMA AND EMBRYONAL
CARCINOMA

	Seminoma	Embryonal Carcinoma
Growth pattern	Diffuse	Papillary, tubular, acinar, solid
Lobular arrangement	Present	Variable
Fibrovascular septa	Present	Variable
Lymphocytes	Present	Variable
Granulomas	Present	Variable
Tumor cell nucleus	Uniform	Pleomorphic
Nuclear chromatin	Fine	Clumping/clearing
Nucleolus	Large, regular	Large, irregular
Mitoses	Frequent	Frequent/atypical
Tumor cell spacing	Evenly spaced	Overlapping
Cell boundary	Distinct	Variable
Cytoplasm	Clear	Amphophilic
Keratin	−*	+
Ki-1	−	+

*May be positive (focal and weak).

Table 10–3

DIFFERENTIAL FEATURES BETWEEN SEMINOMA AND YOLK
SAC TUMOR (YST)

	Seminoma	YST
Growth pattern	Diffuse	Multiple different patterns
Lobular arrangement	Present	Absent
Fibrovascular septa	Present	Absent
Lymphocytes	Present	Variable
Granulomas	Present	Variable
Tumor cell nucleus	Polygonal/round	Cuboidal, flat, round, or oval
Nuclear chromatin	Fine	Fine
Nucleolus	Large, regular	Usually small
Mitoses	Frequent	Variable
Tumor cell spacing	Evenly spaced	Overlapping
Cell boundary	Distinct	Indistinct
Cytoplasm	Clear	Variable
Keratin	−*	+
Alpha-fetoprotein	−	+

*May be positive (focal and weak).

Manivel JC, Jessurun J, Wick MR, et al. Placental alkaline phosphatase immunoreactivity in testicular germ-cell neoplasms. Am J Surg Pathol 11:21–29, 1987.

Percarpio B, Clements JC, McLeod DG, et al. Anaplastic seminoma: An analysis of 77 patients. Cancer 43:2510–2513, 1979.

Stein M, Steiner M, Moshkowitz B, et al. Testicular seminoma: 20-year experience at the Northern Israel Oncology Center (1968–1988). Int Urol Nephrol 26:461–469, 1994.

Suzuki T, Sasano H, Aoki H, et al. Immunohistochemical comparison between anaplastic seminoma and typical seminoma. Acta Pathol Jpn 43:751–757, 1993.

Ulbright TM. Germ cell neoplasms of the testis. Am J Surg Pathol 17:1075–1091, 1993.

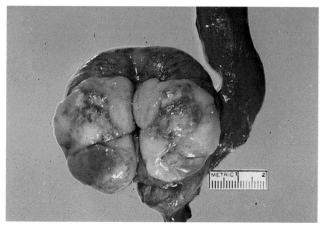

Figure 10–8. Seminoma, gross. This bivalved testis shows a relatively well-delineated tumor. The cut surface is white with a fish flesh bulging appearance. Focal areas of hemorrhage are also present.

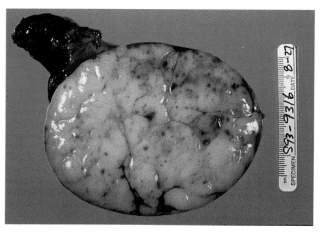

Figure 10–9. Seminoma, gross. This large bulging testicular tumor shows some septation and lobulation.

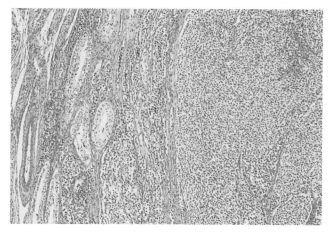

Figure 10–10. Seminoma, low-power view. The tumor is well demarcated from the adjacent compressed testicular parenchyma.

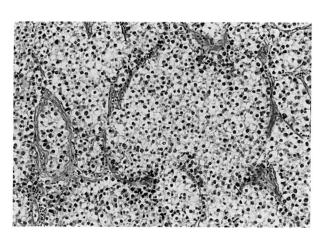

Figure 10–11. Seminoma. Note sheets of large clear cells separated from one another by a delicate cytoplasmic membrane. Thin fibrovascular septa containing lymphocytes divide tumor cells into lobules.

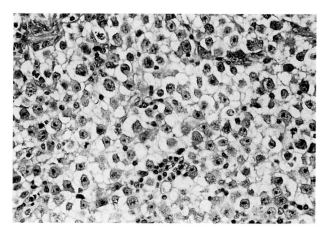

Figure 10–12. Seminoma. In the high-power view the cells of seminoma display a centrally placed round-to-polygonal nucleus which often contains a prominent nucleolus. The cells are relatively monotonous and evenly spaced without nuclear overlapping. Note again delicate cytoplasmic membranes. A few collections of lymphocytes are also seen.

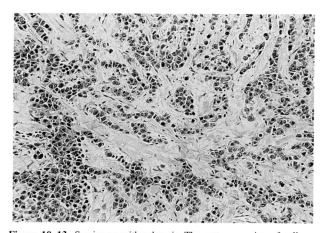

Figure 10–13. Seminoma with sclerosis. The pattern consists of collagenized stroma compressing seminoma cells into cords of cells which sometimes form single file. The key to the recognition of seminoma is based on recognition of characteristic cytologic features.

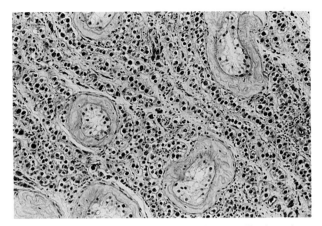

Figure 10–14. Seminoma with interstitial involvement. Classic seminoma cells may infiltrate between seminiferous tubules. This pattern is more commonly seen at the periphery of the tumor than at the center.

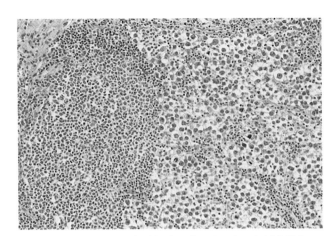

Figure 10–15. Seminoma. In this view there is a lymphoid follicle surrounded by seminomatous cells.

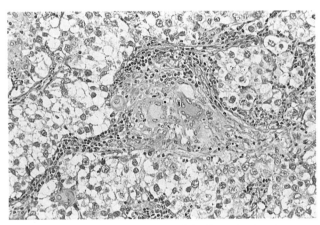

Figure 10–16. Seminoma. In the center of the illustration there is a granuloma with epithelioid histiocytes and multinucleated giant cells.

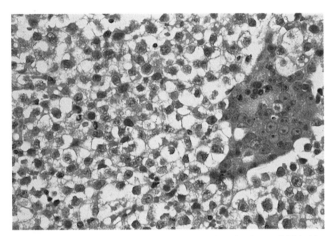

Figure 10–17. Seminoma with a syncytiotrophoblastic giant cell. This histologic finding explains the elevated serum human chorionic gonadotropin level which may be seen in seminoma patients.

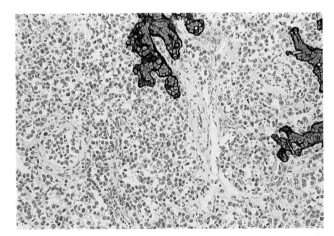

Figure 10–18. Seminoma demonstrating cytokeratin immunoreactivity in syncytiotrophoblastic giant cells. Note negative keratin staining in seminoma cells.

Figure 10–19. Seminoma showing intense PAS staining of the cytoplasm of the tumor cells.

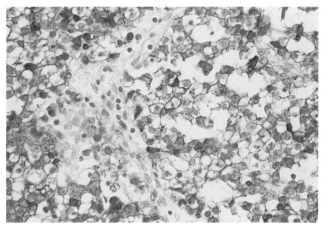

Figure 10–20. Seminoma. There is diffuse membrane immunoreactivity to placental alkaline phosphatase in tumor cells.

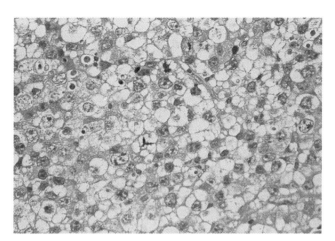

Figure 10–21. Seminoma. In this illustration there are numerous mitotic figures. When such a finding occurs uniformly throughout the tumor, some investigators designate it as the anaplastic variant of seminoma.

Tubular Seminoma

CLINICAL

- A rare variant of seminoma.
- Fewer than 10 cases have been reported in the literature.
- The clinical behavior is similar to classic seminoma, but its recognition is important because it may be confused with an NSGCT or a sex cord–stromal tumor, which has different therapeutic implications.

GROSS

- Not different from that of seminoma

MICROSCOPIC

- Tumor cells forming tubular structures of various sizes and shapes.
- A tubulopapillary growth pattern with central fibrovascular septa containing a sparse lymphocytic infiltrate.
- Areas of classic seminoma always present.
- Tumor cells are cytologically identical to those of classic seminoma.

SPECIAL STAINS AND IMMUNOHISTOCHEMISTRY

- Same as for classic seminoma

DIFFERENTIAL DIAGNOSIS

- Testicular tumors that contain tubular structures, such as Sertoli cell tumor (SCT), embryonal carcinoma (EC), and yolk sac tumor (YST) are in the differential diagnosis. Although morphologic features are critical, immunohistochemistry may be helpful (Table 10–4).
- Spermatocytic seminoma.

References

Damjanov I, Niejadlik DC, Rabuffo JV, et al. Cribriform and sclerosing seminoma devoid of lymphoid infiltrates. Arch Pathol Lab Med 104:527–530, 1980.

Talerman A. Tubular seminoma (letter). Arch Pathol Lab Med 113:1204, 1989.

Ulbright TM. Morphologic variation in seminoma (editorial). Am J Clin Pathol 102:395–396, 1994.

Young RH, Finlayson N, Scully RE. Tubular seminoma: Report of a case. Arch Pathol Lab Med 113:414–416, 1989.

Zavala-Pompa A, Ro JY, El-Naggar AK, et al. Tubular seminoma: An immunohistochemical and DNA flow-cytometric study of four cases. Am J Clin Pathol 102:397–401, 1994.

Table 10–4
DIFFERENTIAL FEATURES OF TUBULAR SEMINOMA AND OTHER TESTICULAR TUMORS (IMMUNOHISTOCHEMISTRY)

	Tubular Seminoma	Embryonal Carcinoma	Yolk Sac Tumor	Sertoli Cell Tumor
PLAP	+	+	+	−
Keratin	−	+	+	+
Alpha-fetoprotein	−	±	+	−
Ki-1	−	+	−	−

PLAP, placental alkaline phosphatase.

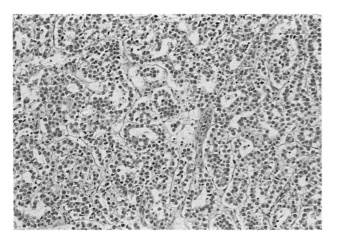

Figure 10–22. Tubular seminoma. In this variant most seminoma cells are attached to connective tissue septa, resulting in a tubular pattern.

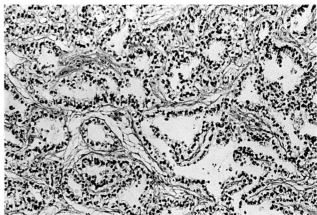

Figure 10–23. Seminoma, tubular pattern. In this interesting growth pattern, which may be a diagnostic pitfall, the cells of seminoma adhere to the connective tissue trabeculae while the central cells are loosely arranged, resulting in a tubular pattern. Cytologically, the cells show abundant clear cytoplasm and a centrally placed nucleus.

Spermatocytic Seminoma

CLINICAL

- This tumor is not a subtype of seminoma, but a distinct clinicopathologic entity with unique morphologic features and biologically indolent course.
- Uncommon tumor (3.5%–7.5% of all seminomas and 1%–2% of all testicular GCTs).
- Germ cell neoplasm unique to the testis; no cases in extratesticular sites, undescended testes, or ovaries.
- Almost always seen in pure form; not associated with ITGCN.
- Frequent in men older than 50 years of age.
- Bilaterality is higher (4%–10%) than seminoma (2%).
- Painless testicular enlargement.
- Indolent clinical behavior in pure forms.
- Rarely associated with malignant mesenchymal tumors such as rhabdomyosarcoma, undifferentiated sarcoma, and chondrosarcoma. The sarcomatous differentiation dictates the clinical course, which is usually poor with distant metastasis.

GROSS

- Small or large, well-circumscribed mass
- Described as yellowish-gray and of soft mucoid and gelatinous consistency; however, in most cases its gross appearance is identical to that of classic seminoma
- Cyst formation and hemorrhage

MICROSCOPIC

- Diffuse proliferation of polymorphic cells with focal microcysts.
- Intratubular and interstitial patterns of growth; intratubular pattern should not be confused with ITGCN as this represents intratubular extension and not preneoplastic lesion.
- Lack of prominent fibrous trabecular stroma.
- Lack of lymphocytic infiltrate and granulomas.
- Three cell types on the basis of size, with intermediate cells predominating:
  - Large cells (50–100 μm): uninucleate or multinucleate; cells and nuclei have a round shape and marked variation in size, and nuclei have filamentous meiotic-type chromatin (spireme-type chromatin).
  - Intermediate cells (10–20 μm): most frequent cell type; have perfectly round nucleus with evenly dispersed granular chromatin and eosinophilic cytoplasm; cells may have distinctive filamentous chromatin (spireme-type chromatin).
  - Small lymphocyte-like cells (6–8 μm): have uniformly hyperchromatic nuclei and scant cytoplasm.
- Numerous mitoses may be evident.
- Lack of PAS-positive clear cytoplasm.
- Not associated with other germ cell neoplasms or ITGCN.
- May be associated with a high-grade sarcoma: approximately a dozen cases have been reported with most sarcomas being high-grade undifferentiated sarcomas. Cases of rhabdomyosarcoma and chondrosarcoma have been

reported. Most patients died of disease in a few months with metastases.

Special Stains and Immunohistochemistry

- Various tumor markers, including the intermediate filaments and PLAP, that are immunoreactive in other types of germ cell tumors are negative in spermatocytic seminoma.
- PAS with and without diastase for glycogen: negative.

Differential Diagnosis

- Seminoma (Table 10–5)
- Malignant lymphoma
- Pure solid embryonal carcinoma

References

Burke AP, Mostofi FK. Spermatocytic seminoma: A clinicopathologic study of 79 cases. J Urol Pathol 1:21–32, 1993.

Cummings OW, Ulbright TM, Eble JN, et al. Spermatocytic seminoma: An immunohistochemical study. Hum Pathol 25:54–59, 1994.

Eble JN. Spermatocytic seminoma. Hum Pathol 25:1035–1042, 1994.

Floyd C, Ayala AG, Logothetis CJ, et al. Spermatocytic seminoma with associated sarcoma of the testis. Cancer 61:409–414, 1988.

Matoska J, Ondrus D, Hornak M. Metastatic spermatocytic seminoma: A case report with light microscopic, ultrastructural and immunohistochemical findings. Cancer 62:1197–1201, 1988.

Talerman A. Spermatocytic seminoma. Clinicopathological study of 22 cases. Cancer 45:2169–2176, 1980.

True LD, Otis CN, Delprado W, et al. Spermatocytic seminoma of testis with sarcomatous transformation. A report of five cases. Am J Surg Pathol 12:75–82, 1988.

Table 10–5
DIFFERENTIAL FEATURES OF SPERMATOCYTIC AND CLASSIC SEMINOMA

	Spermatocytic Seminoma	Classic Seminoma
Incidence	3.5%–7.5%	92.5%–96.5%
Age (yr)	>50	35–45
Site	Testis only	Testis, ovary, mediastinum, retroperitoneum, CNS
Bilaterality	4%–10%	2%
Occurrence of undescended testis	Not documented	8.5%
Associated other germ cell elements	None	25%
Associated sarcoma	5%	None
Prognosis	Excellent	Very good with adequate treatment
Gross appearance	Gray-yellow, soft, gelatinous, mucoid	White-gray, soft, lobulated
Histologic features		
Nuclei	Round and dark, three cell types	Polygonal/round, vesicular
Cytoplasm	Dense, scanty, acidophilic	Clear, abundant
Glycogen	Scant or absent	Abundant
Edema	Present, often marked	Absent
Stroma	Scant and fine	More prominent and dense
Lymphocytes	Absent	Present
Granulomas	Absent	Present
Metastases	Rare	Common

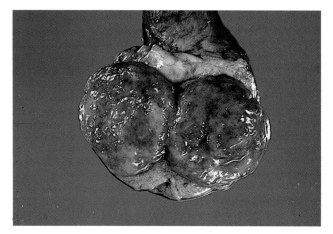

Figure 10–24. Spermatocytic seminoma (SS), gross. This is a bivalved testis exhibiting a bulging brown tumor with focal areas of hemorrhage. In our experience most SS grossly are very similar to classic seminoma, but some cases may have a mucoid and gelatinous, occasionally cystic, appearance. (From Ro JY, Sahin AA, Ayala AG. Tumors and tumorous conditions of the male genital tract. In Fletcher CDM (ed). *Diagnostic Histopathology of Tumors*. Edinburgh, Churchill Livingstone, 1995, p 569.)

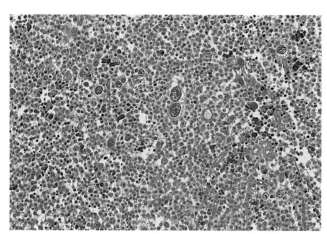

Figure 10–25. Spermatocytic seminoma. In the low-power view there is a solid proliferation of cells with scattered large giant cells demonstrating at least two cell types.

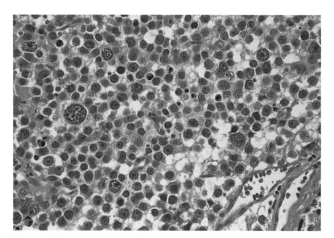

Figure 10–26. Spermatocytic seminoma. All three cell types can be clearly appreciated in this illustration: a few large gigantic cells, a few small dark cells, and a great majority of medium-sized cells.

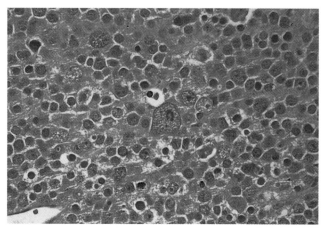

Figure 10–27. Spermatocytic seminoma. A higher magnification than in Figure 10–26 shows morphologic detail of the three cell types. Note spireme-type chromatin in large cells.

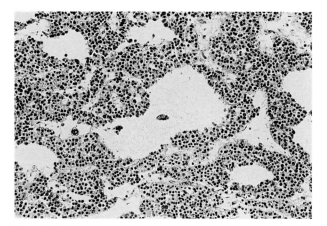

Figure 10–28. Spermatocytic seminoma. This view shows the microcystic pattern of SS, containing edema fluid in cystic cavities. The majority of the cells are of the intermediate type, although there are occasional large cells.

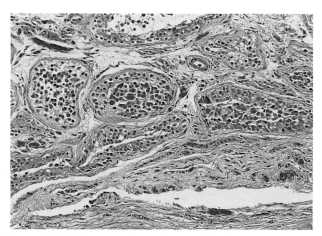

Figure 10–29. Spermatocytic seminoma. This is an illustration of intratubular growth of SS which should not be confused with intratubular germ cell neoplasia.

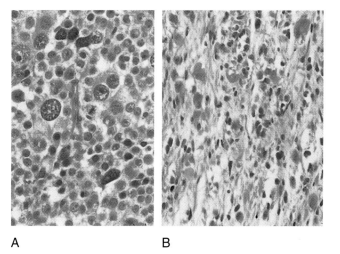

A   B

Figure 10–30. Spermatocytic seminoma and rhabdomyosarcoma. Fields typical of SS (*A*) and embryonal rhabdomyosarcoma (*B*).

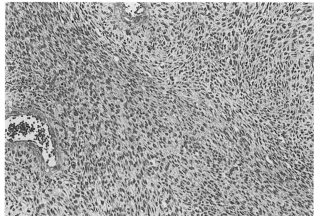

Figure 10–31. Spermatocytic seminoma with unclassified sarcoma.

Nonseminomatous Germ Cell Tumors

GENERAL FEATURES

- Pure or in combination with other germ cell tumor components, including seminoma.
- There are three adverse prognostic factors for stage I nonseminomatous germ cell tumors: (1) 80% or greater of embryonal carcinoma components, (2) presence of vascular or lymphatic invasion (see Fig. 10–42), and (3) AFP serum level 80 ng/mL or greater.
- In the diagnosis list all the components with their relative percentages.

References

Dunphy CH, Ayala AG, Swanson DA, et al. Clinical stage I nonseminomatous and mixed germ cell tumors of the testis. A clinicopathologic study of 93 patients on a surveillance protocol after orchiectomy alone. Cancer 62:1202–1206, 1988.

Moul JW, McCarthy WF, Fernandez EB, et al. Percentage of embryonal carcinoma and of vascular invasion predicts pathological stage in clinical stage I nonseminomatous testicular cancer. Cancer Res 54:362–364, 1994.

Ro JY, Dexeus FH, El-Naggar A, et al. Testicular germ cell tumors: Clinically relevant pathologic findings. Pathol Annu 26:59–87, 1991.

Embryonal Carcinoma (EC)

CLINICAL

- Second most common pure testicular germ cell neoplasm (15%–30%); some authors have reported that pure EC is relatively unusual, accounting for only 2% to 3% of cases, suggesting that a higher incidence of pure EC probably reflects a tendency to underdiagnose foci of YST (correlation with serum AFP is useful).

- Most frequent in third decade; not found in infants and children; very rare after fifth decade.
- Present as painless testicular enlargement, mostly unilateral.
- One third of patients present with metastasis (para-aortic lymph nodes, lungs, liver).
- Occasionally associated with gynecomastia.
- Serum AFP and HCG may be elevated.

GROSS

- Variegated, solid gray-white tumor with poorly demarcated borders
- Large areas of hemorrhage and necrosis
- Invasion of the adjacent epididymis and cord (20%)

MICROSCOPIC

- Acinar, tubular, papillary, or solid pattern.
- Tumor cells with nuclear overlapping (syncytial growth); marked cellular anaplasia (key feature) is evident even at lower power.
- Areas of necrosis and hemorrhage.
- Fibrosis.
- Anaplastic tumor cells with large, irregular nuclei; coarse chromatin with chromatin clumping and clearing; distinct nuclear membrane; prominent macronucleoli; high mitotic activity with frequent atypical forms; abundant finely granular cytoplasm with indistinct cellular borders.
- Intratubular EC or ITGCN (unclassified) may be seen adjacent to invasive EC; intratubular EC often associated with lesional necrosis.
- The presence of undifferentiated cellular spindle stroma should be separately categorized as an immature teratomatous component.
- Vascular invasion is frequent.

SPECIAL STAINS AND IMMUNOHISTOCHEMISTRY

- AFP: may be focally positive
- HCG: positive in syncytiotrophoblastic cells
- PLAP: usually positive
- Ki-1: positive
- Cytokeratin: positive
- Epithelial membrane antigen (EMA): negative
- CEA: negative
- Leu M-1: negative

DIFFERENTIAL DIAGNOSIS

- Seminoma
- Malignant lymphoma (Table 10–6)
- Metastatic carcinoma (Table 10–7)

References

Battifora H, Sheibani K, Tubbs RR, et al. Antikeratin antibodies in tumor diagnosis. Distinction between seminoma and embryonal carcinoma. Cancer 54:843–848, 1984.

Ferreiro JA. Ber-H2 expression in testicular germ cell tumors. Hum Pathol 25:522–524, 1994.

Pierce GB Jr, Abell MR. Embryonal carcinoma of the testis. Pathol Annu 5:27–60, 1970.

Ulbright TM, Goheen MP, Roth LM, et al. The differentiation of carcinomas of teratomatous origin from embryonal carcinoma. A light and electron microscopic study. Cancer 57:257–263, 1986.

Vugrin D, Chen A, Feigl P, et al. Embryonal carcinoma of the testis. Cancer 61:2348–2352, 1988.

Table 10–6
DIFFERENTIAL FEATURES BETWEEN EMBRYONAL CARCINOMA
AND LYMPHOMA

	Embryonal Carcinoma	Lymphoma
Age (yr)	20–30	>60
Bilaterality	Rare	20%
Spermatic cord involvement	20%	50%
Growth pattern	A/T/P/S	Diffuse, interstitial
Tumor cells	Polygonal	Oval/round
Tumor cell nucleus	Pleomorphic	Pleomorphic
Nuclear chromatin	Clumping/clear	Coarse
PLAP	+	−
LCA	−	+
Keratin	+	−
ITGCN	Present	Absent

A/T/P/S, acinar, tubular, papillary, or solid pattern; PLAP, placental alkaline phosphatase; LCA, leukocyte common antigen; ITGCN, intratubular germ cell neoplasia.

Table 10–7
DIFFERENTIAL FEATURES BETWEEN
EMBRYONAL CARCINOMA AND
METASTATIC CARCINOMA

	Embryonal Carcinoma	Metastatic Carcinoma
Age (yr)	20–30	>50
Bilaterality	Rare	15%
History of other cancer	Absent	Present
Interstitial growth pattern	Absent	Present
Vascular invasion	Frequent	More frequent
PLAP	+	−
Ki-1	+	±
EMA	−	+
CEA	−	+
ITGCN	Present	Absent

PLAP, placental alkaline phosphatase; EMA, epithelial membrane antigen; CEA, carcinoembryonic antigen; ITGCN, intratubular germ cell neoplasia.

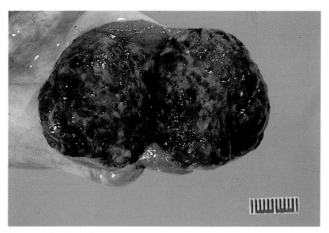

Figure 10–32. Embryonal carcinoma (EC), gross. This bivalved testis shows a hemorrhagic, brownish testicular mass with multifocal necrosis.

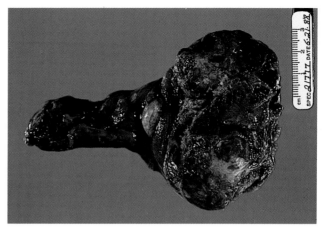

Figure 10–33. Embryonal carcinoma, gross. The hemorrhagic and necrotic nature of EC is depicted in this illustration.

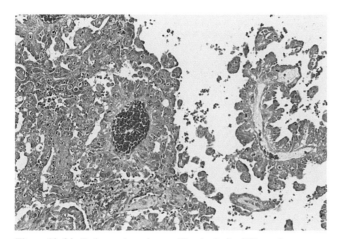

Figure 10–34. Embryonal carcinoma. Histologically, EC may have a papillary pattern, as depicted here.

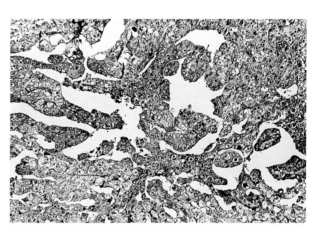

Figure 10–35. Embryonal carcinoma. This illustration shows large anaplastic cells arranged in cords or solid areas with some tubular formation. At this low-power magnification anaplasia is manifested by nuclear variation in size and shape and the presence of large prominent nucleoli.

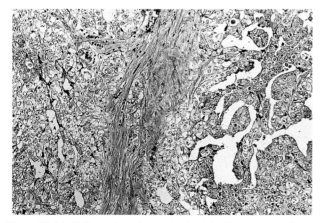

Figure 10–36. Embryonal carcinoma. On the left side there is a solid pattern of EC, with adjacent glandular papillary arrangement of the cells.

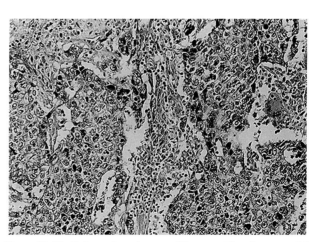

Figure 10–37. Embryonal carcinoma, solid pattern. There is a vague lobulation with a few scattered lymphocytes simulating seminoma.

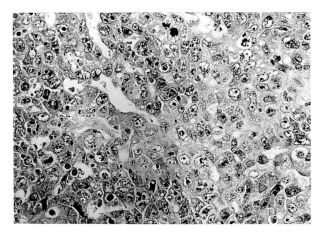

Figure 10–38. Embryonal carcinoma. This high-power view shows the characteristic anaplastic nuclear features of this germ cell tumor. The cells vary in size and in shape, there are numerous mitotic figures, and there are prominent nucleoli. Unlike seminoma, the EC cells show nuclear overlapping and the cell borders are not well defined.

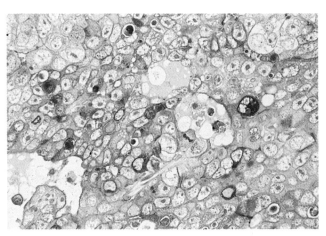

Figure 10–39. Embryonal carcinoma. The cells of EC are positive for keratin immunostaining.

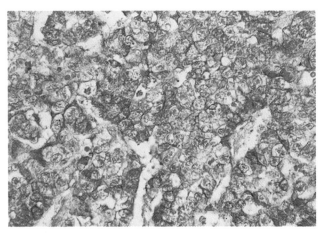

Figure 10–40. Embryonal carcinoma. This view shows positivity for Ki-1 in tumor cells. In the context of germ cell tumors Ki-1 immunostaining is restricted to EC; therefore, Ki-1 is useful in distinguishing EC from other germ cell components in problematic cases.

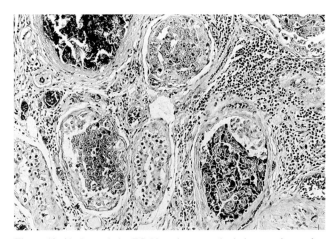

Figure 10–41. Intratubular EC. Note that several tubules contain anaplastic cells of EC. ITGCN is also noted in the remaining two seminiferous tubules.

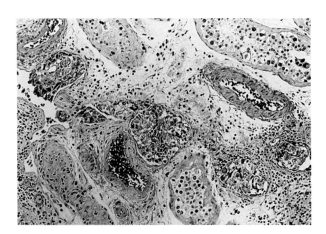

Figure 10–42. Embryonal carcinoma. Vascular and lymphatic invasion is seen in a vessels traversing the illustration. This is an important prognostic factor in this tumor and should be documented in the pathology report.

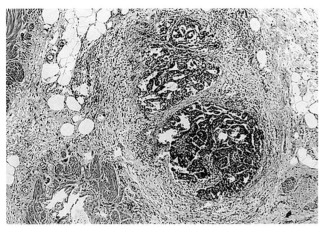
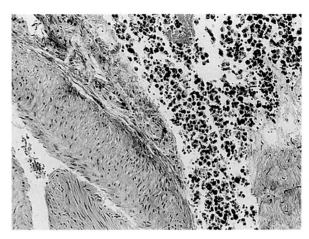

A   B

Figure 10–43. A, Spermatic cord invasion by EC. Note associated desmoplastic tissue reaction around tumor nests signifying true invasion. **B,** Artifactual contamination of the cord. In this illustration of the cord margin there is a collection of dark hyperchromatic malignant cells apparently involving the spermatic cord. These cells represent contamination as there is no desmoplasia. Section of the cord margin should be obtained prior to sectioning the testicular mass to avoid such contamination.

Yolk Sac Tumor (YST)
(Synonym: Endodermal Sinus Tumor [EST])

CLINICAL

- Almost always, in pure form, occurs in infants and young children (birth–5 years).
- Accounts for 75% of all childhood testicular neoplasms.
- In adults, pure form is rare (<1%); it is frequently admixed with other germ cell tumor components (seminoma, EC, teratoma, choriocarcinoma); occurs in 40% to 50% of NSGCTs as a component.
- Present with rapid testicular enlargement.
- Elevated serum AFP.
- In children (pure form) prognosis is excellent.

GROSS

- Enlarged testis (2–6 cm).
- Poorly defined, lobulated, white-gray or gray-yellow.
- Focally cystic, solid mass with variable consistency.
- Hemorrhage and necrosis may be present.

MICROSCOPIC

- Reticular, microcystic pattern: most common pattern (80% of cases); characterized by irregular anastomosing cords of cells forming labyrinthine-like loose spaces or anastomosing tubules, or both, lined by flat or cuboidal cells with ballooning cytoplasm forming microcysts.
- Endodermal sinus pattern (perivascular or festoon): infrequent; a central fibrovascular core is surrounded by cuboidal-to-columnar tumor cells which are housed in a cystic space (glomeruloid structure; Schiller-Duval body).

- Polyvesicular pattern: infrequent; characterized by large constricted vesicles lying in a cellular stroma; lined by flattened-to-cuboidal-to-columnar cells.
- Papillary and tubulopapillary: papillae with central fibrovascular cores.
- Solid pattern: a sheetlike configuration of polygonal tumor cells that may resemble seminoma, but lack the fibrovascular septa containing lymphocytes.
- Glandular-alveolar pattern: simple round glands to anastomosing or branching glands with intervening stroma.
- Macrocystic: usually associated with a microcystic pattern; derives from coalescence of microcysts.
- Myxomatous: consists of island and cords of neoplastic cells in a myxoid stroma; often very vascular (angioblastic mesenchyme).
- Rare patterns include parietal (associated with abundant intercellular basement membrane deposition), enteric or endometrioid (resembling colonic or endometrioid neoplasm), sarcomatoid (spindled), and hepatoid (resembling liver with abundant eosinophilic cytoplasm) patterns.
- The stroma can be cellular and can resemble smooth muscle.
- Tumor cells are usually flat, cuboidal, round to oval with minimal nuclear pleomorphism and therefore can be deceptively benign-appearing; occasionally nuclear pleomorphism may be more pronounced, but does not parallel the extent seen in EC.
- Intra- and extracellular PAS-positive hyaline globules.

SPECIAL STAINS AND IMMUNOHISTOCHEMISTRY

- PAS: positive and diastase-resistant in hyaline globules
- AFP: positive in cytoplasm of tumor cells and usually negative in hyaline globules

Table 10–8

DIFFERENTIAL FEATURES BETWEEN
EMBRYONAL CARCINOMA AND
YOLK SAC TUMOR

	Embryonal Carcinoma	Yolk Sac Tumor
Tumor cells	Pleomorphic	Bland (cuboidal, flat)
Mitoses	Numerous	Less frequent
Nucleolus	Large	Small
Chromatin	Clumping/clearing	Fine
Schiller-Duval body	−	+
Basement membrane	−	+
Hyaline globules	±	+
Alpha-fetoprotein	−	+
Ki-1	+	−

- Cytokeratin: positive (usually stronger than in EC)
- Ki-1: negative
- PLAP: variably positive

DIFFERENTIAL DIAGNOSIS

- EC (Table 10–8)
- Seminoma

- Metastatic carcinoma
- Rete testis hyperplasia

References

Eglen DE, Ulbright TM. The differential diagnosis of yolk sac tumor and seminoma. Usefulness of cytokeratin, alpha-fetoprotein, and alpha-1-antitrypsin immunoperoxidase reactions. Am J Clin Pathol 88:328–332, 1987.

Gonzalez-Crussi F. The human yolk sac and yolk sac (endodermal sinus) tumors. A review. Perspect Pediatr Pathol 5:179–215, 1979.

Griffin GC, Raney RB Jr, Snyder HM, et al. Yolk sac carcinoma of the testis in children. J Urol 137:954–957, 1987.

Harms D, Janig U. Germ cell tumours of childhood. Report of 170 cases including 59 pure and partial yolk sac tumours. Virchows Arch [A] 409:223–239, 1986.

Jacobsen GK, Jacobsen M. Possible liver cell differentiation in testicular germ cell tumours. Histopathology 7:537–548, 1983.

Kaplan GW, Cromie WC, Kelalis PP, et al. Prepubertal yolk sac testicular tumors: Report of the testicular tumor registry. J Urol 140:1109–1112, 1988.

Kramer SA, Wold LE, Gilchrist GS, et al. Yolk sac carcinoma. An immunohistochemical and clinicopathologic review. J Urol 131:315–318, 1984.

Pierce GB, Bullock WK, Huntington RW Jr. Yolk sac tumors of the testis. Cancer 25:644–658, 1970.

Ulbright TM, Roth LM, Brodhecker CA. Yolk sac differentiation in germ cell tumors. A morphologic study of 50 cases with emphasis on hepatic, enteric and parietal yolk sac features. Am J Surg Pathol 10:151–164, 1986.

Wold LE, Kramer SA, Farrow GM. Testicular yolk sac and embryonal carcinomas in pediatric patients: Comparative immunohistochemical and clinicopathologic study. Am J Clin Pathol 81:427–435, 1984.

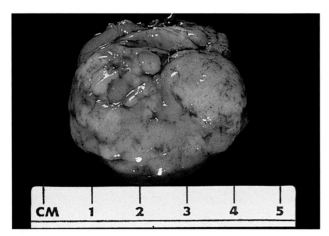

Figure 10–44. Yolk sac tumor (YST), gross. Infantile YST shows a gray-to-yellow myxoid solid cut surface with partial lobulation. (Courtesy of Dr. J. Haas, Detroit.)

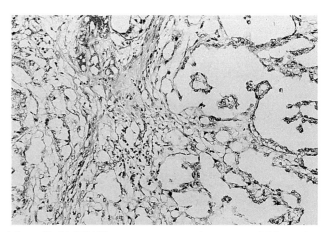

Figure 10–45. YST. There are numerous cystic structures of different sizes lined by a flattened epithelium.

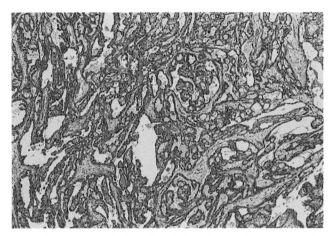

Figure 10–46. YST, reticular pattern. This pattern consists of a reticulated tubular arrangement of the cells.

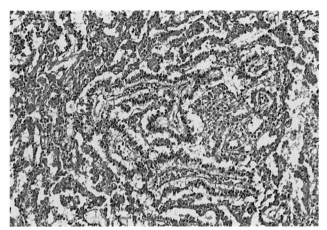

Figure 10–47. YST. Numerous Schiller-Duval bodies cut at different angles.

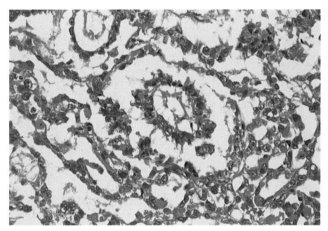

Figure 10–48. YST. In the center of the photomicrograph is a Schiller-Duval body, which consists of a central vessel surrounded by a mantle of cells, a space devoid of cells, and another wall of similar cells. The overall picture suggests a glomeruloid body.

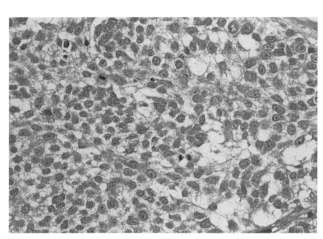

Figure 10–49. YST, solid pattern. Not uncommonly the cells of YST are large and contain abundant cytoplasm. They are seen here forming diffuse sheets.

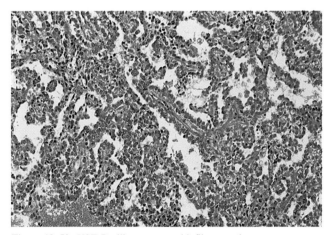

Figure 10–50. YST. Papillary pattern with fibrovascular cores.

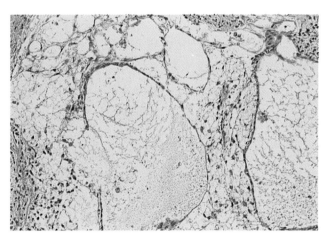

Figure 10–51. YST. Macrocystic and microcystic patterns are depicted in this illustration.

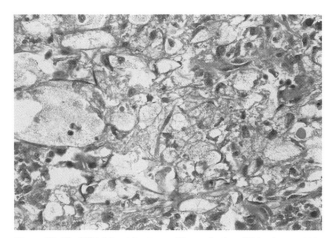

Figure 10–52. YST. Myxoid pattern with neoplastic cell islands set within a myxoid stroma.

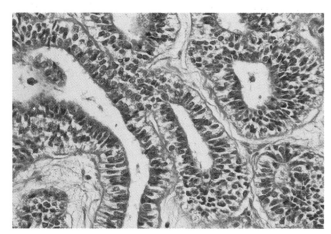

Figure 10–53. YST. Enteric (endometrioid) pattern. The tumor cells are tall columnar with subnuclear vacuoles. This pattern is reminiscent of early secretory endometrium.

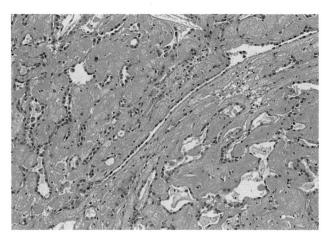

Figure 10–54. YST. Parietal pattern with extensive pericellular basement membrane material deposition.

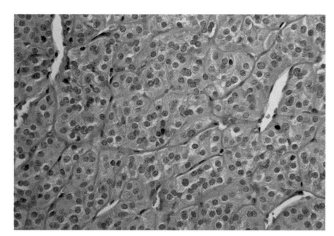

Figure 10–55. YST, hepatoid pattern. Tumor cells contain eosinophilic cytoplasm. This pattern is rare and considered a variant of the solid pattern.

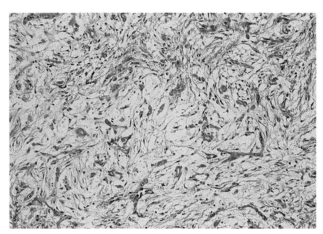

Figure 10–56. YST. Spindle cell pattern. Bland-appearing spindle cells are present in a myxoid stroma.

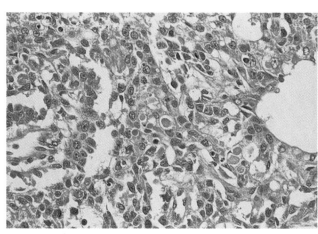

Figure 10–57. YST. Reticular pattern of YST with hyaline globules in the center.

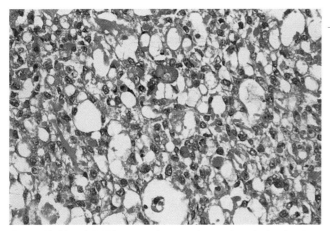

Figure 10–58. YST. This tumor shows a microcystic reticulated pattern. Numerous hyaline globules are present.

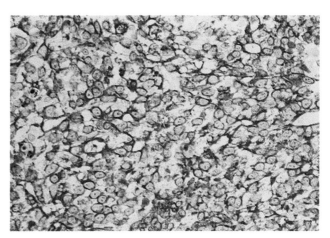

Figure 10–59. YST. Intense immunoreactivity for cytokeratin in tumor cells. YST shows the strongest keratin immunoreactivity of all the germ cell tumors.

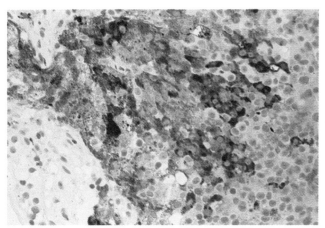

Figure 10–60. YST. This is an illustration of immunoreactivity to alpha-fetoprotein in tumor cells. This immunoreaction may be focal, patchy, and rarely difficult to demonstrate in YST.

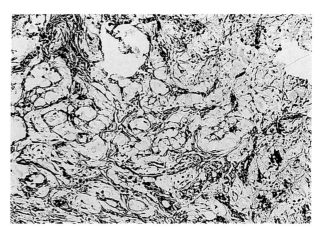

Figure 10–61. YST, microcystic and reticular patterns. Tumor cells are low-cuboidal to flat. Note the bland cytology of tumor cells.

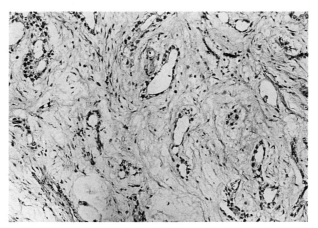

Figure 10–62. YST, polyvitelline pattern. There are irregularly shaped cysts with a central constriction separated by loose connective tissue stroma. The flattened epithelium lines the cystic structures.

Mature Teratoma

CLINICAL

- A common component of mixed germ cell tumor (MGCT).
- Pure form constitutes 4% to 9% of testicular tumors; most common in the first and second decades of life; teratoma is the second most common tumor after YST in childhood germ cell tumors.
- Gradual swelling with or without pain is the commonest presenting symptom.
- Pure teratomas almost always have a benign clinical course in the prepubertal age but have the potential to pursue an aggressive clinical course in the postpubertal age.

GROSS

- Well-demarcated, multicystic, solid mass.
- Cysts, filled with a clear, keratinous, white, flaky, gelatinous, or mucinous substance.
- Cartilage, spicules of bone, or brain tissue may be grossly discernible.

MICROSCOPIC

- Admixture of elements of ectoderm, endoderm, and mesoderm, assembled in either a disorganized or organized pattern.
  - Ectoderm—epidermis, neuronal tissue.
  - Endoderm—gastrointestinal, respiratory mucosa, other mucous glands.
  - Mesoderm—bone, cartilage, muscle.
  - Other somatic components.

- Most common components are nerve, cartilage, and different types of epithelium.
- Respiratory and gastrointestinal epithelium, muscle, and cartilage are more commonly observed in testicular teratomas than in ovarian or extragonadal teratomas; pancreatic, dental, renal, and thyroid tissue are less commonly seen in testicular teratomas than in ovarian or extragonadal teratomas.

SPECIAL STAINS AND IMMUNOHISTOCHEMISTRY

- None

DIFFERENTIAL DIAGNOSIS

- Epidermoid cyst: absence of adnexal structures of the skin and other tissue elements

References

Colodny AH, Hopkins TB. Testicular tumors in infants and children. Urol Clin North Am 4:347–358, 1977.

Fraley EE, Ketcham AS. Teratoma of testis in an infant. J Urol 100:659–660, 1968.

Hawkins EP. Pathology of germ cell tumors in children. Crit Rev Oncol Hematol 10:165–179, 1990.

Leibovitch I, Foster RS, Ulbright TM, et al. Adult primary pure teratoma of the testis. The Indiana experience. Cancer 75:2244–2250, 1995.

Mahour GHJ, Wooley MM, Trivedi SN, et al. Teratomas in infancy and childhood: Experience with 81 cases. Surgery 76:309–318, 1974.

Mosli HA, Carpenter B, Schillinger JF. Teratoma of the testis in a pubertal child. J Urol 133:105–106, 1985.

Tapper D, Lack EE. Teratomas in infancy and childhood: A 54 year experience at the Children's Hospital Medical Center. Ann Surg 198:398–410, 1983.

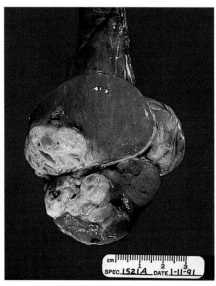

Figure 10–63. Teratoma, gross. In this bivalved testicle there is a relatively small tumor showing cystic areas and glistening tissue suggestive of cartilaginous tissue.

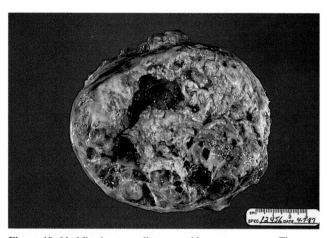

Figure 10–64. Mixed germ cell tumor with teratoma, gross. There are numerous cystic cavities representing teratomatous cysts and there are solid areas of white-gray tissue with necrosis, which histologically were EC.

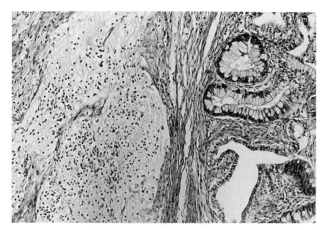

Figure 10–65. Mature teratoma. In this illustration there are glandular structures of gastrointestinal lineage, and neuroectodermal tissue within a fibrillar background.

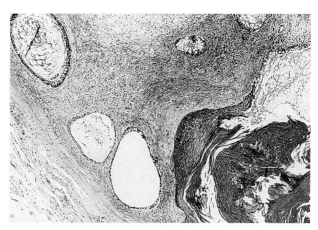

Figure 10–66. Mature teratoma. This view shows cystic spaces lined by gastrointestinal glandular epithelium with goblet cells, and focally by squamous epithelium. Note keratinous debris within the cyst.

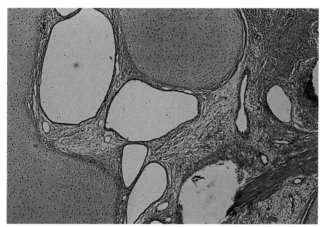

Figure 10–67. Mature teratoma. Histologically, there are several dilated glands intermixed with nodules of cellular hyaline cartilage.

Immature Teratoma

CLINICAL

- A common component of MGCT
- Does not occur in pure form but mixed with mature teratoma

GROSS

- See mature teratoma and MGCT.

MICROSCOPIC

- Primitive mesoderm: undifferentiated spindle cell proliferation (the most common immature teratoma component in the testis).
- Primitive endoderm.
- Primitive neuroectodermal tissue.
- Peripheral neuroectodermal tumor:
  - Considered as a monodermal immature teratoma (three cases have been reported: patients aged 20, 30, 51 years).

- Aggressive behavior.
- Small cells arranged in diffuse sheets, tubules, and ependymal-type rosettes.
- Can be seen in MGCTs as an immature teratomatous component.
- Stromal overgrowth with foci of Wilms' tumor–like component, embryonal rhabdomyosarcoma, or angiosarcoma.
- Carcinomatous elements of teratomatous type: have invasive growth pattern and stromal desmoplasia; EMA positivity.

SPECIAL STAINS AND IMMUNOHISTOCHEMISTRY

- Cytokeratin: positive in epithelial tissue
- Vimentin: usually positive in stromal tissue
- AFP: may be positive in enteric and hepatoid tissue
- HCG: positive in syncytiotrophoblastic cells
- PLAP: positive in glandular components in a few cases
- EMA: positive in carcinomatous elements of teratomatous type

DIFFERENTIAL DIAGNOSIS

- Primary or metastatic sarcoma: not associated with other somatic or germ cell components; more pleomorphic; usually involves the paratesticular structure
- Metastatic carcinoma
- Embryonal carcinoma

References

Harms D, Janig U. Immature teratomas of childhood. Report of 21 cases. Pathol Res Pract 179:388–400, 1985.

Hughes DF, Allen DC, O'Neill JJ. Angiosarcoma arising in a testicular teratoma. Histopathology 18:81–83, 1991.

Kooijman CD. Immature teratomas in children. Histopathology 12:491–502, 1988.

Serrano-Olmo J, Tang CK, Seidmon EJ, et al. Neuroblastoma as a prominent component of a mixed germ cell tumor of testis. Cancer 72:3271–3276, 1993.

Ulbright TM, Clark SA, Einhorn LH. Angiosarcoma associated with germ cell tumors. Hum Pathol 16:268–272, 1985.

Ulbright TM, Goheen MP, Roth LM, et al. The differentiation of carcinomas of teratomatous origin from embryonal carcinoma. A light and electron microscopic study. Cancer 57:257–263, 1986.

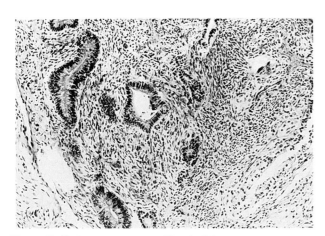

Figure 10–68. Immature teratoma. The glandular component represents mature teratoma, but the spindle cellular mesenchymal component is no longer recognizable as representing any lineage of mature tissue, thus representing immature teratoma. This spindle cellular stromal component is the most common pattern of immature teratoma in the testis.

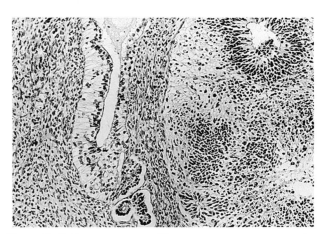

Figure 10–69. Immature teratoma. The teratomatous component consists of neuroectodermal small dark cells attempting to form neural tubes.

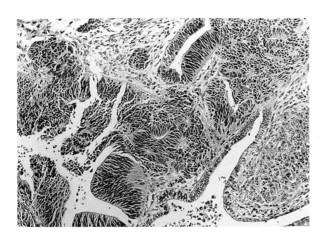

Figure 10–70. Immature teratoma. Neuroectodermal differentiation as seen here is occasionally seen in testicular teratoma.

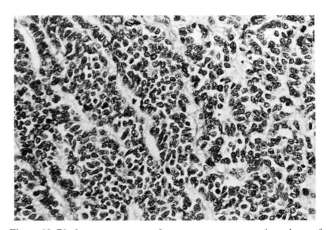

Figure 10–71. Immature teratoma. Immature teratoma may show sheets of undifferentiated small cells no different from the pattern of peripheral neuroectodermal tumor (PNET).

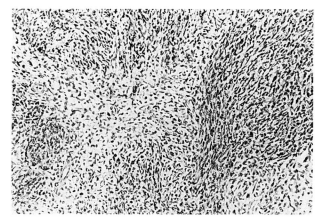

Figure 10–72. Immature teratoma with sarcomatous overgrowth. When the immature spindle cell component becomes diffuse and there is clear malignant cellular change, the tumor is interpreted as a sarcoma arising in teratoma.

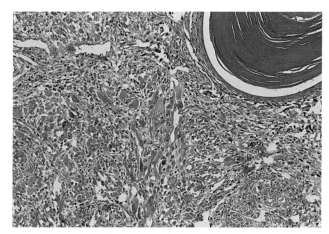

Figure 10–73. Immature teratoma with rhabdomyosarcoma. A keratinous cyst is present in one corner of the illustration; the remainder of the tissue displays spindle cell proliferation with occasional large "strap" cells containing eosinophilic cytoplasm.

Choriocarcinoma

CLINICAL

- Extremely rare in its pure form (0.3% of cases); more commonly a component of MGCT (7% of cases).
- Pure form occurs commonly in second and third decades.
- Highly malignant testis tumor owing to its vascular invasiveness and tendency to disseminate subclinically.
- Presentation due to hormonal symptoms, that is, gynecomastia (10%) or symptoms of metastases.
- Elevated serum HCG.
- A common germ cell neoplasm found in brain metastases.

GROSS

- The testis is usually normal in size; may be enlarged and firm, depending on the extent of hemorrhage.
- Hemorrhagic mass with grayish-white viable tissue at periphery.
- In patients with widespread metastasis no apparent tumor may be present; serial sections may show stigmas in the form of scar.

MICROSCOPIC

- Hemorrhage and necrosis.
- Two cell components: syncytiotrophoblast and cytotrophoblast with syncytiotrophoblasts wrapping around aggregates of cytotrophoblasts.
  - Syncytiotrophoblasts: large, vacuolated, and multinucleated cells with dark eosinophilic cytoplasm.
  - Cytotrophoblasts: uniform, medium-sized polygonal cells with abundant clear cytoplasm and distinct cytoplasmic borders.

- Solid nests and sheets with vague villus-like arrangement.
- Choriocarcinoma-like lesions (CCLLs): (1) unusual proliferation of teratomatous epithelium (teratomatous CCLL) and (2) nonbiphasic and cystic form of choriocarcinoma similar to atypical choriocarcinoma (consists of mononucleated cytotrophoblastic cells) seen in treated patients. The former is regarded as a teratoma component and the latter as a trophoblastic neoplastic component.

SPECIAL STAINS AND IMMUNOHISTOCHEMISTRY

- HCG: positive in syncytiotrophoblasts
- Human placental lactogen: positive in syncytiotrophoblasts and intermediate trophoblasts but not in cytotrophoblasts
- CEA: may be positive (25%)
- Cytokeratin: positive in both cytotrophoblasts and syncytiotrophoblasts
- PLAP: positive (50%)
- Vimentin: negative

DIFFERENTIAL DIAGNOSIS

- Collections of syncytiotrophoblastic giant cells in other germ cell tumors
- MGCT with choriocarcinoma components

References

Azzopardi JG, Mostofi FK, Theiss EA. Lesions of testes observed in certain patients with widespread choriocarcinoma and related tumors. The significance and genesis of hematoxylin-staining bodies in the human testis. Am J Pathol 38:207–225, 1961.

Bredael JJ, Vugrin D, Whitmore WF Jr. Autopsy findings in 154 patients with germ cell tumors of the testis. Cancer 50:548–551, 1982.

Henry SC, Walsh PC, Rotner MB. Choriocarcinoma of the testis. J Urol 112:105–108, 1974.

Manivel JC, Niehans G, Wick MR, et al. Intermediate trophoblast in germ cell neoplasms. Am J Surg Pathol 11:693–701, 1987.

Ulbright TM, Loehrer PJ. Choriocarcinoma-like lesions in patients with testicular germ cell tumors. Two histologic variants. Am J Surg Pathol 12:531–541, 1988.

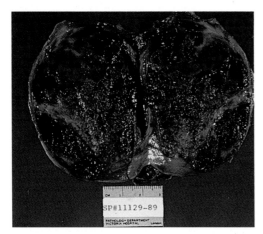

Figure 10–74. Choriocarcinoma, gross. Testicular tumor with extensive hemorrhage and necrosis. (Courtesy of Dr. D.I. Turnbull, London, Ontario, Canada.)

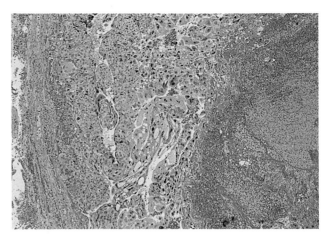

Figure 10–75. Choriocarcinoma. A lower power shows central hemorrhagic necrosis and viable tumor cells at the periphery.

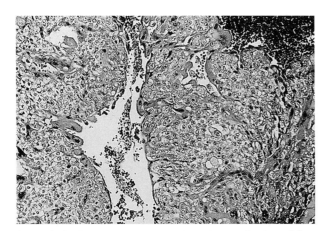

Figure 10–76. Choriocarcinoma. This view shows collections of large clear cells (cytotrophoblast) covered by syncytiotrophoblastic cells.

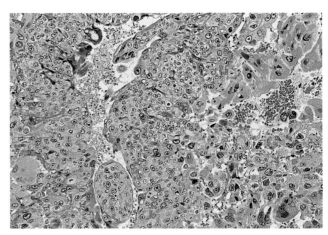

Figure 10–77. Choriocarcinoma. The cytologic detail of both cytotrophoblasts and syncytiotrophoblasts is depicted. The syncytiotrophoblasts are capping the cytotrophoblastic cells, which are together arranged in a villous configuration.

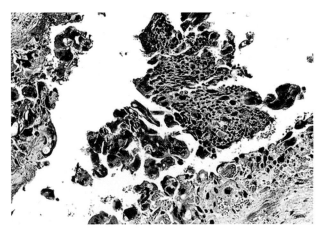

Figure 10–78. Choriocarcinoma-like lesion (CCLL). This is a teratomatous CCLL with a cystic area showing a lacelike arrangement of eosinophilic cells with squamoid appearance. This lesion is associated with typical teratomatous elements.

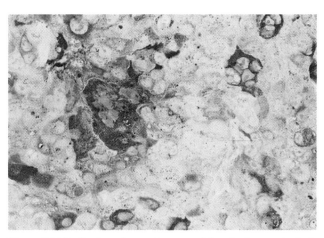

Figure 10–79. Choriocarcinoma. Immunostaining for human chorionic gonadotropin is positive in syncytiotrophoblastic cells.

Mixed Germ Cell Tumor (MGCT)

CLINICAL

- Forty percent to 45% of all primary testicular germ cell tumors.
- Teratoma-EC (25%); EC-seminoma (15%); teratoma-EC-seminoma (15%); other combinations may occur rarely.
- Foci of YST in 40% to 50% of MGCTs.
- Most frequent during third and fourth decades.
- Presentation: testicular enlargement and pain.
- Distinct forms of MGCTs include polyembryoma and diffuse embryoma (discussed below).

GROSS

- Largest testis tumor.
- Testis often entirely replaced by the tumor.
- Variegated appearance; cystic and solid, hemorrhage and necrosis.
- Cannot distinguish the different components grossly except for seminoma.
- Large areas of hemorrhage and necrosis should raise suspicion of choriocarcinoma.

MICROSCOPIC

- Various histologic combinations depending on the tumor components
- Features of seminoma, EC, YST, mature and immature teratoma, choriocarcinoma, polyembryoma

SPECIAL STAINS AND IMMUNOHISTOCHEMISTRY (TABLE 10–9)

DIFFERENTIAL DIAGNOSIS

- None

References

Burke AP, Mostofi FK. Placental alkaline phosphatase immunohistochemistry of intratubular malignant germ cells and associated testicular germ cell tumors. Hum Pathol 19:663–670, 1988.

Czaja JT, Ulbright TM. Evidence for the transformation of seminoma to yolk sac tumor, with histogenetic considerations. Am J Clin Pathol 97:468–477, 1992.

Dunphy CH, Ayala AG, Swanson DA, et al. Clinical stage I nonseminomatous and mixed germ cell tumors of the testis. A clinicopathologic study

Table 10–9
IMMUNOHISTOCHEMISTRY OF GERM CELL TUMORS

Component	K	AFP	Ki-1	PLAP	HCG
Seminoma	±	−	−	+	−*
Spermatocytic seminoma	−	−	−	−	−
Embryonal carcinoma	+	−	+	+	−*
YST	+	+	−	±	−*
Choriocarcinoma	+	−	−	+	+
Teratoma	±	−	−	±	−*

*Positive in syncytiotrophoblasts.

YST, yolk sac tumor; PLAP, placental alkaline phosphatase; AFP, alpha-fetoprotein; K, cytokeratin; HCG, human chorionic gonadotropin.

of 93 patients on a surveillance protocol after orchiectomy alone. Cancer 62:1202–1206, 1988.

Fraley EE, Lange PH, Kennedy BJ. Germ-cell testicular cancer in adults. N Engl J Med 301:1370–1377, 1420–1426, 1979.

Javadpour N. The National Cancer Institute experience with testicular cancer. J Urol 120:651–659, 1978.

Moriyama N, Daly JJ, Keating MA, et al. Vascular invasion as a prognosticator of metastatic disease in nonseminomatous germ cell tumors of the testis. Importance in "surveillance only" protocols. Cancer 56:2492–2498, 1985.

Mostofi FK, Sesterhenn IA, Davis CJ Jr. Immunopathology of germ cell tumors of the testis. Semin Diagn Pathol 4:320–341, 1987.

Raghavan D, Vogelzang NJ, Bosl GJ, et al. Tumor classification and size in germ-cell testicular cancer. Influence on the occurrence of metastases. Cancer 50:1591–1595, 1982.

Ulbright TM, Loehrer PJ, Roth LM, et al. The development of non-germ-cell malignancies within germ cell tumors. A clinicopathologic study of 11 cases. Cancer 54:1824–1833, 1984.

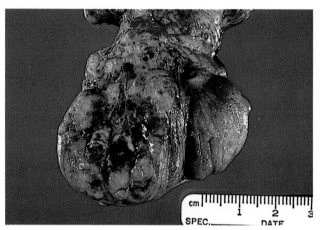

Figure 10–80. Mixed germ cell tumor, gross. White-gray necrotic tumor with variegated cut surface.

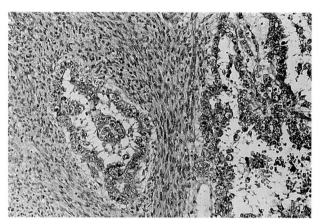

Figure 10–81. Mixed germ cell tumor. This illustration exhibits EC embedded on the spindle cells of an immature teratoma.

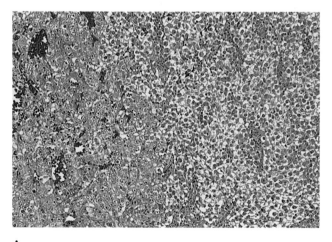

A

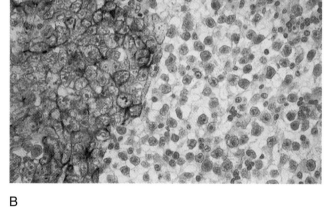

B

Figure 10–82. A, Embryonal carcinoma and seminoma. This illustration shows seminoma (*right*) and EC (*left*) components. Note the cytologic difference between these germ cell elements: the cytoplasm of the seminoma cells is clear, whereas the EC cells have granular, pink, amphophilic cytoplasm. **B,** In this keratin immunostain the cells of EC are strongly immunoreactive, whereas the seminoma cells are nonreactive.

Polyembryoma

CLINICAL

- A distinct form of MGCT; pure form is extremely rare; composed of EC and EST, in which embryoid bodies are set in a myxoid stroma
- Usually associated with other germ cell tumors
- The same malignant biologic potential and outcome as other MGCTs

GROSS

- Solid, soft, and somewhat edematous

MICROSCOPIC

- Numerous embryoid bodies; three components: (1) amniotic-like cavity on the dome; (2) central embryonic disk composed of cells identical to EC; (3) yolk sac structure immediately adjacent to embryonic disk composed of cells constituting YST
- Surrounded by primitive extraembryonic mesenchyme and loose myxomatous tissue

SPECIAL STAINS AND IMMUNOHISTOCHEMISTRY

- AFP: usually positive in yolk sac structure
- Cytokeratin: positive in entire embryoid bodies
- Vimentin: positive in surrounding mesenchyme and myxomatous stroma
- Ki-1: negative, but may be positive in cells of embryonic disks
- CEA: negative
- PLAP: can be positive

DIFFERENTIAL DIAGNOSIS

- Metastatic carcinoma
- Embryonal carcinoma
- Yolk sac tumor
- Teratoma
- Diffuse embryoma

References

Evans RW. Developmental stages of embryo-like bodies in teratoma testis. J Clin Pathol 10:31–39, 1957.

Gaillard JA: Yolk sac tumour patterns and entoblastic structure in polyembryomas. Acta Pathol Microbiol Scand [A] 233:18–25, 1972.

Jacobsen GK. Histogenetic considerations concerning germ cell tumours. Morphological and immunohistochemical comparative investigation of human embryo and testicular germ cell tumours. Virchows Arch [A] 408:509–525, 1986.

Marin-Padilla M. Origin, nature and significance of the "embryoids" of human teratomas. Virchows Arch [A] 340:105–121, 1965.

Nakashima N, Murakami S, Fukatsu T, et al. Characteristics of "embryoid body" in human gonadal germ cell tumors. Hum Pathol 19:1144–1154, 1988.

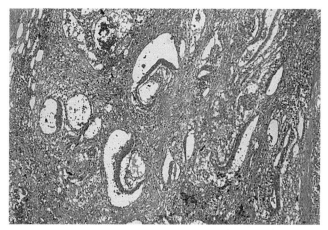

Figure 10–83. Polyembryoma. This rare lesion is characterized by the presence of numerous embryoid bodies randomly arranged in a myxoid stroma.

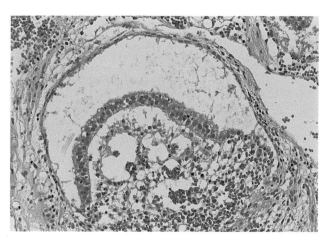

Figure 10–84. Polyembryoma. In the high-power view an embryoid body consists of a plate of primitive cells covered by epithelium (embryonic disk), an amniotic-like cavity (*top*), and a yolk sac (*bottom*).

Diffuse Embryoma

CLINICAL

- A rare form of MGCT.
- Four cases have been reported, with ages ranging from 22 to 38 years (mean 31.5 years).
- Present most commonly with nonpainful testicular mass or enlargement.
- Elevated serum AFP and HCG.
- Three patients are alive and well; one died of disease.

GROSS

- Yellow-gray-to-tan, firm nodular mass with areas of hemorrhage and necrosis

MICROSCOPIC

- Diffuse orderly arrangement of equal amounts of EC and YST components; reticular pattern of YST encircles the glandular structure formed by EC in necklace-like fashion
- Scattered syncytiotrophoblasts or small areas of choriocarcinoma

SPECIAL STAINS AND IMMUNOHISTOCHEMISTRY

- AFP: positive in YST component
- Cytokeratin: positive in both EC and YST; staining intensity is much stronger in YST than in EC component
- Ki-1: positive in EC component
- HCG: positive in syncytiotrophoblasts
- CEA: negative
- PLAP: positive

DIFFERENTIAL DIAGNOSIS

- Embryonal carcinoma
- Yolk sac tumor
- Polyembryoma

References

Cardoso de Almeida PC, Scully RE. Diffuse embryoma of the testis: A distinctive form of mixed germ cell tumor. Am J Surg Pathol 7:633–642, 1983.

de Peralta-Venturina MN, Ro JY, Ordonez NG, et al. Diffuse embryoma of the testis: An immunohistochemical study of two cases. Am J Clin Pathol 101:402–405, 1994.

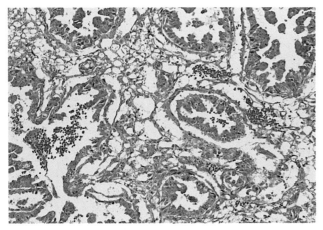

Figure 10–85. Diffuse embryoma. This pattern consists of central nodules of EC surrounded by YST epithelium. The EC forms small nodules with papillary infolding and central cystic areas. The YST epithelium is delicate and covers the EC. Note the presence of areas of YST between the nodules of EC.

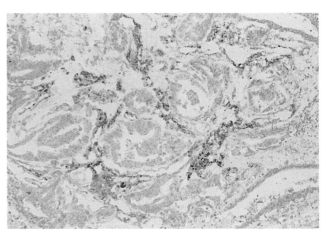

Figure 10–86. Diffuse embryoma. Alpha-fetoprotein immunostain. This illustration shows the staining of YST cells, not EC cells.

▪ Regression of Germ Cell Tumors

CLINICAL

- Occurs in patients who receive therapy before orchiectomy; may occur de novo in cases of seminoma and choriocarcinoma.
- Testis may show scar associated with ITGCN, intratubular calcification, or hematoxylin-staining bodies (burntout primary tumors).
- Patients with isolated retroperitoneal germ cell tumors most likely represent retroperitoneal metastasis with tumor regression in testis.
- Germ cell tumors in retroperitoneum below the renal vessels are considered metastasis from the ipsilateral testis. This testis is removed even if it is clinically negative.

GROSS

- Localized fibrous scar, calcifications, or no gross abnormalities

MICROSCOPIC

- Fibrosis, hemosiderin-laden macrophages, chronic inflammatory cells, calcifications.

- ITGCN in adjacent seminiferous tubules.
- Mature teratomatous elements may be seen.

SPECIAL STAINS AND IMMUNOHISTOCHEMISTRY

- PLAP positive in ITGCN

DIFFERENTIAL DIAGNOSIS

- Nonspecific scar; clinical history; no association with ITGCN

References

Azzopardi JG, Mostofi FK, Theiss EA. Lesions of testes observed in certain patients with widespread choriocarcinoma and related tumors: The significance and genesis of hematoxylin-staining bodies in the human testis. Am J Pathol 38:207–225, 1961.

Bar W, Hedinger C. Comparison of histologic types of primary testicular germ cell tumors with their metastases: Consequences for the WHO and the British Nomenclatures. Virchows Arch [A] 370:41–54, 1976.

Daugaard G, von der Maase H, Olsen J, et al. Carcinoma-in-situ testis in patients with assumed extragonadal germ-cell tumors. Lancet 2:528–530, 1987.

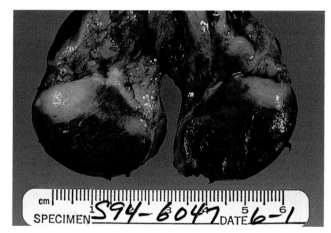

Figure 10–87. Burnt-out germ cell tumor. Fibrous scar without discrete nodule is seen.

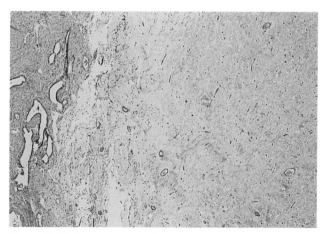

Figure 10–88. Burnt-out germ cell tumor. Fibrous collagenous tissue and blood vessels. No residual germ cell tumor is seen.

■ Other Germ Cell Tumors

Primary Carcinoid Tumor

CLINICAL

- Majority of patients 40–60 years old.
- Present with testicular enlargement, which may be painful or asymptomatic.
- Nearly always unilateral, but bilaterality has been reported.
- Occurs mostly in pure form; rare cases with mature teratoma.
- Benign clinical course in majority; metastases rare.
- There must be absence of a carcinoid tumor in another site (e.g., lung, gastrointestinal tract, etc.) as a prerequisite before labeling tumor as a primary carcinoid tumor.

GROSS

- Three to 5 cm in diameter
- Gray-tan to yellow, solid, and lobulated
- Usually devoid of necrosis and hemorrhage
- Shows typical gross features of teratoma when associated with teratoma

MICROSCOPIC

- Insular, acinar, or trabecular pattern.
- Cords, nests, aggregates of uniform tumor cells.
- Fine or wide fibrous strands.
- Tumor cells have round nuclei containing finely dispersed chromatin (salt and pepper); acidophilic, finely granular, usually abundant cytoplasm.

SPECIAL STAINS AND IMMUNOHISTOCHEMISTRY

- Grimelius: usually positive
- Fontana-Masson: may be positive
- NSE: positive
- Chromogranin: positive
- Cytokeratin: usually positive

DIFFERENTIAL DIAGNOSIS

- Metastatic carcinoid tumor
- Brenner tumor
- Granulosa cell tumor
- Sertoli-Leydig cell tumor

References

Hosking DH, Bowman DM, McMorris SL, et al. Primary carcinoid of the testis with metastases. J Urol 125:255–256, 1981.

Kaufman JJ, Waisman J. Primary carcinoid tumor of testis with metastasis. Urology 25:534–536, 1985.

Sullivan JL, Packer JT, Bryant M. Primary malignant carcinoid of the testis. Arch Pathol Lab Med 105:515–517, 1981.

Talerman A, Gratama S, Miranda S, et al. Primary carcinoid tumor of the testis: Case report, ultrastructure and review of the literature. Cancer 42:2696–2706, 1978.

Zavala-Pompa A, Ro JY, El-Naggar AK, et al. Primary carcinoid tumor of testis: Immunohistochemical, ultrastructural, and DNA flow cytometric study of three cases with a review of the literature. Cancer 72: 1726–1732, 1993.

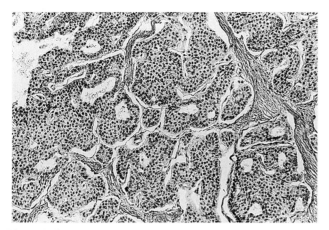

Figure 10–89. Testicular carcinoid. This view displays islands of medium-sized cytoplasmic cells arranged in an insular pattern. The nuclei are monotonous and oval to round.

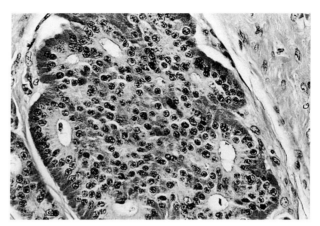

Figure 10–90. Testicular carcinoid. The cells of carcinoid show monotonous round-to-oval nuclei with small nucleoli and relatively abundant cytoplasm. The cells at the periphery show eosinophilic granular cytoplasm. Note focal glandular formation.

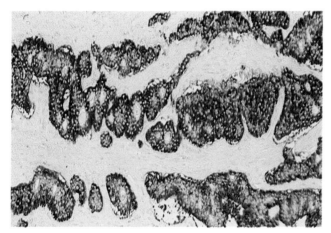

Figure 10–91. Testicular carcinoid. A chromogranin immunostain displays marked reactivity of the cells with this antibody.

CHAPTER 11

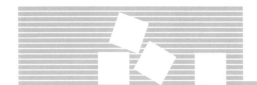

Sex Cord–Stromal Tumors

■ Leydig (Interstitial) Cell Tumor

CLINICAL

- One percent to 3% of all testicular neoplasms.
- Usually unilateral; 3% bilateral.
- Any age from second to sixth decades.
- Presentation in adults: testicular swelling, decreased libido (20%), gynecomastia (15%).
- Presentation in prepubertal patients: sexual precocity (neoplasms are usually nonpalpable).
- Malignant clinical behavior in approximately 10%.
- Malignant behavior not reported in children and typically not associated with endocrine abnormalities.
- There are no reliable pathologic features that separate benign from malignant tumors. Metastasis is only criterion for malignancy: malignant tumors tend to be larger (>5 cm); have infiltrative margins, vascular invasion, nuclear atypia, necrosis, high mitotic rate (more than three mitoses per 10 high-power fields); and lack lipofuscin pigment.

GROSS

- Three to 5 cm in diameter
- Sharply circumscribed, solid nodule
- Homogeneous, soft, intraparenchymal mass
- Usually yellow to mahogany-brown, but rarely gray-white
- Occasionally lobulated
- Focal hemorrhage or necrosis in one fourth of cases
- Extraparenchymal tumor extension in 10% to 15%

MICROSCOPIC

- Diffuse (most common), insular, trabecular, tubular, ribbonlike, and pseudofollicular patterns.
- Sheets or broad cords of tumor cells separated by fibrous stroma.
- The fibrous stroma typically inconspicuous but rarely may be hyalinized, edematous, and myxoid.
- Numerous thin-walled blood vessels.

- Large polygonal tumor cells with round nuclei, single prominent nucleolus, and abundant eosinophilic or vacuolated cytoplasm.
- Abundant lipid within the cytoplasm gives a clear cell appearance.
- Spindle cells may be present, and predominate in rare cases.
- Rare nuclear grooves, mimicking granulosa cells.
- Variable number of mitoses; typically rare or absent.
- Pleomorphism rare, but may occur.
- Pathognomonic crystalloids of Reinke (25%–40%).
- Lipofuscin pigment (10%–15%).
- Psammoma bodies rare.
- Electron microscopy (EM): Reinke crystalloids (hexagonal prismlike structure with periodicity); membranous whorls; abundant rough endoplasmic reticulum (RER).

SPECIAL STAINS AND IMMUNOHISTOCHEMISTRY

- Cytokeratin: negative, rarely focally positive
- Vimentin: positive
- S-100 protein: negative
- HMB-45: negative
- PLAP: negative
- Smooth muscle actin (SMA): positive

DIFFERENTIAL DIAGNOSIS

- Malignant melanoma
- Malignant lymphoma
- Metastatic carcinoma
- Malacoplakia
- Other sex cord–stromal tumors: Sertoli cell tumor, large cell calcifying Sertoli cell tumor, and tumor of adrenogenital syndrome

References

Bertram KA, Bratloff B, Hodges GF, et al. Treatment of malignant Leydig cell tumor. Cancer 68:2324–2329, 1991.

Caldamone AA, Altebarmakian V, Frank IN, et al. Leydig cell tumor of testis. Urology 14:39–43, 1979.

Grem JL, Robins HI, Wilson KS, et al. Metastatic Leydig cell tumor of the testis. Report of three cases and review of the literature. Cancer 58:2116–2119, 1986.

Kim I, Young RH, Scully RE. Leydig cell tumors of the testis. A clinico-pathological analysis of 40 cases and review of the literature. Am J Surg Pathol 9:177–192, 1985.

Sasano H, Nakashima N, Matsuzaki O, et al. Testicular sex cord–stromal lesions: Immunohistochemical analysis of cytokeratin, vimentin and steroidogenic enzymes. Virchows Arch [A] 421:163–169, 1992.

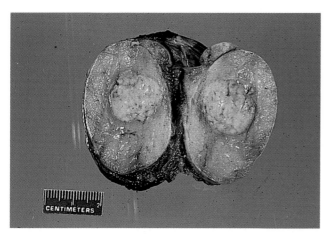

Figure 11–1. Leydig (interstitial) cell tumor (LCT), gross. Sharply circumscribed yellow-to-brown mass.

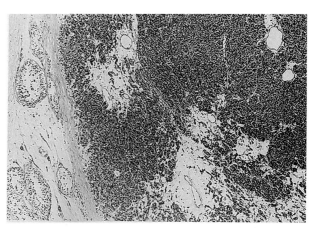

Figure 11–2. LCT of testis. This low-power view displays a well-circumscribed tumor separated from the uninvolved testis by a band of collagenous connective tissue. The tumor cells show a solid pattern, although focal acellular areas around vessels are also present.

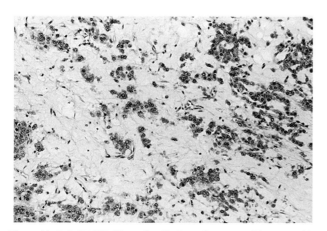

Figure 11–3. LCT. This illustration displays a loose myxoid pattern with a few cells and a loose edematous and myxoid stroma.

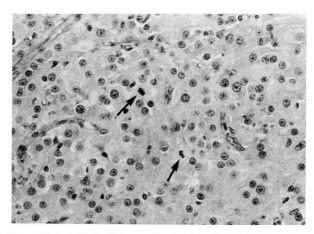

Figure 11–4. LCT. On high magnification the cells of LCT show absent-to-minimal variation in nuclear size and abundant, pink, granular cytoplasm. Small prominent nucleoli may be seen. Also note that there is mitotic activity (*arrows*) in this tumor.

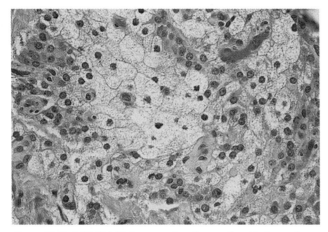

Figure 11–5. LCT. This high-power view shows cells with clear and vacuolated cytoplasm in the center of the picture. More typical eosinophilic granular cells are also present.

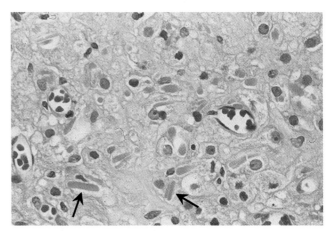

Figure 11–6. LCT. Note crystalloids of Reinke (*arrows*) seen as intracytoplasmic small eosinophilic rods.

■ Sertoli Cell Tumor

CLINICAL

- Less than 1% of all testicular neoplasms
- All ages; 30% in the first decade
- Scrotal mass
- Most unilateral, but bilateral cases have been reported
- May have gynecomastia; this is more commonly associated with malignant forms (approximately 20%)
- May be seen in patients with undescended testes, Peutz-Jeghers syndrome, and testicular feminization
- Majority benign; malignant behavior in less than 10%

GROSS

- Small, well-delineated, usually homogeneous, sometimes lobulated, yellow-gray or orange-tan tumor
- Rarely cystic
- Hemorrhage and necrosis unusual

MICROSCOPIC

- Uniform cuboidal or columnar cells arranged in tubules (well-differentiated), solid cords and nests (intermediate differentiation), and solid sheets (poorly differentiated); the tumor cells have large vesicular nuclei with prominent, centrally located nucleoli and abundant eosinophilic cytoplasm; cytologic pleomorphism rare
- Delicate fibrous stroma surrounding the tumor nests
- Tubules with well-developed basement membranes occasionally
- Vascular invasion, increased mitoses, necrosis, pleomorphism, lesser tendency to form tubules, spindle cell differentiation are more commonly found in malignant forms. About 20 cases of malignant Sertoli cell tumor have been reported (<10% of Sertoli cell tumors are malignant)
- EM: basal lamina around solid tubules; Charcot-Böttcher crystals; desmosomes; lipid; abundant smooth endoplasmic reticulum

SPECIAL STAINS AND IMMUNOHISTOCHEMISTRY

- Cytokeratin: usually positive
- Vimentin: positive
- PLAP: negative

DIFFERENTIAL DIAGNOSIS

- Carcinoma, primary, of rete testis or metastatic (Table 11–1)
- Leydig cell tumor
- Tubular seminoma

Table 11–1
DIFFERENTIAL FEATURES BETWEEN SERTOLI CELL TUMOR AND CARCINOMA

	Sertoli Cell Tumor	Carcinoma
Size of glands	Usually small, uniform	Mixture of small and large
Pattern	May show a mixture—glandular, spindled, trabecular, retiform	Only glandular
Solid tubules	Frequent	Rare
Pleomorphism	Absent to mild	Marked
Mitoses	Rare	Frequent
Mucin	Absent	Present

References

Dubois RS, Hoffman WH, Krishnan TH, et al. Feminizing sex cord tumor with annular tubules in a boy with Peutz-Jeghers syndrome. J Pediatr 101:568–571, 1982.

Gabrilove JL, Freiberg EK, Leiter E, et al. Feminizing and non-feminizing Sertoli cell tumors. J Urol 124:757–767, 1980.

Godec CJ. Malignant Sertoli cell tumor of testicle. Urology 26:185–188, 1985.

Jacobsen GK. Malignant Sertoli cell tumors. J Urol Pathol 1:233–255, 1993.

Kaplan GW, Cromie WJ, Kelalis PP, et al. Gonadal stromal tumors: A report of the prepubertal testicular tumor registry. J Urol 136:300–302, 1986.

Nielsen K, Jacobsen GK. Malignant Sertoli cell tumour of the testis. An immunohistochemical study and a review of the literature. APMIS 96:755–760, 1988.

Weitzner S, Gropp A. Sertoli cell tumor of testis in childhood. Am J Dis Child 128:541–543, 1974.

Wilson DM, Pitts WC, Hintz RL, et al. Testicular tumors with Peutz-Jeghers syndrome. Cancer 57:2238–2240, 1986.

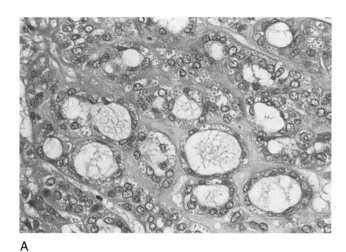

A

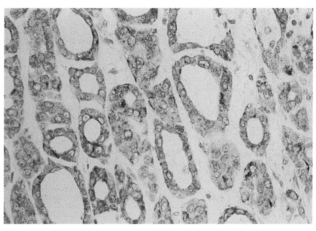

B

Figure 11–7. Sertoli cell tumor (SCT). **A,** On this medium-power view there is tubular differentiation. The tubules contain fibrillar proteinaceous material. **B,** Keratin immunostain displays positivity in tumor cells.

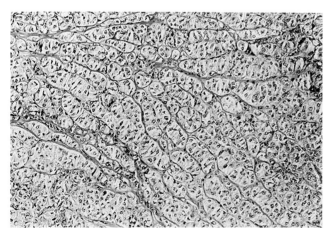

Figure 11–8. SCT. This illustration shows solid tubules containing large cytoplasmic elongated cells that have a tendency to align themselves at 90-degree angles from the sustaining connective tissue.

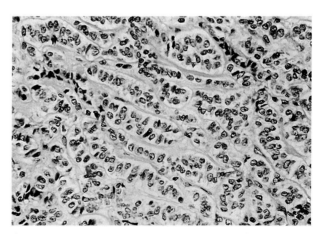

Figure 11–9. SCT. Trabecular arrangement in SCT manifested by cords of one, two, or more cells held together by a thin basement membrane-like band of connective tissue. The nuclei are round to oval, occasionally elongated, and contain small prominent nucleoli. The cytoplasm is clear.

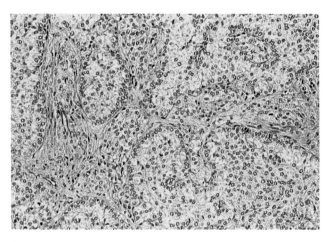

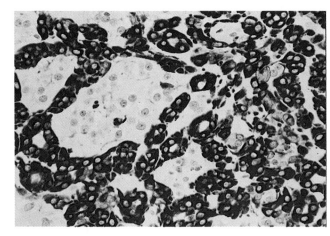

A   B

Figure 11–10. SCT. **A,** This illustration shows solid sheets of clear cells limited by a darker-staining basal cell layer. The palisading arrangement of the cells to the connective tissue trabeculae is retained. **B,** Immunostaining with keratin shows strong immunoreactivity for the tumor cells.

■ Large Cell Calcifying Sertoli Cell Tumors

CLINICAL

- A subtype of Sertoli cell tumor.
- Most common in second decade (range 5–45 years; average 16 years).
- Presentation: testicular mass.
- High frequency of bilaterality (40%) and multifocality (60%).
- Clinical association with gynecomastia, sexual precocity, acromegaly, sudden death, Carney's complex, and Peutz-Jeghers syndrome.
- In 50% of the cases, other lesions, such as pituitary adenoma, cardiac myxoma, nodular hyperplasia of adrenal cortex, and pigmentation of skin, have been reported.
- Rarely malignant.

GROSS

- Less than 4 cm in diameter
- Firm, yellow to tan
- Well-circumscribed
- May be gritty on cut section (variable consistency due to interspersed areas of calcification)

MICROSCOPIC

- Large (15–35 μm) neoplastic cells with abundant eosinophilic, ground-glass, or finely granular cytoplasm; very similar to cells of Leydig cell tumor; rarely spindle-shaped; round or oval nuclei with stippled chromatin and small nucleoli; mitoses are rare.
- Diffuse sheets or nests, trabeculae, cords, tubules, or clusters of tumor cells separated by fibrous stroma.

- Calcification with formation of large, basophilic, laminated nodules; may be spotty or markedly prominent, including psammoma bodies.
- Mixed inflammatory infiltrate usually accompanies the neoplastic cells.
- Foci of intratubular tumor growth with hyalinization of basement membranes in 50%.
- Association with areas of tumor resembling a sex cord tumor with annular tubules was reported in a boy with Peutz-Jeghers syndrome.
- EM: Charcot-Böttcher crystals (rare); other features in keeping with Sertoli cells; Reinke crystalloids absent.

SPECIAL STAINS AND IMMUNOHISTOCHEMISTRY

- Cytokeratin: may be positive
- Vimentin: positive
- PLAP: negative
- SMA: positive

DIFFERENTIAL DIAGNOSIS

- Leydig cell tumor
- Tumor of adrenogenital syndrome

References

Horn T, Jao W, Keh PC. Large-cell calcifying Sertoli tumor of the testis: A case report with ultrastructural study. Ultrastruct Pathol 4:359–364, 1983.

Niewenhuis JC, Wolf MC, Kass EJ. Bilateral asynchronous Sertoli cell tumor in a boy with the Peutz-Jeghers syndrome. J Urol 152:1246–1248, 1994.

Nogales FF, Andujar M, Zuluaga A, et al. Malignant large-cell calcifying Sertoli cell tumor of the testis. J Urol 153:1935–1937, 1995.

Perez-Atayde AR, Nunez AE, Carroll WL, et al: Large-cell calcifying Sertoli cell tumor of the testis. An ultrastructural, immunocytochemical, and biochemical study. Cancer 51:2287–2292, 1983.

Proppe KH, Dickersin GR. Large-cell calcifying Sertoli cell tumor of the testis: Light microscopic and ultrastructural study. Hum Pathol 13:1109–1114, 1982.

Proppe KH, Scully RE. Large-cell calcifying Sertoli cell tumor of the testis. Am J Clin Pathol 74:607–619, 1980.

Redgrave NG, Allan P, Johnson WF. Large-cell calcifying Sertoli cell

tumor of the testis. Br J Urol 75:411–412, 1995.

Tetu B, Ro JY, Ayala AG. Large-cell calcifying Sertoli cell tumor of the testis: A clinicopathologic, immunohistochemical, and ultrastructural study of two cases. Am J Clin Pathol 96:717–722, 1991.

Waxman M, Damjanov I, Khapra A, et al. Large cell calcifying Sertoli tumor of the testis: Light microscopic and ultrastructural study. Cancer 54:1574–1581, 1984.

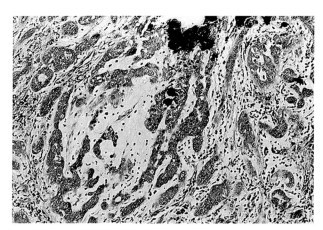

Figure 11–11. Large cell calcifying SCT. Cords, nests, and tubules of large cells separated by a loose connective tissue stroma with foci of calcifications.

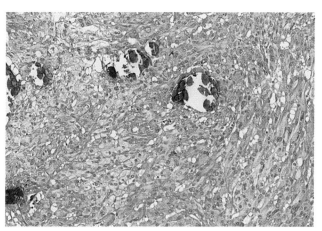

Figure 11–12. Large cell calcifying SCT. This view shows cords sometimes forming tubules of large cells with eosinophilic granular cytoplasm and prominent areas of calcification. Areas of prominent calcification are pathognomonic and helpful in the differential diagnosis of cells with abundant eosinophilic and granular cytoplasm.

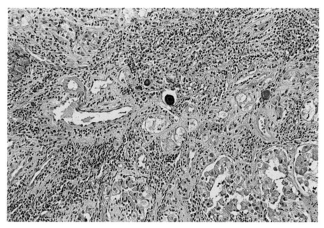

Figure 11–13. Large cell calcifying SCT. This tumor may show intratubular neoplastic cells and calcifications; the intratubular location of the cells argues for Sertoli cell origin of the tumor as these cells are constituents of the seminiferous tubules.

■ Sclerosing Sertoli Cell Tumor

CLINICAL

- Recently described rare variant of Sertoli cell tumor.
- Age range 18 to 80 years with a mean of 35 years.
- Presentation: painless testicular mass.
- Unlike conventional Sertoli cell tumors, there are no hormonal manifestations.
- Indolent clinical course.
- Malignancy and metastasis not reported.
- Not associated with Peutz-Jeghers syndrome.
- Not reported in prepubertal age group.

GROSS

- Usually less than 1.5 cm
- Well-circumscribed, firm, white-to-tan-to-yellow mass

MICROSCOPIC

- Solid or hollow tubules, cords, and nests of cells in the background of hypocellular, fibrous, often collagenized, stroma; the latter feature is hallmark of this neoplasm.
- Tumor cells have pale cytoplasm with occasional lipid vacuoles.
- Nuclei are variable, ranging from small and hyperchromatic to large and vesicular.
- May have significant cytologic atypia and mitotic activity.

IMMUNOHISTOCHEMISTRY

- Cytokeratin: positive
- Vimentin: positive
- PLAP: negative
- SMA: positive

DIFFERENTIAL DIAGNOSIS

- Adenomatoid tumor
- Metastatic carcinoma

Reference

Zukerberg LR, Young RH, Scully RE: Sclerosing Sertoli cell tumor of the testis: A report of 10 cases. Am J Surg Pathol 15:829–834, 1991.

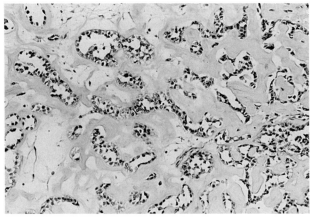

Figure 11–14. Sclerosing SCT. This variant contains cords or tubules lined by a single cell layer of flat-to-cuboidal epithelium set amid a characteristic acellular collagenous stroma.

■ Granulosa Cell Tumor (GCT)

CLINICAL

- Juvenile form:
  - Predominantly in infants.
  - Most common neoplasm of the neonatal testes.
  - May be associated with undescended testes or gonadal dysgenesis with chromosomal abnormality affecting Y chromosome.
  - Presents as a scrotal mass; unlike the ovarian counterpart it is not associated with endocrine manifestations.
  - Clinically benign.
- Adult form:
  - Very rare.
  - Age range 20 to 53 years.
  - May be associated with gynecomastia.
  - Although the majority are benign, cases with metastasis have been reported; long-term follow-up is warranted.

GROSS

- Juvenile form:
  - From 0.8 to 6.0 cm in diameter
  - Mostly cystic, partially solid
  - Usually thin cystic wall, containing viscid fluid
- Adult form:
  - From 2 to 10 cm
  - Homogeneous, yellow to yellow-gray, lobulated

MICROSCOPIC

- Juvenile form:

- Cystic areas interspersed with solid areas or may have a predominantly cystic or solid component
- Variably sized follicles; may be quite large forming large cysts
- Basophilic to faintly eosinophilic fluid within follicles; stains positively with mucicarmine
- Round-to-polyhedral cells with hyperchromatic nuclei and abundant pale-to-eosinophilic cytoplasm; mitotic activity can be high; nuclear grooves absent
- Adult form:
  - Microfollicular pattern with Call-Exner bodies
  - Diffuse pattern
  - Trabecular, cordlike, and nested patterns
  - Uniform cells with scant cytoplasm and typical angular nuclei containing nuclear grooves; focal cytologic atypia may be seen; mitoses are rare

SPECIAL STAINS AND IMMUNOHISTOCHEMISTRY

- Mucicarmine: negative in adult tumors; may be positive in cystic spaces of juvenile GCT
- Cytokeratin: variable reports in literature; up to 25% to 30% positive
- Vimentin: positive
- LCA: negative
- SMA: positive

DIFFERENTIAL DIAGNOSIS

- Lymphoma
- Small cell carcinoma
- Carcinoid
- Leydig cell tumor
- Sertoli cell tumor

References

Jimenez-Quintero LP, Ro JY, Zavala-Pompa A, et al. Granulosa cell tumour of the adult testis: A clinicopathologic study of seven cases and a review of the literature. Hum Pathol 24:1120–1126, 1993.

Lawrence WD, Young RH, Scully RE. Juvenile granulosa cell tumor of the infantile testis. A report of 14 cases. Am J Surg Pathol 9:87–94, 1985.

Matoska J, Ondrus D, Talerman A. Malignant granulosa cell tumor of the testis associated with gynecomastia and long survival. Cancer 69:1769–1772, 1992.

Nistal M, Lazaro R, Garcia J, et al. Testicular granulosa cell tumor of the adult type. Arch Pathol Lab Med 115:284–287, 1992.

Talerman A. Pure granulosa cell tumour of the testis: Report of a case and review of the literature. Appl Pathol 3:117–122, 1985.

Tanaka Y, Sasaki Y, Tachibana K, et al. Testicular juvenile granulosa cell tumor in an infant with X/XY mosaicism clinically diagnosed as true hermaphroditism. Am J Surg Pathol 18:316–322, 1994.

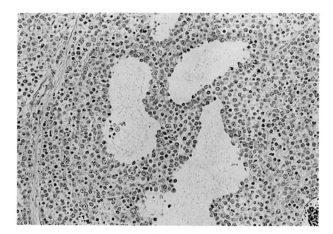

Figure 11–15. Juvenile GCT. This tumor shows medium-sized cells with round-to-oval nuclei and small prominent nucleoli. There is also abundant cytoplasm. Note follicles of varying sizes and shapes containing eosinophilic, watery mucicarminophilic fluid. The cells do not have nuclear grooves.

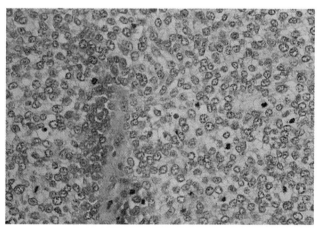

Figure 11–16. Juvenile GCT. Besides the microcystic and macrocystic patterns, the tumor may be arranged as solid sheets of cells of medium to large size. Note numerous mitotic figures.

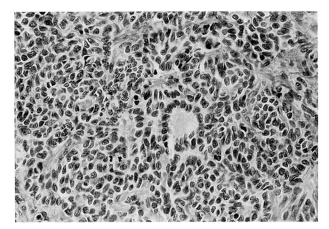

Figure 11–17. Granulosa cell tumor (GCT). This illustration displays medium-sized cells attempting to form tubules or rosettes. The cytoplasm of the cells is ill defined; the nuclei are round to oval and show distinct nuclear grooves.

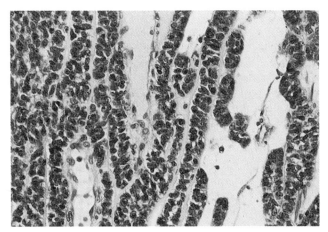

Figure 11–18. GCT. This tumor shows cords and occasional trabeculae of hyperchromatic cells. The nuclear details are similar to those described in Figure 11–17.

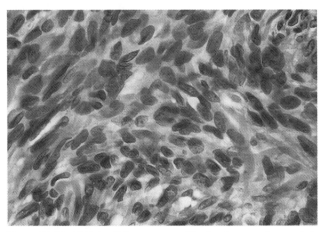

Figure 11–19. GCT. On high-power magnification there are characteristic nuclear grooves in the spindle cells.

■ Tumors of Adrenogenital Syndrome Type

CLINICAL

- Synchronously bilateral
- Associated with salt-losing form of adrenogenital syndrome; 21-hydroxylase deficiency
- Family history of adrenogenital syndrome
- Controversy whether it is a neoplastic or a hyperplastic process; latter favored because of bilaterality, presence of seminiferous tubules within the lesions, nonautonomous growth, response to medical treatment, and no reports of malignant outcome

GROSS

- Well-circumscribed, dark-brown, lobulated mass traversed by fibrous septa
- May be small, multiple, and bilateral and as large as 10 cm
- Most commonly originates in hilar region

MICROSCOPIC

- Diffuse proliferation of large cells or broad cords of tumor cells separated by thin fibrovascular septa.
- Seminiferous tubules scattered throughout the proliferation.

- Large polyhedral-to-polygonal cells resembling Leydig cells.
- Abundant eosinophilic cytoplasm containing lipofuscin pigment.
- Central nuclei with prominent nucleoli.
- Lack of crystalloids of Reinke.
- Fibrosis may be prominent.
- Focal nuclear atypia and mitotic figures may be found.
- EM: features of Leydig and adrenocortical cells; believed to arise from pluripotential cell of hilar region.

SPECIAL STAINS AND IMMUNOHISTOCHEMISTRY

- Cytokeratin: negative
- Vimentin: positive

DIFFERENTIAL DIAGNOSIS

- Leydig cell tumor
- Large cell calcifying Sertoli cell tumors

References

Knudsen JL, Savage A, Mobb GE. The testicular "tumour" of adrenogenital syndrome: A persistent diagnostic pitfall. Histopathology 19: 468–470, 1991.

Newell ME, Lippe BM, Ehrlich RM. Testis tumors associated with congenital adrenal hyperplasia: A continuing diagnostic and therapeutic dilemma. J Urol 117:256–258, 1977.

Rutgers JL, Young RH, Scully RE. The testicular "tumor" of the adrenogenital syndrome: A report of six cases and review of the literature on testicular masses in patients with adrenocortical disorders. Am J Surg Pathol 12:503–513, 1988.

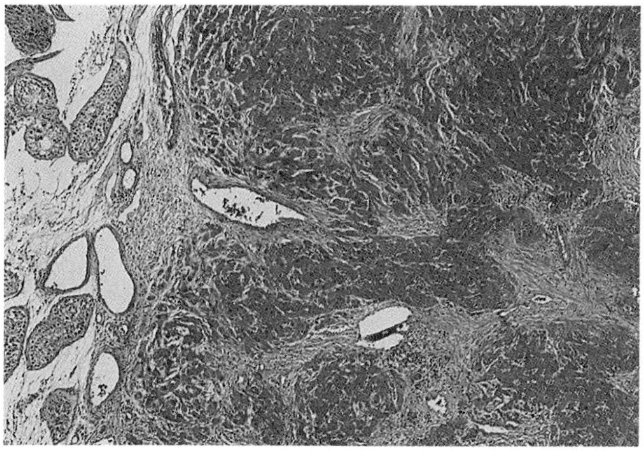

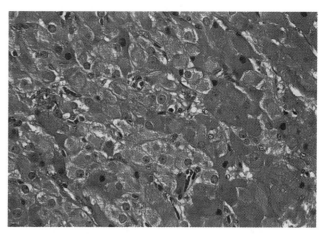

Figure 11–20. Testicular tumor of the adrenogenital syndrome (TTAGS). This lesion is made up of large eosinophilic granular cells arranged in a diffuse fashion. The pattern is indistinguishable from an LCT. Clinical information is important for the appropriate diagnosis.

Figure 11–21. TTAGS. High-power view shows the striking resemblance of this lesion to LCT.

■ Mixed or Unclassified Gonadal-Stromal Tumor

CLINICAL

- All ages, most common in children (30% <1 year old).
- Presentation: painless testicular enlargement.
- Gynecomastia may be present.
- Mostly benign in prepubertal children; can pursue a malignant clinical course in adults.
- Histologically, a combination of recognizable sex cord–stromal components (mixed gonadal-stromal tumor) or predominantly undifferentiated spindle cells (unclassified gonadal-stromal tumor), classified together because of similar prognosis.

GROSS

- Well-circumscribed, lobulated, white-yellow nodules.
- Variable size; may be large and replace the entire testis.
- Cystic areas can be seen.
- Hemorrhage and necrosis uncommon.

MICROSCOPIC

- Mixture of patterns; readily recognizable tumor components: Leydig cell tumor, Sertoli cell tumor, GCT in varying proportions (mixed).
- Admixture of epithelioid and spindle components or predominantly spindle component (unclassified):

- Epithelioid component: well-formed solid or hollow tubules, or cords in well-differentiated tumors; irregular aggregates or anastomosing trabeculae of sex cord–type cells embedded in a fibrous stroma in less differentiated tumors; tumor cells usually have eosinophilic, amphophilic, or vacuolated cytoplasm which may contain abundant lipid; usually have round-to-oval, vesicular nuclei; may have prominent nucleoli; mitotic figures rare or absent.
- Stromal component: hypercellular or less cellular with fibrous background; may form fascicles of spindle cells which may show nuclear pleomorphism depending on the degree of differentiation; mitotic figures can be frequent; spindle cells may have nuclear grooves; myofibroblastic differentiation by EM.
- Call-Exner bodies-like arrangement may be seen.

SPECIAL STAINS AND IMMUNOHISTOCHEMISTRY

- Staining patterns of mixed tumors depend on the different components. See individual tumor types (Leydig cell, Sertoli cell, and granulosa cell tumors).
- Unclassified tumors:

- Vimentin: positive
- Desmin: may be positive
- SMA: usually positive
- Cytokeratin: may be positive (usually focal)

DIFFERENTIAL DIAGNOSIS

- Metastatic melanoma (spindle cell type)
- Sarcoma
- Mixed germ cell tumor with immature teratoma component

References

Campbell CM, Middleton AW Jr. Malignant gonadal stromal tumor: Case report and review of the literature. J Urol 125:257–259, 1981.

Eble JN, Hull MT, Warfel KA, et al. Malignant sex cord-stromal tumor of testis. J Urol 131:546–550, 1984.

Gohji K, Higuchi A, Fujii A, et al. Malignant gonadal stromal tumor. Urology 43:244–247, 1994.

Lawrence WD, Young RH, Scully RE. Sex cord–stromal tumor. In Talerman A, Roth LM (eds). *Pathology of the Testis and Its Adnexa. Contemporary issues in surgical pathology.* New York, Churchill Livingstone, 1986.

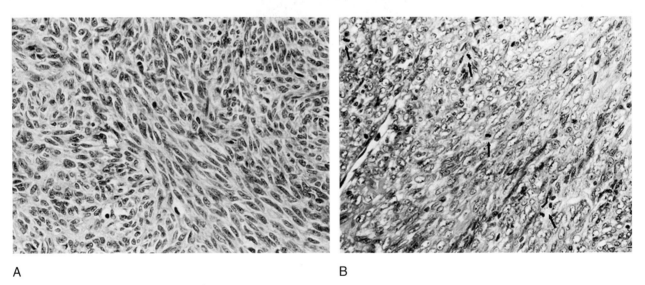

A   B

Figure 11–22. A, Unclassified sex cord–stromal tumor (SCST). This tumor shows closely packed cells with oval-to-spindled nuclei and indistinct cytoplasm. The features are undifferentiated, although there is a hint that this tumor may be demonstrating granulosa cell differentiation. **B,** Numerous mitoses *(arrows)* may be present in some areas of the tumor.

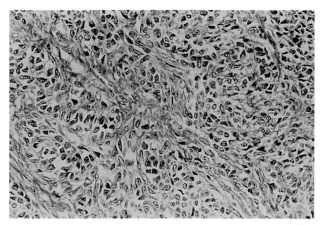

Figure 11–23. Unclassified SCST. This undifferentiated tumor pattern, like Figure 11–22, shows a feeble attempt to form cords or tubules, suggesting Sertoli cell differentiation. Occasional cells with nuclear grooves are apparent.

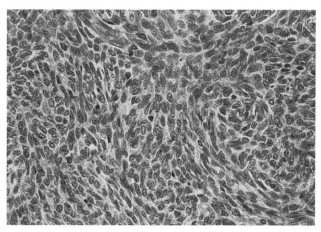

Figure 11–24. Unclassified SCST. This illustration shows a tumor composed of closely packed oval-to-spindled cells containing indistinct cytoplasm and lack of a specific pattern of growth.

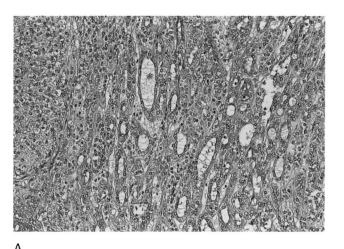

A

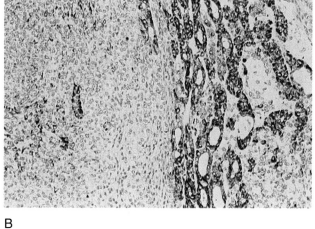

B

Figure 11–25. Combined LCT and SCT. **A,** In this illustration one sees the juxtaposition of the Sertoli cell component (right tubular area) contrasting with the Leydig cell tumor component (left solid area). **B,** Immunostaining with keratin demonstrates marked immunoreactivity in the tubular area, proving Sertoli cell differentiation.

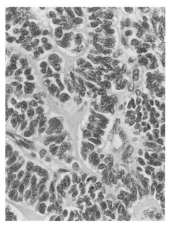
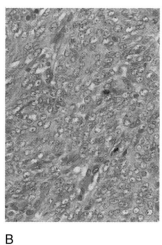

A

B

Figure 11–26. GCT and unclassified SCST. This composite picture shows the cordlike arrangement of the granulosa cell tumor *(A)* contrasting with the solid growth of the unclassified stromal tumor component *(B).*

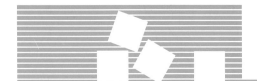

CHAPTER 12

Germ Cell and Sex Cord–Stromal Tumors

■ Gonadoblastoma

CLINICAL

- Almost always occurs in dysgenetic gonads or in an undescended testis; very rare in a normal gonad.
- Tumor composed of sex cord–stromal and germ cells.
- Eighty percent in phenotypic females, 20% in phenotypic males.
- Patients usually have cryptorchidism, hypospadias, and internal female sex organs.
- Intraabdominal or inguinal location.
- Bilateral in about one third.
- Majority younger than 20 years.
- Sixty percent of clinically detectable cases are associated with malignant germ cell tumors, most commonly seminoma, but occasionally with embryonal carcinoma (EC), yolk sac tumor (YST), or teratoma; gonadoblastoma may be considered a premalignant lesion.

GROSS

- Gray to yellow-brown, very small mass; size ranging from microscopic foci in dysgenetic gonad to several centimeters in diameter.
- Soft and fleshy or firm and may resemble cartilage; may be speckled due to granules of calcification, or may be almost totally calcified.
- Larger tumors are usually due to superimposition by other malignant germ cell tumors.

MICROSCOPIC

- Nests of tumor cells: nests composed of germ cells (seminoma-like) and sex cord–stromal cells (Sertoli or granulosa cells).
- Germ cells are large and round with vacuolated cytoplasm, closely admixed with small round-to-oval sex cord derivatives.
- Sex cord–stromal cells are present at the periphery of nests, around groups of individual germ cells, or around

small spaces with hyaline PAS-positive material resembling Call-Exner bodies.
- Connective tissue stroma.
- Marked hyalinization or calcification (calcification may be present within the nests or in stroma).
- The overgrowth of other neoplastic germ cells, usually seminoma, may lead to distortion and obliteration of gonadoblastomatous foci.
- Malignant form: increased mitotic activity or invasion of the nontumorous portions of the gonad.

SPECIAL STAINS AND IMMUNOHISTOCHEMISTRY

- None

DIFFERENTIAL DIAGNOSIS

- Unclassified mixed germ cell and sex cord–stromal tumor (Table 12–1)
- Germ cell tumor

References

Hughesdon PE, Kumarasamy T. Mixed germ cells tumours (gonadoblastomas) in normal and dysgenetic gonads. Case reports and review. Virchows Arch [A] 349:258–280, 1970.

Ishida T, Tagatz GE, Okagaki T. Gonadoblastoma: Ultrastructural evidence for testicular origin. Cancer 37:1770–1781, 1976.

Scully RE. Gonadoblastoma. A review of 74 cases. Cancer 25:1340–1356, 1970.

Talerman A. The pathology of gonadal neoplasms composed of germ cells and sex cord stroma derivatives. Pathol Res Pract 170:24–38, 1980.

■ Unclassified Mixed Germ Cell and Sex Cord–Stromal Tumor

CLINICAL

- Extremely rare tumor; occurs in adults (30–70 years).
- Presentation: testicular mass.
- Unlike gonadoblastoma, no association with gonadal dysgenesis or an intersex syndrome.
- Malignant behavior not reported.

Table 12–1

DIFFERENTIAL FEATURES BETWEEN GONADOBLASTOMA AND UNCLASSIFIED
MIXED GERM CELL SEX CORD–STROMAL TUMOR (UMGCSCST)

	Gonadoblastoma	UMGCSCST
Growth patterns	Nestlike	Cordlike, tubular, patternless
Hyalinization	+	–
Calcification	+	–
Gonads	Dysgenetic	Normal
Bilaterality	One third	Rare
Associated germ cell tumors	60%	None
Extragonadal location	+	–

- Overgrowth of germ cell resulting in a germ cell tumor is not reported.

GROSS

- Gray-white, solid to partly cystic mass of variable size.

MICROSCOPIC

- The two cell components, the large germ cells (seminoma–like cells) and sex cord–stromal cells (granulosa or Sertoli cells), are intimately admixed with each other: mitoses can be seen in both germ cells and sex cord cells.
- Three different histologic patterns: cordlike, tubular, and patternless (devoid of any specific arrangement).

- No calcification or hyalinization.
- Call-Exner-like hyaline bodies are rarely seen.

DIFFERENTIAL DIAGNOSIS

- Gonadoblastoma

References

Bolen JW. Mixed germ cell–sex cord stromal tumor: A gonadal tumor distinct from gonadoblastoma. Am J Clin Pathol 75:565–573, 1981.

Matoska J, Talerman A. Mixed germ cell–sex cord stroma tumor of the testis. A report with ultrastructural findings. Cancer 64:2146–2153, 1989.

Talerman A. The pathology of gonadal neoplasms composed of germ cells and sex cord stroma derivatives. Pathol Res Pract 170:24–38, 1980.

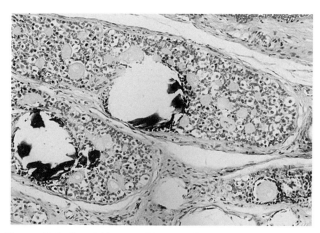

Figure 12–1. Gonadoblastoma. Note two large nests containing cells attempting to form rosettes or Call-Exner bodies (sex cord–stromal cells) and large single cells with clear cytoplasm (germ cells). Areas of calcification are also present.

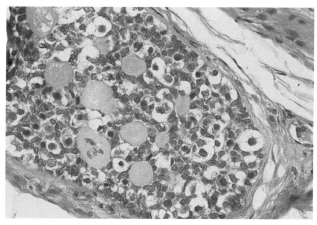

Figure 12–2. Gonadoblastoma. In this high–power view the two cell types are closely admixed: sex cord–stromal cells with eosinophilic hyaline material–forming Call-Exner bodies and germ cells with abundant vacuolated cytoplasm.

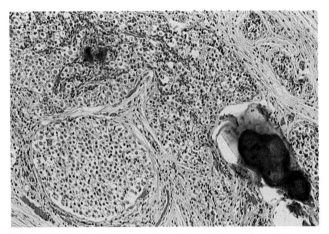

Figure 12–3. Gonadoblastoma with seminoma. The seminoma has overgrown and obliterated the gonadoblastoma component. Only residual calcification is observed.

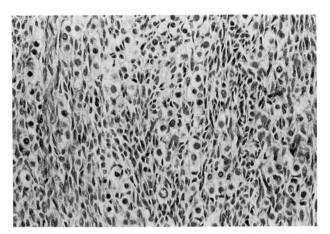

Figure 12–4. Unclassified germ cell–sex cord tumor. This lesion shows closely packed oval-to-spindle–shaped sex cord–stromal cells and some haphazardly arranged large cells with clear cytoplasm (germ cells).

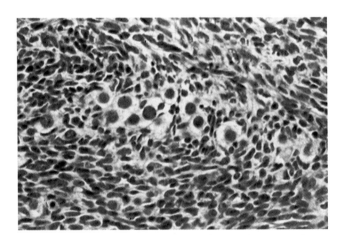

Figure 12–5. Unclassified germ cell–sex cord tumor. Aggregates of germ cells intermingled with sex cord derivatives are arranged as solid sheets.

CHAPTER 13

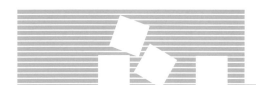

Lymphoreticular
and Metastatic Neoplasms

■ Lymphoma

CLINICAL

- Primary malignant lymphoma of the testis is rare; it is more commonly a late manifestation of disseminated disease (20%).
- Accounts for about 5% of all testicular neoplasms.
- The most common malignant tumor of the testis after 60 years of age.
- Most frequent secondary malignant neoplasm of testis.
- Presentation: testicular enlargement, usually painless; may have systemic symptoms (fever, weight loss).
- Greater than 90% are of B-cell lineage.
- Propensity to be associated with lymphoma of skin, CNS, and Waldeyer's ring.
- Bilaterality: 6% to 38% (average 20%).
- Overall survival: 15% to 30% at 2 years; stage is most important prognostic parameter (prognosis is better if testis is primary site with no evidence of nodal disease at time of diagnosis).

GROSS

- Replacement of part or all of the parenchyma by diffuse involvement or multiple nodules within testis
- Firm or soft, fleshy homogeneous mass
- Cream-colored, tan or slightly pink (closely resembles a seminoma)
- Necrosis: uncommon
- Extension to spermatic cord or epididymis in up to 50%

MICROSCOPIC

- Predominant interstitial infiltration of neoplastic cells between seminiferous tubules, but there may be infiltration of the wall and lumen of seminiferous tubules.
- Central portions may have a more diffuse arrangement with effacement of seminiferous tubules.

- Variable sclerosis: presence of any sclerosis is associated with a more favorable outcome.
- Most commonly non-Hodgkin's lymphoma, diffuse type; nodular lymphoma and Hodgkin's disease only rarely reported.
- Diffuse large cell lymphoma in 70% to 90%.
- Small cell, cleaved and noncleaved; Burkitt type can occur.
- Lymphoblastic lymphoma has propensity to involve testis, and is recognized by characteristic convoluted nuclei with delicate chromatin and inconspicuous nucleoli.
- Classification according to cell type: Working formulation or Lukes-Collins classification has been shown to have prognostic significance.

SPECIAL STAINS AND IMMUNOHISTOCHEMISTRY

- LCA: usually positive
- Cytokeratin: negative
- PLAP: negative
- Subtyping for T-cell and B-cell markers

DIFFERENTIAL DIAGNOSIS

- Seminoma
- Orchitis
- Spermatocytic seminoma
- Embryonal carcinoma
- Leukemic infiltrate
- Metastatic Merkel cell carcinoma

References

Baldetorp LA, Brunkvall J, Cavallin-Stahl E, et al. Malignant lymphoma of the testis. Br J Urol 56:525–530, 1984.

Doll DC, Weiss RB. Malignant lymphoma of the testis. Am J Med 81:515–524, 1986.

Ferry JA, Harris NL, Young RH, et al. Malignant lymphoma of the testis, epididymis, and spermatic cord. A clinicopathologic study of 69 cases with immunophenotypic analysis. Am J Surg Pathol 18:376–390, 1994.

Paladugu RR, Bearman RM, Rappaport H. Malignant lymphoma with primary manifestation in the gonad. A clinicopathologic study of 38 patients. Cancer 45:561–571, 1980.

Sussman EB, Hajdu SI, Lieberman PH, et al. Malignant lymphoma of the testis: A clinicopathologic study of 37 cases. J Urol 118:1004–1007, 1977.

Wilkins BS, Williamson JM, O'Brien CJ. Morphological and immunohistological study of testicular lymphomas. Histopathology 15:147–156, 1989.

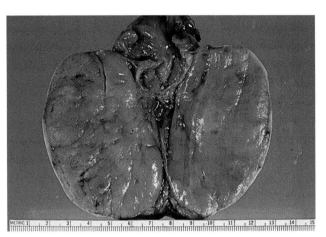

Figure 13–1. Large cell lymphoma (LCL). Light-tan fleshy homogeneous tissue replaces the testicular parenchyma. Tumor also invades the epididymis.

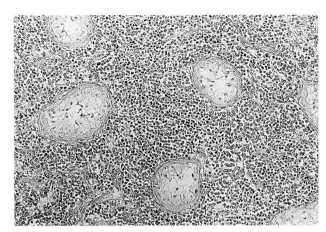

Figure 13–2. LCL. On low-power magnification LCL has a striking proclivity to infiltrate the interstitium sparing a significant number of tubules. The tubules present in this illustration are atrophic and contain Sertoli cells only.

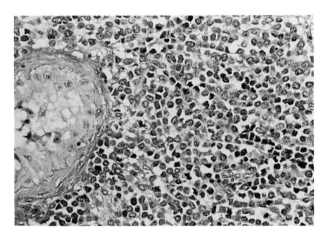

Figure 13–3. LCL. High-power view with characteristic cytologic features of neoplastic cells.

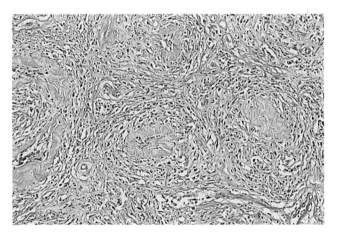

Figure 13–4. LCL. Large cell lymphoma with sclerosis.

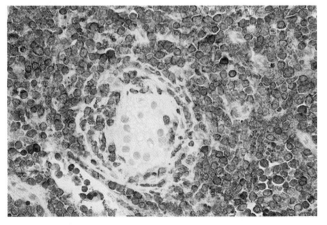

Figure 13–5. LCL. Leukocyte common antigen immunostaining shows positive immunoreactivity in tumor cells.

■ Leukemic Infiltration

CLINICAL

- History of acute leukemia.
- Invariably bilateral and usually asymmetric.
- Symptomatic testicular enlargement rare.
- Testis is considered to be a harbinger of systemic relapse, especially lymphoblastic leukemia.
- Testis is an important "protected site" in childhood leukemic patients.

GROSS

- Testis is seldom removed for leukemia but may be biopsied.
- Rarely, appreciable testicular enlargement (4.5%).
- In gross tumors: bulging cut surface above the confining tunica albuginea.

MICROSCOPIC

- Interstitial pattern of infiltration
- Seminiferous tubule invasion rare
- Testicular vessel wall infiltration
- Features dependent on type of leukemia:
  - Lymphoid and myeloid cells
  - Acute lymphoblastic leukemia (ALL)
  - Acute myelogenous leukemia
  - Chronic lymphocytic leukemia
  - Chronic myelogenous leukemia

SPECIAL STAINS AND IMMUNOHISTOCHEMISTRY

- NASD (naphthol-ASD-chloroacetate esterase): usually positive in myeloid leukemia; negative in lymphoid type
- Lysozyme: usually positive
- LCA: may be positive
- Leu M-1: may be positive
- Terminal deoxynucleotidyl transferase (TdT): positive in ALL (requires fresh or frozen tissue)

DIFFERENTIAL DIAGNOSIS

- Orchitis
- Seminoma
- Spermatocytic seminoma
- Embryonal carcinoma
- Lymphoma

References

Eden OB, Hardisty RM, Innes EM, et al. Testicular disease in acute lymphoblastic leukaemia in childhood. Report on behalf of the Medical Research Council's Working Party on Leukaemia in Childhood. Br Med J 1:334–338, 1978.

Givler RL: Testicular involvement in leukemia and lymphoma. Cancer 23:1290–1295, 1969.

Layfield LJ, Hilborne LH, Ljung BM, et al. Use of fine needle aspiration cytology for the diagnosis of testicular relapse in patients with acute lymphoblastic leukemia. J Urol 139:1020–1022, 1988.

Reid H, Marsden HB. Gonadal infiltration in children with leukemia and lymphoma. J Clin Pathol 33:722–729, 1980.

■ Plasmacytoma (Multiple Myeloma)

CLINICAL

- Involves testes in 2% of patients with multiple myeloma
- May represent an extramedullary manifestation of multiple myeloma
- Testicular enlargement alone (primary) or in association with systemic manifestations of multiple myeloma
- Fifth to seventh decades (75%)
- Bilateral in 30%

GROSS

- Pink-to-tan, lobulated, firm, ill-defined, or discrete nodules
- Fleshy cut section
- No hemorrhage, necrosis, or cyst formation

MICROSCOPIC

- Predominantly interstitial growth pattern of plasma cells: the plasma cells may be mature and immature and may have numerous binucleated forms.
- Commonly involves the tubules, blood vessels, and tunica albuginea.
- Histiocytes, lymphocytes, and neutrophils are absent.

SPECIAL STAINS AND IMMUNOHISTOCHEMISTRY

- Immunoglobulins and κ and λ light chains. Positive in monoclonal pattern
- LCA: may be positive (LCA positivity is more likely to indicate plasmacytoid lymphoma)
- L26: negative
- Cytokeratin: negative

DIFFERENTIAL DIAGNOSIS

- Seminoma
- Orchitis
- Spermatocytic seminoma
- Embryonal carcinoma
- Lymphoma
- Leukemia

References

Chica G, Johnson DE, Ayala AG. Plasmacytoma of testis presenting as primary testicular tumor. Urology 11:90–92, 1978.

Oppenheim PI, Cohen S, Anders KH. Testicular plasmacytoma. A case report with immunohistochemical studies and literature review. Arch Pathol Lab Med 115:629–632, 1991.

Terzian N, Blumenfrucht MJ, Yook CR, et al. Plasmacytoma of the testis. J Urol 137:745–746, 1987.

White J, Chan YF. Solitary testicular plasmacytoma. Br J Urol 75:107–108, 1995.

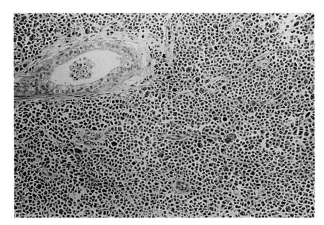

Figure 13–6. Plasmacytoma. Surrounding a tubule is diffuse proliferation of plasma cells with large and pleomorphic forms.

■ Metastatic Tumors

CLINICAL

- Tumors metastatic to the testis are relatively rare.
- More common over the age of 50 years (mean 55 years).
- Testicular enlargement associated with single or multiple intratesticular nodules or masses; bilateral in 15%; presentation is usually late in the course of disease.
- Paratesticular involvement: earlier presentation, as lesions are more easily palpable.
- Primary tumor sites: prostate, lung, malignant melanoma, colon, kidney.
- Although the majority have a history of a primary tumor elsewhere, the metastasis to the testis may be the initial manifestation in 10% of testicular metastases.
- Survival after diagnosis is usually less than 1 year.

GROSS

- Usually single or multiple nodules
- Rarely diffuse effacement of the entire parenchyma

MICROSCOPIC

- Single or multiple nodules
- Areas of necrosis or hemorrhage
- Desmoplastic reaction around tumor nests
- Three distinctive patterns: (1) predominant interstitial location with relative sparing of seminiferous tubules; (2) predominant intratubular growth; (3) formation of nodules that replace the normal structures
- Frequent lymphatic and blood vessel invasion
- Histologic characteristics of metastatic tumor similar to those of primary tumor

SPECIAL STAINS AND IMMUNOHISTOCHEMISTRY

Note: Immunoprofile of the tumor depends on the origin of the tumor

- Mucin: may be positive in adenocarcinoma
- Cytokeratin: positive in carcinoma
- EMA: usually positive in carcinoma
- CEA: may be positive in carcinoma
- Leu-M1: may be positive in carcinoma
- PSA: positive (prostate primary)
- PAP: positive (prostate primary)
- AFP: negative
- HCG: negative
- S-100 and HMB-45: positive in melanoma

DIFFERENTIAL DIAGNOSIS

- Seminoma
- Embryonal carcinoma
- Yolk sac tumor
- Sertoli cell tumor
- Rete testis adenocarcinoma
- Mesothelioma
- Tumors of müllerian origin

References

Almagro UA. Metastatic tumors involving testis. Urology 32:357–360, 1988.

Grignon DJ, Shum DT, Hayman WP. Metastatic tumours of the testes. Can J Surg 29:359–361, 1986.

Haupt HM, Mann RB, Trump DL, et al. Metastatic carcinoma involving the testis. Clinical and pathologic distinction from primary testicular neoplasms. Cancer 54:709–714, 1984.

Meares EM Jr, Ho TL. Metastatic carcinomas involving the testis: A review. J Urol 109:653–655, 1973.

Muir GH, Fisher C. Gastric carcinoma presenting with testicular metastasis. Br J Urol 73:713–714, 1994.

Ro JY, Sahin AA, Ayala AG, et al. Lung carcinoma with metastasis to testicular seminoma. Cancer 66:347–353, 1990.

Tiltman AJ. Metastatic tumours in the testis. Histopathology 3:31–37, 1979.

Young RH, Van Patter HT, Scully RE. Hepatocellular carcinoma metastatic to the testis. Am J Clin Pathol 87:117–120, 1987.

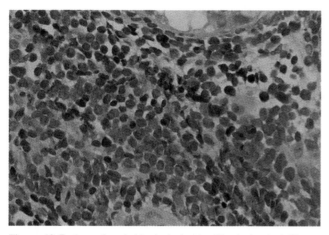

Figure 13–7. Acute lymphoblastic leukemia. The leukemic infiltrates expand the interstitium with relative preservation of the seminiferous tubules.

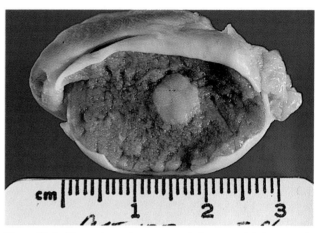

Figure 13–8. Metastatic carcinoma, gross. A discrete nodule is present in the testicular parenchyma.

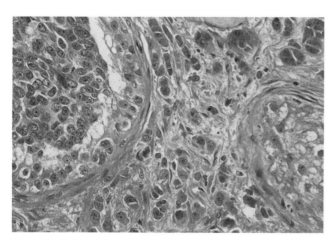

Figure 13–9. Metastatic carcinoma. Tumor cells are present in both interstitium and seminiferous tubules (primary in the lung).

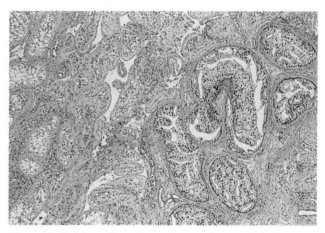

Figure 13–10. Metastatic carcinoma. Tumor cells are exclusively present within the seminiferous tubules (primary in the prostate).

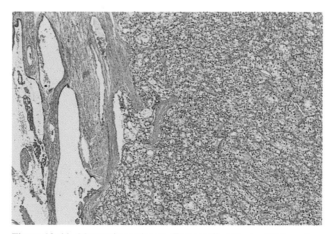

Figure 13–11. Metastatic carcinoma. Tumor cell nests completely replace the normal structure (primary in the kidney).

CHAPTER 14

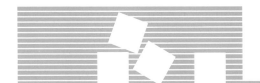

Tumors and Tumorous Conditions of the Testis and Paratesticular Area

■ Tumorous Conditions

Epidermoid Cyst

CLINICAL

- One percent of testicular masses
- All ages, but most common in second to fourth decades
- Right testis affected more than left
- Benign

GROSS

- Average 2 cm in diameter, up to 10 cm
- Round to oval
- Soft and well-demarcated cystic mass
- Laminated cheesy material within a thin fibrous cystic wall.

MICROSCOPIC

- A discrete squamous cell–lined cyst within the testis
- Keratin and necrotic material within cyst
- No associated skin appendages; designated teratoma if skin appendages present

- Focal ulceration and foreign body giant cell reaction
- No other germ cell component or intratubular germ cell neoplasia (ITGCN) in the seminiferous tubules surrounding the cysts: these are key features to differentiate it from mature teratoma

SPECIAL STAINS AND IMMUNOHISTOCHEMISTRY

- None

DIFFERENTIAL DIAGNOSIS

- Mature cystic teratoma

References

Dieckmann KP, Loy V. Epidermoid cyst of the testis: A review of clinical and histogenetic considerations. Br J Urol 73:436–441, 1994.

Manivel JC, Reinberg Y, Niehans GA, et al. Intratubular germ cell neoplasia in testicular teratomas and epidermoid cysts. Correlation with prognosis and possible biologic significance. Cancer 64:715–720, 1989.

Price EB. Epidermoid cysts of the testis: A clinical and pathologic analysis of 69 cases from the testicular tumor registry. J Urol 102:708–713, 1969.

Shah KH, Maxted WC, Chun B. Epidermoid cysts of the testis: A report of three cases and analysis of 141 cases from the world literature. Cancer 47:577–582, 1981.

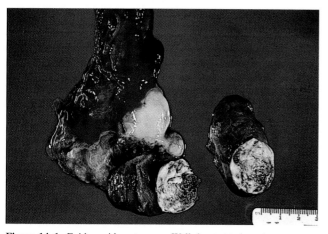

Figure 14–1. Epidermoid cyst, gross. Well-demarcated cystic mass containing laminated, cheesy, keratinous material. (From Ro JY, Sahin AA, Ayala AG. Tumors and tumorous conditions of the male genital tract. In Fletcher CDM (ed). *Diagnostic Histopathology of Tumors.* Edinburgh, Churchill Livingstone, 1995, p 587.)

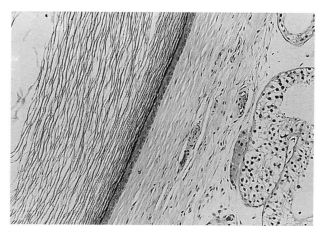

Figure 14–2. Epidermoid cyst. The cyst is lined by squamous epithelium and the cystic lumen contains keratinous debris. Skin adnexal structures are not seen.

Fibrous Periorchitis (Inflammatory Pseudotumor)

CLINICAL

- Diffuse or localized reactive, fibromatous proliferation involving the tunica vaginalis or tunica albuginea
- Age range 15 to 75 years
- May be associated with idiopathic retroperitoneal fibrosis

GROSS

- Firm white thickening of the tunics
- Diffuse form: diffuse induration and thickening
- Localized form: single or multiple nodules

MICROSCOPIC

- Hypercellular spindle cells arranged in fascicles or as in granulation tissue; may be paucicellular or variably cellular
- The spindle cell proliferation is cytologically bland: minimal or no cellular atypia; rare or absent mitosis (early lesion may be mitotically active), no atypical mitosis, and no infiltration of surrounding tissue
- May have an admixture of inflammatory cell components: plasma cells, lymphocytes, histiocytes, or neutrophils
- Typically hyalinized and collagenized background in longstanding lesions
- Focal calcification

SPECIAL STAINS AND IMMUNOHISTOCHEMISTRY

- None

DIFFERENTIAL DIAGNOSIS

- Sarcoma
- Malacoplakia

References

Begin LR, Frail D, Brzezinski A. Myofibroblastoma of the tunica testis: Evolving phase of so-called fibrous pseudotumor? Hum Pathol 21:866–868, 1990.

Benisch B, Peison B, Sobel HJ, et al. Fibrous mesotheliomas (pseudofibroma) of the scrotal sac: A light and ultrastructural study. Cancer 47:731–735, 1981.

Lam KY, Chan KW, Ho MH. Inflammatory pseudotumor of the epididymis. Br J Urol 75:255–257, 1995.

Parveen T, Fleischmann J, Petrelli M. Benign fibrous tumor of the tunica vaginalis testis. Report of a case with light, electron microscopic, and immunocytochemical study, and review of the literature. Arch Pathol Lab Med 116:277–280, 1992.

Young RH, Scully RE. Miscellaneous neoplasms and non-neoplastic lesions. In Talerman A, Roth LM (eds). *Pathology of the Testis and Its Adnexa. Contemporary issues in surgical pathology.* New York, Churchill Livingstone, 1986.

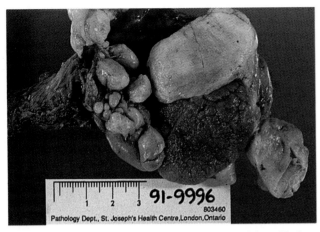

Figure 14–3. Fibrous periorchitis, gross. Multiple nodules with firm, white cut surface involve the tunica vaginalis. (Courtesy of Dr. J.G. Heathcote, London, Ont., Canada.)

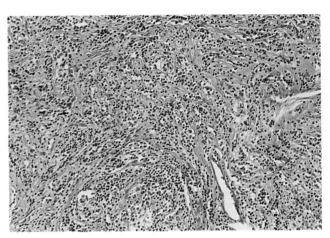

Figure 14–4. Fibrous periorchitis. This lesion contains spindle cells and inflammatory cells associated with granulation tissue type of vascularity.

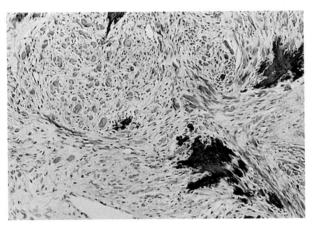

Figure 14–5. Fibrous periorchitis with calcification. This lesion represents an advanced stage with thick bundles of collagen and ill-defined calcifications.

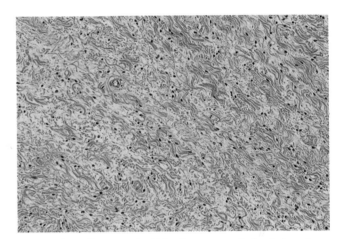

Figure 14–6. Fibrous periorchitis. Late stage of the lesion shows decreased cellularity with increased collagen deposition and decrease in inflammatory component.

■ Malacoplakia

CLINICAL

- Involves testis (60%), epididymis, or both
- Any age, usually 40 to 69 years (75%)
- Almost always unilateral; more commonly involves the right side
- Nonspecific symptoms; usually presents as an enlarged testis which may be fixed to surrounding tissue owing to fibrous adhesions

GROSS

- Replacement of testicular parenchyma by a yellow, tan-to-brown, soft-to-firm nodular mass.
- Fibrosis may be prominent.
- Areas of necrosis.

MICROSCOPIC

- Destructive inflammatory lesion which is usually polymorphous but may contain aggregates of monomorphous inflammatory cell types

- One or more abscesses
- Replacement of the tubules and interstitial tissue by large histiocytes with abundant granular eosinophilic cytoplasm (Hansemann cells)
- Intracytoplasmic targetoid basophilic inclusions (Michaelis-Gutmann bodies)
- Polymorphous infiltrates with acute (neutrophils) and chronic (lymphocytes, plasma cells, histiocytes) inflammatory cells, granulation tissue, and fibrosis
- EM: Phagolysosomes that have ingested the breakdown products of bacteria such as *Escherichia coli*

SPECIAL STAINS AND IMMUNOHISTOCHEMISTRY

- von Kossa's: positive in Michaelis-Gutmann bodies (indicating calcium)
- PAS: positive in Michaelis-Gutmann bodies (indicating mucopolysaccharide substances)
- Prussian blue: positive in Michaelis-Gutmann bodies (indicating iron)

DIFFERENTIAL DIAGNOSIS

- Sclerosing lipogranulomas
- Sperm granuloma
- Granulomatous orchitis
- Inflammatory pseudotumor

References

Damjanov I, Katz SM. Malakoplakia. Pathol Annu 16:103–126, 1981.
McClure J. Malakoplakia of the testis and its relationship to granulomatous orchitis. J Clin Pathol 33:670–678, 1980.
McClure J. Malakoplakia. J Pathol 140:275–330, 1983.
Stevens SA. Malakoplakia of the testis. Br J Urol 75:111–112, 1995.

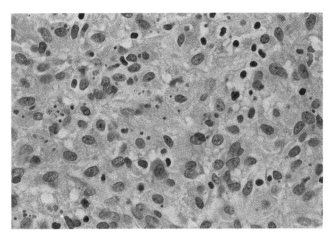

Figure 14–7. Malacoplakia. Histiocytes with abundant granular eosinophilic cytoplasm contain intracytoplasmic targetoid basophilic inclusions.

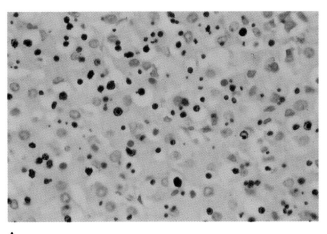

A

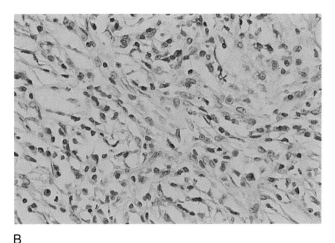

B

Figure 14–8. Malacoplakia. *A,* von Kossa's stain shows positivity of the inclusions indicating that the bodies contain calcium substance. *B,* Iron stain (Prussian blue) is also positive.

Sperm Granuloma

CLINICAL

- Age: 18 to 74 years (>50%, third decade).
- Almost always involves epididymis or vas deferens.
- Painful, firm-to-hard nodule.
- History of vasectomy (15%–40%), trauma, or epididymitis.
- Ninety percent of cases associated with vasectomy are located in vas deferens.
- Vasitis nodosa (proliferation of vas deferens epithelium with inflammation in the wall) in 30%.

GROSS

- Typically firm, well-demarcated nodule
- Small, soft-yellow to white-cream foci on sectioning
- Usually 2 to 3 mm, can be up to 1 cm

MICROSCOPIC

- Early stage: neutrophils predominate which are gradually replaced by epithelioid histiocytes with granuloma formation
- Later stage: progressive fibrosis and hyalinization, prominent accumulation of lipofuscin pigment
- Aggregates of sperm with inflammatory infiltrates; phagocytosis of sperm by histiocytes; occasionally aggregates of sperm are present amid the inflammatory infiltrates
- Ducts showing intense infiltrate of neutrophils and histiocytes, with ulceration and necrosis; occasional squamous metaplasia of the ductal epithelium
- Rare multinucleated giant cells

SPECIAL STAINS AND IMMUNOHISTOCHEMISTRY

- Acid-fast stain: negative
- Gomori's methenamine silver (GMS): negative
- Gram stain: negative

DIFFERENTIAL DIAGNOSIS

- Granulomatous orchitis
- Malacoplakia
- Lipogranuloma (also see Chapter 17)

References

Glassy FJ, Mostofi FK. Spermatic granulomas of the epididymis. Am J Clin Pathol 26:1303–1313, 1956.
Schmidt SS. Spermatic granuloma: An often painful lesion. Fertil Steril 31:178–181, 1979.
Schmidt SS, Morris RR. Spermatic granuloma: The complication of vasectomy. Fertil Steril 24:941–947, 1973.

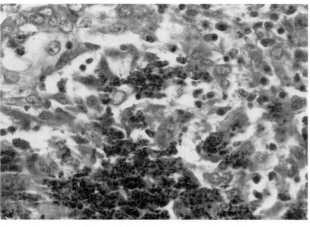

Figure 14–9. Sperm granuloma. Inflammatory cells, which are predominantly neutrophils and histiocytes, surround aggregates of sperm.

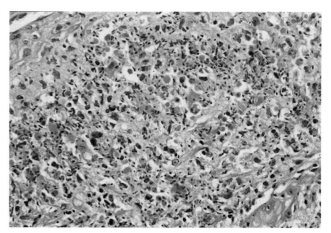

Figure 14–10. Sperm granuloma. This view shows scattered sperm, histiocytes, and neutrophils.

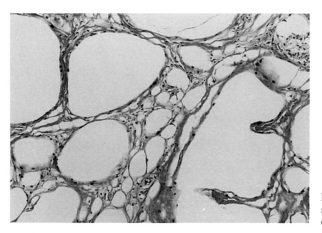

Figure 14–11. Lipogranuloma. Note multicystic change representing dissolved fat (alcohol processing dissolves fat). Histiocytic cells line the empty cavitary spaces.

Vasitis Nodosa

CLINICAL

- Age: 18 to 50 years.
- History of vasectomy (most common), hernia repair, infection, or de novo.
- A nodular thickening of the vas deferens.
- Sperm granuloma is seen with vasitis nodosa in 30%.
- Usually asymptomatic, but localized pain and tenderness may occur, occasionally during intercourse.
- Usually detected at vasovasostomy to restore fertility.
- Bilaterality in 16%.

GROSS

- Typically firm, well-demarcated nodule
- Small, soft-yellow to white-cream foci on sectioning
- Usually 2 to 3 mm, can be up to 1 cm

MICROSCOPIC

- Proliferation of vas deferens epithelium forming ductules with inflammatory cells (predominantly lymphocytes) in the wall.
- Ductules usually confined to the wall of the vas deferens, but may extend into adjacent fibroconnective tissue; desmoplastic response is lacking.
- The ductules are lined by low columnar to cuboidal epithelium without cytologic atypia; mitoses are rare and nucleolus is small or inconspicuous (may rarely be prominent).
- The ductules contain spermatozoa.

- Perineural and vascular wall invasion is seen in up to 20% of cases resembling a malignant neoplasm (nerve involvement may also be seen in other benign conditions such as sclerosing adenosis of the breast, normal and hyperplastic prostatic tissue, and sclerosing pancreatitis).
- Vasitis nodosa can extend to skin and form a vasocutaneous fistula.
- An epididymal lesion similar to vasitis nodosa has been reported as "epididymitis nodosa."

SPECIAL STAINS AND IMMUNOHISTOCHEMISTRY

- None

DIFFERENTIAL DIAGNOSIS

- Adenocarcinoma
- Adenomatoid tumor

References

Balogh K, Travis WD. The frequency of perineurial ductules in vasitis nodosa. Am J Clin Pathol 82:710–713, 1984.

Balogh K, Travis WD. Benign vascular invasion in vasitis nodosa. Am J Clin Pathol 83:426–430, 1985.

Ralph DJ, Lynch MJ, Pryor JP. Vasitis nodosa due to torture. Br J Urol 72:515–516, 1993.

Schned AR, Selikowitz SM. Epididymitis nodosa. An epididymal lesion analogous to vasitis nodosa. Arch Pathol Lab Med 110:61–64, 1986.

Taxy JB, Marshall FF, Erlichman RJ. Vasectomy: Subclinical pathologic changes. Am J Surg Pathol 5:767–772, 1981.

Zimmerman KG, Johnson PC, Paplanus SH. Nerve invasion by benign proliferating ductules in vasitis nodosa. Cancer 51:2066–2069, 1983.

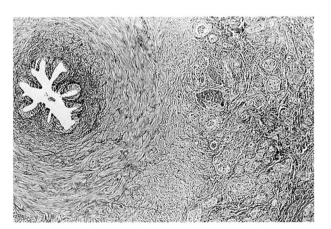

Figure 14–12. Vasitis nodosa. Within the wall of the vas deferens there are numerous round tubules lined by large cells with amphophilic cytoplasm.

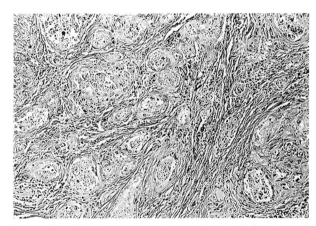

Figure 14–13. Vasitis nodosa. On high magnification the nodule shows tubular proliferation associated with inflammatory reaction.

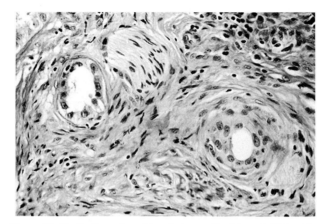

Figure 14–14. Vasitis nodosa. The tubules are lined by cuboidal epithelium lacking features of malignancy. Note the close apposition of a tubule to a nerve trunk.

■ Tumors of Rete Testis

Adenomatous Hyperplasia of Rete Testis

CLINICAL

- Age range from 30 to 74 years (mean 59 years).
- Most are incidental finding: may present as a solid and cystic testicular hilar mass.
- No local recurrence or metastasis.
- Possible pathogenesis includes hormonal imbalance or stimulatory influence, as by germ cell neoplasm.

GROSS

- Spherical cystic structure (up to 0.9 cm) containing jelly-like material
- Diffuse thickening and focal calcification

MICROSCOPIC

- Tubulopapillary epithelial proliferation of rete testis.
- The lining cells are cuboidal to low columnar.
- Lacks nuclear pleomorphism or mitotic activity.
- Atrophic seminiferous tubules are frequent finding.

- Hyaline globules may be seen in association with rete testis hyperplasia in patients with germ cell tumors.
- Pagetoid spread by germ cell neoplasm may accompany rete testis epithelial hyperplasia.

IMMUNOHISTOCHEMISTRY

- Cytokeratin and EMA: positive
- S-100 protein, SMA, desmin, vimentin: negative

DIFFERENTIAL DIAGNOSIS

- Rete testis adenocarcinoma
- Yolk sac tumor

References

Hartwick RW, Ro JY, Srigley JR, et al. Adenomatous hyperplasia of the rete testis. A clinicopathologic study of nine cases. Am J Surg Pathol 15:350–357, 1991.

Lee AH, Theaker JM. Pagetoid spread into rete testis by testicular tumours. Histopathology 24:385–389, 1994.

Ulbright TM, Gersell DJ. Rete testis hyperplasia with hyaline globule formation. A lesion simulating yolk sac tumor. Am J Surg Pathol 15:66–74, 1991.

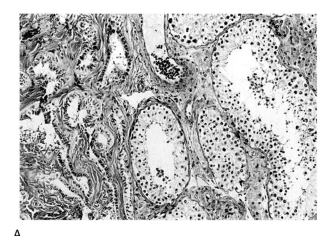

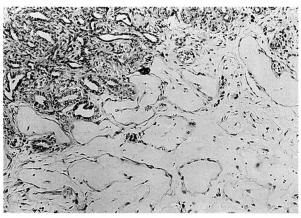

A   B

Figure 14–15. Rete testis hyperplasia. *A,* This photomicrograph displays rete testis showing adenomatous hyperplasia. The lining cells are cuboidal to low columnar without atypia. *B,* Rete testis hyperplasia may be associated with testicular atrophy.

Adenocarcinoma of Rete Testis

CLINICAL

- More common over the age of 60 years (range 20–90 years).
- Twenty-five percent associated with hydrocele.
- Scrotal mass associated with pain: most common presenting symptom.
- Testicular hilar location.
- Variable clinical course.
- The tumor is a high-grade tubulopapillary adenocarcinoma, and because of its rarity the possibility of a mesothelioma or a metastasis, which is more frequent, should be excluded.

GROSS

- Solid; occasionally cystic mass with or without necrosis or hemorrhage.
- Mass is hilar in location.

MICROSCOPIC

- Tubular, papillary, and solid epithelial proliferation.
- Stroma: desmoplastic or hyalinized.
- Morphologic transition between non-neoplastic rete and carcinoma (useful diagnostic feature).
- Tumor cells are large, pleomorphic, and cuboidal with scanty cytoplasm.
- Nuclear stratification within tubulopapillary structures.
- Moderate-to-marked nuclear pleomorphism.
- Sarcomatoid variant has been reported.
- Mitotic activity, irregular chromatin, prominent nucleoli.

SPECIAL STAINS AND IMMUNOHISTOCHEMISTRY

- PAS with diastase treatment: usually positive
- Alcian blue: usually positive
- Mucicarmine: usually positive
- Cytokeratin: positive
- CEA: usually positive
- EMA: usually positive
- AFP: negative
- HCG: negative
- PLAP: negative

DIFFERENTIAL DIAGNOSIS

- Metastatic carcinoma
- Embryonal carcinoma
- Yolk sac tumor
- Tumors of müllerian origin
- Malignant mesothelioma

References

Crisp-Lindgren N, Travers H, Wells MM, et al. Papillary adenocarcinoma of rete testis. Autopsy findings, histochemistry, immunohistochemistry, ultrastructure, and clinical correlations. Am J Surg Pathol 12:492–501, 1988.

Nochomovitz LE, Orenstein JM. Adenocarcinoma of the rete testis: Consolidation and analysis of 31 reported cases with a review of miscellaneous entities. J Urol Pathol 2:1–38, 1994.

Sarma DP, Weilbaecher TG. Adenocarcinoma of the rete testis. J Surg Oncol 30:67–71, 1985.

Stein JP, Freeman JA, Esrig D, et al. Papillary adenocarcinoma of the rete testis: A case report and review of the literature. Urology 44:588–594, 1994.

Visscher DW, Talerman A, Rivera LR, et al. Adenocarcinoma of the rete testis with a spindle cell component. A possible metaplastic carcinoma. Cancer 64:770–775, 1989.

Watson PH, Jacob VC. Adenocarcinoma of the rete testis with sertoliform differentiation. Arch Pathol Lab Med 113:1169–1171, 1989.

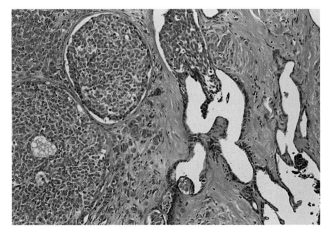

Figure 14–16. Rete testis carcinoma. Rete testis carcinoma arranged in solid nests and papillae. There is vague evidence of transition from hyperplastic rete epithelium to carcinoma (an important histologic clue).

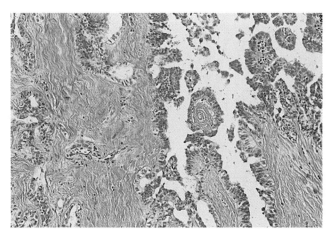

Figure 14–17. Rete testis carcinoma. Apparent transition of hyperplastic rete epithelium into carcinoma. The tumor shows a tubulopapillary growth pattern.

■ Tumors of Tunica and Mesothelium

Mesothelioma of the Tunica Vaginalis

CLINICAL

- Usually associated with a hydrocele, may form a firm mass
- Age: 20 to 75 years; bimodal; third to fourth and sixth to seventh decades
- May involve a history of asbestos exposure

GROSS

- A solid or partly cystic tumor
- From 0.6 to 6.0 cm in diameter
- Forms multiple shaggy or papillary nodules on the surface of the tunica vaginalis; the tumor may coat the entire surface of the tunica vaginalis

MICROSCOPIC

- Pure epithelial, spindle cell–sarcomatoid, or biphasic patterns.
- Epithelial component: papillary, glandular (tubuloalveolar), or solid; typically cuboidal neoplastic cells with oval, vesicular nuclei and moderate amounts of eosinophilic cytoplasm in well-differentiated tumors.
- Spindle cell–sarcomatoid component: poorly defined fascicles of spindle cells with elongated nuclei and scant cytoplasm.
- Biphasic pattern rare.

- Transition from mesothelial (tunica vaginalis) lining to neoplasm (helpful feature).
- Marked cellular pleomorphism and bizarre cells present.
- Psammoma bodies in mesothelioma with papillary component.
- High mitotic rate, significant nuclear atypia, and invasion of adjacent structures in some cases.
- EM: presence of tall slender microvilli, glycogen, tonofilaments, desmosomes, and perinuclear location of mitochondria.
- Well-differentiated (benign) papillary mesothelioma has been reported.

SPECIAL STAINS AND IMMUNOHISTOCHEMISTRY

- PAS: negative
- Alcian blue: positive and hyaluronidase-sensitive
- Mucicarmine: negative
- Cytokeratin: positive
- EMA: usually positive
- CEA: negative
- Leu-M1: negative
- Factor VIII: negative
- B72.3: negative
- Ber-EP4: negative

DIFFERENTIAL DIAGNOSIS

- Carcinoma of rete testis
- Metastatic carcinoma
- Serous papillary carcinoma (müllerian carcinoma)
- Embryonal carcinoma
- Benign papillary mesothelioma (Table 14–1)

Table 14–1
DIFFERENTIAL FEATURES BETWEEN
MESOTHELIOMA AND BENIGN PAPILLARY
MESOTHELIOMA

	Mesothelioma	Benign Papillary Mesothelioma
Size	Large	Small
Mitoses	+	−
Nuclear pleomorphism	+	−
Stromal invasion	+	−
Clinical course	Malignant	Benign

References

Carp NZ, Petersen RO, Kusiak JF, et al. Malignant mesothelioma of the tunica vaginalis testis. J Urol 144:1475–1478, 1990.

Chetty R. Well differentiated (benign) papillary mesothelioma of the tunica vaginalis. J Clin Pathol 45:1029–1030, 1992.

Eden CG, Bettochi C, Coker CB, et al. Malignant mesothelioma of the tunica vaginalis. J Urol 153:1053–1054, 1995.

Grove A, Jensen ML, Donna A. Mesotheliomas of the tunica vaginalis testis and hernial sacs. Virchows Arch [A] 415:283–292, 1989.

Kamiya M, Eimoto T. Malignant mesothelioma of the tunica vaginalis. Pathol Res Pract 186:680–684, 1990.

Morikawa Y, Ishihara Y, Yanase Y, et al. Malignant mesothelioma of the tunica vaginalis with squamous differentiation. J Urol Pathol 2:95–102, 1994.

Reynard JM, Hasan N, Baithun SI, et al. Malignant mesothelioma of the tunica vaginalis testis. Br J Urol 74:389–390, 1994.

Saw KC, Barker TH, Khalil KH, et al. Biphasic malignant mesothelioma of the tunica vaginalis testis. Br J Urol 74:381–382, 1994.

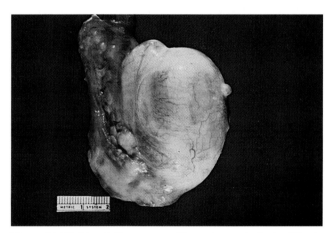

Figure 14–18. Mesothelioma, gross. The tunica vaginalis is diffusely thickened.

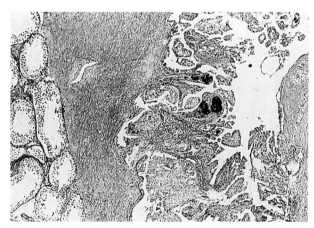

Figure 14–19. Mesothelioma. On the left side there are normal seminiferous tubules; the remainder of the picture shows a papillary tumor apparently arising from the tunica vaginalis. Few calcifications are noted.

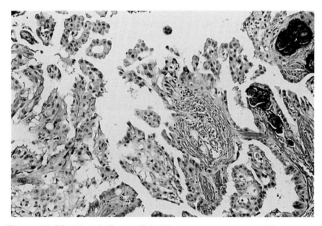

Figure 14–20. Mesothelioma. This illustration shows a papillary tumor with a few psammoma bodies.

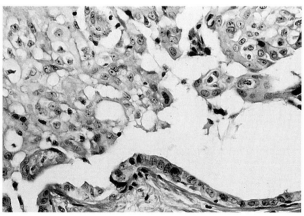

Figure 14–21. Mesothelioma. This view shows an atypical hyperplastic mesothelial lining with transition into the tumor.

■ Tumors of Müllerian Origin

Brenner Tumor

CLINICAL

- Very rare lesion; infrequently associated with an adenomatoid tumor
- No clinical significance

GROSS

- Small (6 mm–2.7 cm), gray-white to yellow lesions
- Nodules in paratesticular tissues, tunica albuginea, or tunica vaginalis; testis involvement rare

MICROSCOPIC

- Well-defined nests, mostly solid and occasionally cystic.
- Polygonal cells (transitional cell type) with characteristic longitudinal nuclear grooves and bland nuclear features; focal mucinous differentiation may be seen.
- Collagenous stroma in the background in which the epithelial nests are embedded.
- Malignant form with a component of transitional and squamous carcinoma has been reported.

SPECIAL STAINS AND IMMUNOHISTOCHEMISTRY

- None

DIFFERENTIAL DIAGNOSIS

- Carcinoid tumor
- Metastatic carcinoma

References

Caccamo D, Socias M, Truchet C. Malignant Brenner tumor of the testis and epididymis. Arch Pathol Lab Med 115:524–527, 1991.

Goldman RL. A Brenner tumor of the testis. Cancer 26:853–856, 1970.

Nogales FF Jr, Matilla A, Ortega I, et al. Mixed Brenner and adenomatoid tumor of the testis. An ultrastructural study and histogenetic considerations. Cancer 43:539–543, 1979.

Ross L. Paratesticular Brenner-like tumor. Cancer 21:722–726, 1968.

Uzoaru I, Ray VH, Nadimpalli V. Brenner tumor of the testis. J Urol Pathol 3:249–253, 1995.

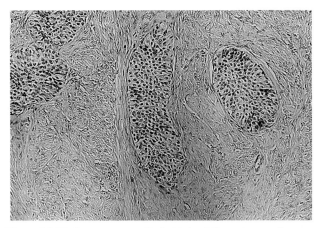

Figure 14–22. Brenner tumor. Embedded within a dense collagenous stroma are nests of monotonous epithelial cells typical of Brenner tumor.

Other Tumors

- A range of tumors histologically resembling ovarian epithelial neoplasms: papillary serous tumor of low malignant potential and invasive carcinoma, serous cystadenoma, papillary cystadenofibroma, mucinous cystadenoma, and clear cell carcinoma have been reported in the testicular tunics.
- These are thought to occur as a result of müllerian metaplasia.
- Intratesticular presentation is possible.
- Immunohistochemical findings: positive for CEA, Leu-M1, B72.3, S-100 protein, CA-125, cytokeratin, and vimentin.

References

Axiotis CA. Intratesticular serous papillary cystadenoma of low malignant potential: An ultrastructural and immunohistochemical study suggesting müllerian differentiation. Am J Surg Pathol 12:56–63, 1988.

De Nictolis M, Tommasoni S, Fabris G, et al. Intratesticular serous cystadenoma of borderline malignancy. A pathological, histochemical and DNA content study of a case with long-term follow-up. Virchows Arch [A] 423:221–225, 1993.

Remmele W, Kaiserling E, Zerban U, et al. Serous papillary cystic tumor of borderline malignancy with focal carcinoma arising in testis: Case report with immunohistochemical and ultrastructural observations. Hum Pathol 23:75–79, 1992.

Young RH, Scully RE. Testicular and paratesticular tumors and tumor-like lesions of ovarian common epithelial and müllerian types. A report of four cases and review of the literature. Am J Clin Pathol 86:146–151, 1986.

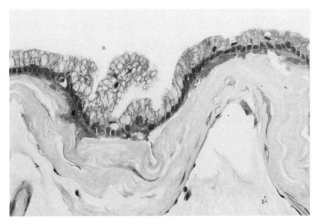

Figure 14–23. Mucinous tumor. This illustration shows the lining of a mucinous tumor consisting of tall columnar cells with basally located nuclei. There is no nuclear stratification, atypia, or stromal invasion.

■ Tumors of Paratesticular Region

Adenomatoid Tumor

CLINICAL

- Most common benign neoplasm of the paratesticular tissues
- Almost always presents as an asymptomatic, unilateral, solitary mass which does not transilluminate
- Occurs in all age groups, but is most commonly seen in third to fifth decades
- Typically located in the epididymis and most commonly in the lower pole
- May also be found in the tunica albuginea and spermatic cord
- Benign clinical outcome

GROSS

- Usually less than 5 cm in diameter (majority <2 cm).
- Typically single, gray-white, well-demarcated, firm nodule.
- Rarely may form a plaquelike lesion.
- Cut surfaces resemble seminoma when testis is involved.

MICROSCOPIC

- Two major elements: epithelial-like cells and fibrous stroma.
- Epithelial-like cells arranged in network of tubules (round, oval, or slitlike); numerous irregular cysts, small cords and clusters.
- Fibrous stroma, sometimes hyalinized, may contain smooth muscle.
- Can have infiltrative borders.
- Tubules lined by flat to cuboidal or low-columnar cells with round or oval nuclei and abundant dense cytoplasm.
- Large intracytoplasmic vacuoles may be present mimicking signet ring cells or fat cells; may also resemble an adipose tissue or vascular neoplasm.
- Lymphoid aggregates may be prominent throughout tumor or at its periphery.
- EM: numerous microvilli on the luminal surface and well-developed desmosomes on the lateral cell surface (mesothelial origin).

SPECIAL STAINS AND IMMUNOHISTOCHEMISTRY

- PAS with diastase: negative
- Mucicarmine: negative
- Alcian blue: may be positive, but hyaluronidase digests it
- Fat stain: negative
- Cytokeratin: positive
- CEA: negative
- Leu-M1: negative
- Factor VIII and ulex europaeus agglutinin I: negative
- S-100 protein: negative

DIFFERENTIAL DIAGNOSIS

- Metastatic carcinoma
- Carcinoma of rete testis
- Malignant mesothelioma
- Histiocytoid (epithelioid) hemangioma
- Embryonal carcinoma

References

Banks ER, Mills SE. Histiocytoid (epithelioid) hemangioma of the testis. The so-called vascular variant of "adenomatoid tumor." Am J Surg Pathol 14:584–589, 1990.

Barwick KW, Madri JA. An immunohistochemical study of adenomatoid tumors utilizing keratin and factor VIII antibodies. Evidence for a mesothelial origin. Lab Invest 47:276–280, 1982.

Mackay B, Bennington JL, Skoglund RW. The adenomatoid tumor. Fine structural evidence for a mesothelial differentiation. Cancer 27:109–115, 1971.

Nakamura Y, Tanimura A, Itoh Y, et al. Elastin in adenomatoid tumor. Light microscopic and electron microscopic study. Arch Pathol Lab Med 116:143–145, 1992.

Taxy JB, Battifora H, Oyasu R. Adenomatoid tumors. A light microscopic, histochemical, and ultrastructural study. Cancer 34:306–316, 1974.

Urdiales-Viedma M, Martos-Padilla S, Caballero-Morales T. Adenomatoid tumors. Immunohistochemical study and histogenesis. Arch Pathol Lab Med 109:636–638, 1985.

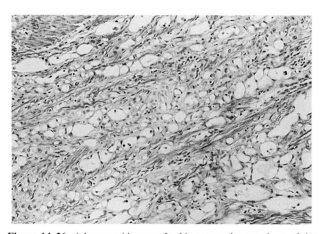

Figure 14–24. Adenomatoid tumor, gross. A well-defined, firm, gray nodule in the epididymis.

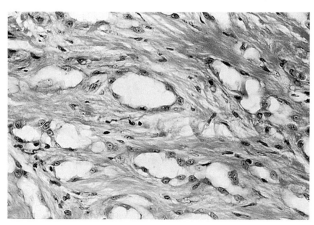

Figure 14–25. Adenomatoid tumor. Glandular type composed of tubules lined by flattened-to-cuboidal cells.

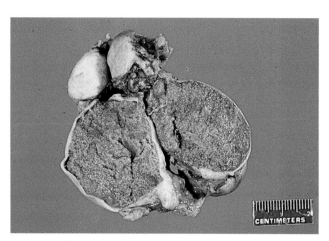

Figure 14–26. Adenomatoid tumor. In this pattern the cytoplasm of the tumor cells is vacuolated, simulating adipocytes.

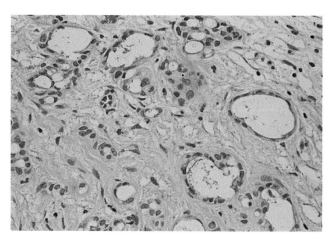

Figure 14–27. Adenomatoid tumor. This pattern, manifested by tubules lined by flattened cells, simulates a vascular tumor.

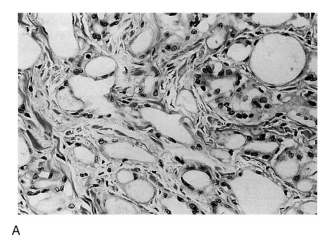

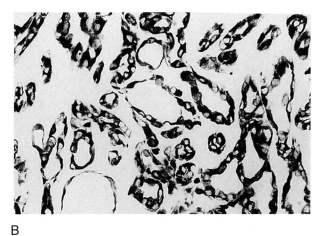

A

B

Figure 14–28. Adenomatoid tumor. *A,* In this view there are tubules lined by flattened cells as well as tubules lined by cuboidal cells. *B,* This is a positive immunoreaction to an anticytokeratin cocktail.

Papillary Cystadenoma of Epididymis

CLINICAL

- Wide age range (mean age 35 years).
- Most frequent presentation is a scrotal mass.
- Association with von Hippel-Lindau syndrome, particularly in cases with bilateral involvement.
- Benign clinical course.
- Rare cases of papillary cystadenocarcinoma have been reported.

GROSS

- Bilateral in 40%.
- Cystic and solid.
- Papillary fronds of gray-brown tissue project into cystic spaces.

MICROSCOPIC

- Cuboidal-to-columnar cells line papillary cores.
- Cytoplasm is abundant and clear, containing glycogen.
- Bland cytologic features.
- Eosinophilic colloid-like material in cystic spaces.

DIFFERENTIAL DIAGNOSIS

- Metastatic renal cell carcinoma
- Papillary serous tumor of müllerian origin
- Mesothelioma
- Rete testis adenocarcinoma

References

Calder CJ, Gregory J. Papillary cystadenoma of the epididymis: A report of two cases with an immunohistochemical study. Histopathology 23:89–91, 1993.

Kragel PJ, Pestaner J, Travis WD, et al. Papillary cystadenoma of the epididymis: A report of three cases with lectin histochemistry. Arch Pathol Lab Med 114:672–675, 1993.

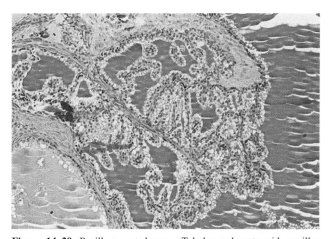

Figure 14–29. Papillary cystadenoma. Tubules and cysts with papillae projecting into the lumina. The cells are bland and contain abundant clear cytoplasm.

Retinal Anlage Tumor of Epididymis or Testis (Synonyms: Melanotic Neuroectodermal Tumor, Melanotic Progonoma, Melanotic Hamartoma)

CLINICAL

- Fewer than 10 cases reported involving testis or epididymis.
- Most cases occur at 10 months of age or less.
- Chiefly epididymal lesions, but rarely may involve testicular parenchyma.
- Scrotal enlargement most common presenting symptom.
- Usually benign, but one case with malignant behavior reported.

GROSS

- Usually less than 4 cm in diameter.
- Well-circumscribed, round-to-oval, solid nodule.
- Closely apposed to the testis, but does not invade the parenchyma.
- Cut section is typically brown, black, or predominantly gray with areas of dark pigmentation.

MICROSCOPIC

- Irregularly shaped nests, cords, and, in places, cleftlike or glomeruloid-like spaces composed of or lined by two types of cells: melanin-containing cells and neuroblastoma-like cells
- Two cell types:
  - Small, undifferentiated, round-to-oval, dark-staining cells with small hyperchromatic nuclei and scant cytoplasm, resembling the cells of a neuroblastoma
  - Large columnar or cuboidal epithelial-like cells with abundant eosinophilic cytoplasm containing melanin pigment, and large vesicular nuclei containing small nucleoli
- Typically prominent fibrous and hyalinized stroma
- High mitotic rate in malignant tumors

SPECIAL STAINS AND IMMUNOHISTOCHEMISTRY

- HMB-45: usually positive in larger cells
- S-100 protein: usually positive in larger cells
- NSE: usually positive in smaller cells
- Cytokeratin: negative in both cells

DIFFERENTIAL DIAGNOSIS

- Malignant melanoma
- Neuroblastoma

References

Cutler LS, Chaudhry AP, Topazian R. Melanotic neuroectodermal tumor of infancy: An ultrastructural study, literature review, and reevaluation. Cancer 48:257–270, 1981.

Johnson RE, Scheithauer BW, Dahlin DC. Melanotic neuroectodermal tumor of infancy. A review of seven cases. Cancer 52:661–666, 1983.

Pettinato G, Manivel JC, d'Amore ES, et al. Melanotic neuroectodermal tumor of infancy. A reexamination of a histogenetic problem based on immunohistochemical, flow cytometric, and ultrastructural study of 10 cases. Am J Surg Pathol 15:233–245, 1991.

Ricketts RR, Majmudar B. Epididymal melanotic neuroectodermal tumor of infancy. Hum Pathol 16:416–420, 1985.

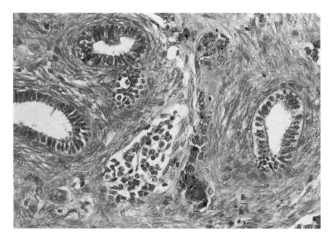

Figure 14–30. Melanotic progonoma. Nests of small, darkly staining cells are associated with larger cells containing eosinophilic cytoplasm, large nuclei, and melanin pigment.

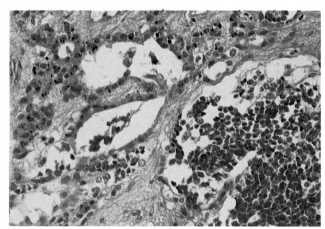

Figure 14–31. Melanotic progonoma. A higher-power view shows the two different cellular populations: small cells (*right*) and large cells containing pigment (*left*).

Rhabdomyosarcoma

CLINICAL

- Age: 7 to 36 years with 60% in first two decades.
- Most common type of sarcoma in children; 20% of rhabdomyosarcoma in boys are paratesticular; the paratesticular region is the most common site of rhabdomyosarcoma in the Armed Forces Institute of Pathology (AFIP) files.
- Presentation: mass in the scrotum (95%).
- Common in spermatic cord and paratesticular tissue.
- Frequent local recurrence and pelvic lymph node metastases.
- Most common type is embryonal rhabdomyosarcoma.
- Recently described variant—leiomyomatous (spindle cell) rhabdomyosarcoma—has a unique predilection for this site.
- Multimodal therapeutic approach has markedly improved survival rates (currently overall 85% 5-year survival).
- Prognosis depends on type and stage.
- Leiomyomatous (spindle cell) rhabdomyosarcoma has better prognosis than embryonal rhabdomyosarcoma and represents the most differentiated end of the spectrum of embryonal rhabdomyosarcoma.

GROSS

- Lobulated, smooth, gray-white, glistening mass (leiomyomatous rhabdomyosarcoma may be firm and fleshy)
- Displaces the testicle without replacing it

MICROSCOPIC

- Markedly variable histologic pattern
- Embryonal rhabdomyosarcoma most frequent (90%): myxoid background with hypo- and hypercellular areas
- Leiomyomatous (spindle cell) rhabdomyosarcoma:
  - Fascicles of spindle cells
  - Abundant eosinophilic fibrillary cytoplasm
  - Cross-striations and areas of classic embryonal rhabdomyosarcoma always present
- Strap cells, with or without cross striations
- Bizarre "tadpole" cells
- Primitive rhabdomyoblast-type cells with intense eosinophilic cytoplasm

SPECIAL STAINS AND IMMUNOHISTOCHEMISTRY

- Myoglobin: usually positive
- Desmin: positive
- Titin: positive (usually positive in leiomyomatous [spindle cell] rhabdomyosarcoma, indicating a more differentiated form)
- Muscle-specific actin: positive
- Vimentin: positive
- Cytokeratin: negative
- SMA: usually negative

DIFFERENTIAL DIAGNOSIS

- Other sarcomas
- Immature teratoma
- Unclassified sex cord–stromal tumor

References

Arean VM, Kreager JA. Paratesticular rhabdomyosarcoma. Am J Clin Pathol 43:418–427, 1965.

Cavazzana AO, Schmidt D, Ninfo V, et al. Spindle cell rhabdomyosarcoma. A prognostically favorable variant of rhabdomyosarcoma. Am J Surg Pathol 16:229–235, 1992.

Cecchetto G, G. Grotto P, De Bernardi B, et al. Paratesticular rhabdomyosarcoma in childhood: Experience of the Italian Cooperative Study. Tumori 74:645–647, 1988.

Hughes LL, Baruzzi MJ, Ribeiro RC, et al. Paratesticular rhabdomyosarcoma: Delayed effects of multimodality therapy and implications for current management. Cancer 73:476–482, 1994.

Leuschner I, Newton WA Jr, Schmidt D, et al. Spindle cell variants of embryonal rhabdomyosarcoma in the paratesticular region: A report of the Intergroup Rhabdomyosarcoma Study. Am J Surg Pathol 17:221–230, 1993.

Loughlin KR, Retik AB, Weinstein HJ, et al. Genitourinary rhabdomyosarcoma in children. Cancer 63:1600–1606, 1989.

Stewart LH, Lioe TF, Johnston SR. Thirty-year review of intrascrotal rhabdomyosarcoma. Br J Urol 68:418–420, 1991.

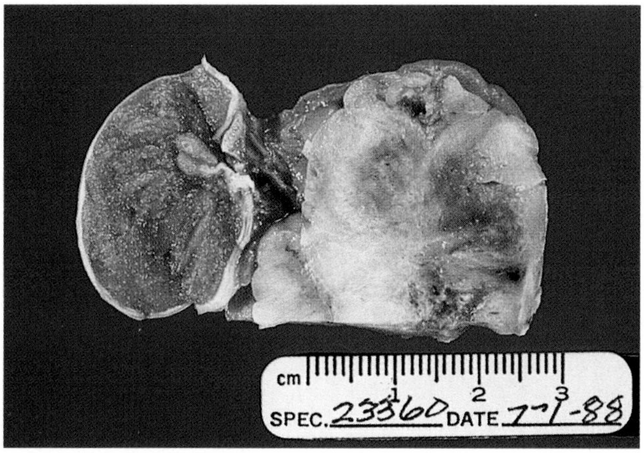

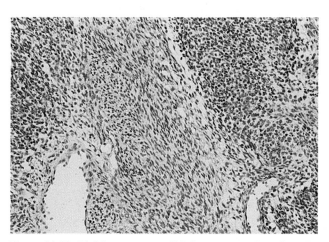

Figure 14–32. Rhabdomyosarcoma, gross. Grayish-white fleshy tumor involving paratesticular tissue (From Ro JY, Sahin AA, Ayala AG. Tumors and tumorous conditions of the male genital tract. In Fletcher CDM (ed). *Diagnostic Histopathology of Tumors.* Edinburgh, Churchill Livingstone, p 592.)

Figure 14–33. Rhabdomyosarcoma. Cellular areas are alternating with myxoid areas, a characteristic feature of embryonal rhabdomyosarcoma.

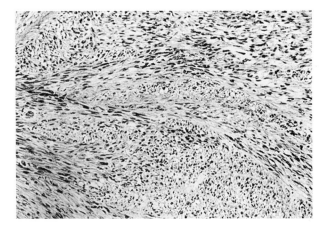

Figure 14–34. Leiomyomatous (spindle cell) rhabdomyosarcoma of the spermatic cord. The fascicular pattern of the spindle cells with abundant fibrillar eosinophilic cytoplasm simulates a smooth muscle tumor. The presence of cross striations and the invariable presence of areas of classic embryonal rhabdomyosarcoma (not shown here) within the tumor are important features to be recognized in order to arrive at the correct diagnosis.

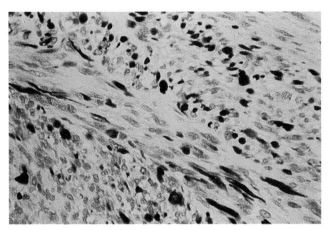

Figure 14–35. Rhabdomyosarcoma. Desmin immunoreactivity in tumor cells.

Other Soft Tissue Tumors

CLINICAL

- Typically in paratesticular tissue with secondary involvement of testis, but rarely occur within the testis.
- Spermatic cord and epididymis most common sites of involvement.
- Most common benign tumor: leiomyoma.
- Most common malignant tumor: rhabdomyosarcoma in children (see Rhabdomyosarcoma).
- Liposarcoma is the most common sarcoma (sclerosing liposarcoma also known as atypical lipomatous tumor and dedifferentiated liposarcoma) in adults. Other sarcomas include leiomyosarcoma, malignant fibrous histiocytoma, and a variety of others.

GROSS AND MICROSCOPIC

- Features are similar to those observed in these neoplasms in more common sites.

SPECIAL STAINS AND IMMUNOHISTOCHEMISTRY

- Features are similar to those observed in these neoplasms in more common sites.

DIFFERENTIAL DIAGNOSIS

- Rhabdomyosarcoma
- Sarcoma arising in teratoma
- Sex cord–stromal tumor

References

Eltorky MA, O'Brien TF, Walzer Y. Primary paratesticular malignant fibrous histiocytoma: Case report and review of the literature. J Urol Pathol 1:425–429, 1993.

Enzinger FM, Weiss SW. *Soft Tissue Tumors*, ed 2. St Louis, Mosby–Year Book, 1988.

Hargreaves HK, Scully RE, Richie JP. Benign hemangioendothelioma of the testis: Case report with electron microscopic documentation and review of the literature. Am J Clin Pathol 77:637–642, 1982.

Hartwick RWJ, Srigley JR, Burns B, et al. A clinicopathologic review of 112 paratesticular tumors (abstr. 173). Lab Invest 56:30A, 1987.

Kinjo M, Hokamura K, Tanaka K, et al. Leiomyosarcoma of the spermatic cord. A case report and a brief review of literature. Acta Pathol Jpn 36:929–934, 1986.

Matthew T, Prabhakaran K. Osteosarcoma of the testis. Arch Pathol Lab Med 105:38–39, 1981.

Yachia P, Auslaender L. Primary leiomyosarcoma of the testis. J Urol 141:955–956, 1989.

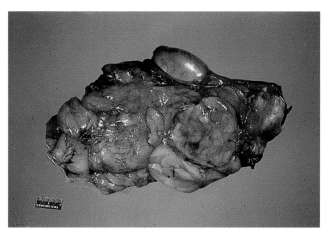

Figure 14–36. Liposarcoma, gross. A relatively well-circumscribed, oval, gold-yellow mass, suggesting adipose tissue derivation.

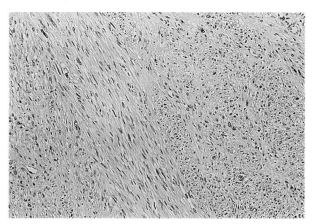

Figure 14–37. Leiomyosarcoma of spermatic cord. Compare with Figure 14–35. The two lesions have in common a fascicular arrangement and elongated nuclei.

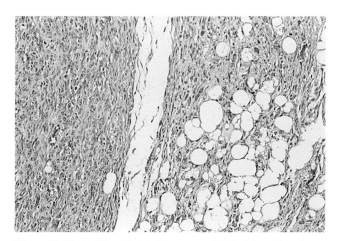

Figure 14–38. Dedifferentiated liposarcoma. Atypical lipomatous tumor (*right*) is associated with a high-grade nonlipogenic sarcoma (MFH; *left*) representing a dedifferentiated liposarcoma.

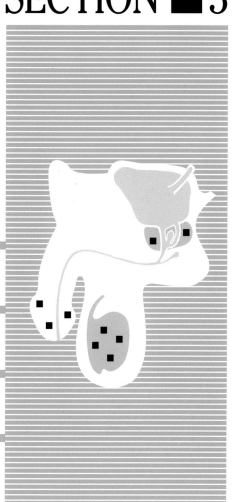

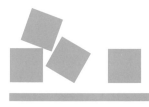

THE PENIS
AND SCROTUM

CHAPTER 15

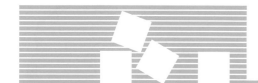

Normal Anatomy and Histology of the Penis

- The penis consists of three parts: (1) the root, (2) the body, and (3) the glans covered by the foreskin.
  - The root lies in the superficial perineal pouch and provides stability and fixation.
  - The body constitutes the major part of the penis and is composed of three cylinders of spongy erectile tissues: the paired corpora cavernosa and the single corpus spongiosum.
    - The two corpora cavernosa form the dorsum of the penis and are surrounded by a double layer of dense, partially hyalinized fibrous connective tissue—Buck's fascia and the thicker (and inner) tunica albuginea.
    - The corpus spongiosum is located on the ventral aspect of the penis and surrounds the urethra in the center.
    - The corpus spongiosum is composed of variable-caliber interconnected venous sinuses surrounded by smooth muscle. The intercorporal tissue is fibroconnective and abundant, with numerous nerve endings.
    - The corpora cavernosa are important for erection. They consist of numerous irregular and wide vascular lumina lined by a single layer of endothelium and surrounded by smooth muscle.
    - The balanopreputial sulcus is a cul-de-sac on the lateral and dorsal aspects behind the glans penis. It is the most common site for Tyson's glands, which produce smegma.
    - The frenulum is a mucosal fold that attaches the foreskin to the glans, immediately below the urethral meatus.
  - The glans is the distal expansion of the corpus spongiosum; it is conical and covered by the loose skin of the prepuce (foreskin).
    - Uncircumcised male: five to six layers of stratified nonkeratinizing squamous epithelium.
    - Circumcised male: keratinized squamous epithelium.
- The foreskin is thin, dark, and loosely connected to the tunica albuginea.
  - Histologically, it has features of true skin but is devoid of subcutaneous tissue. There are sebaceous glands without associated hair follicles and sweat glands in superficial dermis.
  - The foreskin has five layers: (1) epidermis, (2) dermis, (3) dartos, (4) lamina propria, and (5) squamous mucosa, which is a prolongation of the squamous mucosa of the glans and balanopreputial sulcus.
- Penile urethra
  - Navicular fossa: stratified squamous epithelium or stratified columnar or ciliated epithelium.
  - Penile, bulbomembranous, and prostatic urethra: stratified ciliated columnar or transitional epithelium.
  - The lamina propria of the urethra is a thin layer of fibrous and elastic tissue containing mucous-secreting Littré's glands.
  - The penile urethra is enveloped by the corpus spongiosum.
- Blood supply
  - Arterial
    - Internal pudendal artery (three branches): (1) deep artery, (2) bulbar artery, (3) urethral artery
  - Venous
    - Cavernous veins
    - Deep veins
    - Superficial dorsal veins
- Lymphatic drainage
  - Superficial and deep inguinal nodes that drain into external and common iliac nodes
- Embryology
  - Corpora cavernosa are derived from genital tubercles, urethra and corpus spongiosum from urogenital sinus and urogenital folds.

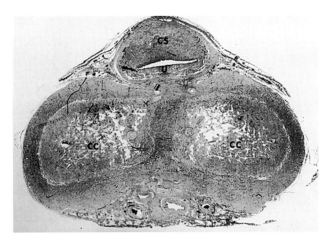

Figure 15–1. Cross section through the body of the penis. Three cylindrical structures form the body: the paired corpora cavernosa *(CC)*, the ventral corpus spongiosum *(CS)*, and the central urethra *(U)*.

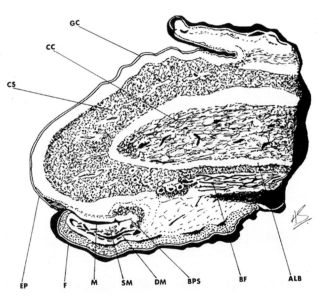

Figure 15–2. Schematic representation of longitudinal section of penis. *GC,* glans corona; *CC,* corpora cavernosa; *CS,* corpus spongiosum; *EP,* epidermis; *F,* foreskin; *M,* mucosa; *SM,* submucosa; *DM,* dartos muscle; *BPS,* balanopreputial sulcus; *BF,* Buck's fascia; *ALB,* albuginea covering corpora cavernosa. (Drawn by Dr. A. Savera, Senior Resident, Department of Pathology, Henry Ford Hospital, Detroit.)

CHAPTER 16

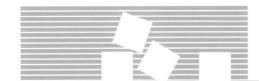

Inflammatory and Infectious Diseases of the Penis

■ Balanoposthitis

- Inflammation of the glans penis and prepuce occurring most commonly in uncircumcised men.
- Most common cause is poor hygiene—failure to retract and clean the foreskin leads to accumulation of desquamated epithelial cells and smegma, which incites an inflammatory response, and may subsequently lead to phimosis.

Classification of Balanoposthitis

Balanoposthitis NOS
Candidal balanitis
Plasma cell balanitis (Zoon's balanitis)
Balanitis xerotica obliterans (lichen sclerosus et atrophicus)
Papulosquamous diseases
    Lichen planus
    Psoriasis
    Balanitis circinata of Reiter's disease
Contact dermatitis
    Allergic
    Irritant
Vesiculobullous diseases (may simulate balanitis clinically)
    Cicatricial pemphigoid
    Fixed drug eruption

- Zoon's or plasma cell balanitis and balanitis xerotica obliterans are frequently encountered lesions for surgical pathologists and are discussed below; papulosquamous and vesiculobullous diseases are beyond the scope of this Atlas. Excellent descriptions are available in dermatologic textbooks.

Plasma Cell Balanitis (Synonyms: Zoon's Balanitis, Balanitis Circumscripta Plasmacellularis)

CLINICAL

- Disorder first described by Zoon (1952).
- It is not rare, and is clinically important because it resembles erythroplasia of Queyrat or Bowen's disease.

- It is a benign disorder of unknown cause which is thought to represent a reaction to a multitude of diverse stimuli.
- Its vulvar counterpart, vulvitis circumscripta plasmacellularis, has identical clinical and histologic features.
- Biopsy is mandatory as clinical appearance overlaps with erythroplasia of Queyrat or Bowen's disease.
- Treatment of choice is circumcision, but laser surgery, topical application of tretinoin (Retin-A) preparations, or steroids have been used with variable success.

GROSS/CLINICAL APPEARANCE

- Zoon's balanitis seems to chiefly affect uncircumcised males.
- A single bright-red and moist patch usually 2 cm or greater situated on glans or inner prepuce.
- In rare instances multiple patches are present.
- In severe cases extensive visibly eroded lesions may be visualized.

MICROSCOPIC

- The histologic hallmark is a distinct bandlike infiltrate in the upper dermis containing numerous plasma cells.
- In some cases plasma cells may be scant or moderate and the histologic findings need to be correlated with clinical presentation to arrive at the diagnosis.
- Additional histologic features include dermal vascular ectasia, extravasated red blood cells, and hemosiderin pigment deposition. Other inflammatory cells include lymphocytes, neutrophils, and macrophages.
- The epidermis is thinned-out, ulcerated, or partially separated. Another distinctive feature is the presence of diamond, rhomboid, or flattened keratinocytes, which are separated from one another by uniform intercellular edema.

DIFFERENTIAL DIAGNOSIS

- Clinical
- Bowen's disease

- Erythroplasia of Queyrat
- Candidal balanitis
- Histology
  - Syphilis

References

Brodin M. Balanitis circumscripta plasmacellularis. J Am Acad Dermatol 2:33–35, 1980.

Jolly BB, Krishnamurty S, Vaidyanathan S. Zoon's balanitis. Urol Int 50:182–184, 1993.

Vohra S, Badlani G. Balanitis and balanoposthitis. Urol Clin North Am 9:143–147, 1992.

Zoon JJ. Balano-posthite chronique circonscrite bénigne à plasmocytes. Dermatologica 105:1–7, 1952.

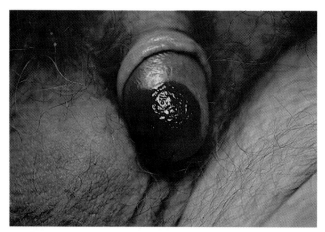

Figure 16–1. Zoon's balanitis. Bright-red moist patch on the glans penis. (Courtesy of Dr. Hans Stricker, Department of Urology, Henry Ford Hospital, Detroit.)

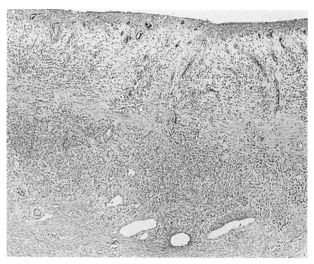

Figure 16–2. Zoon's balanitis. Low-power view depicting ulceration and bandlike dermal inflammatory infiltrate.

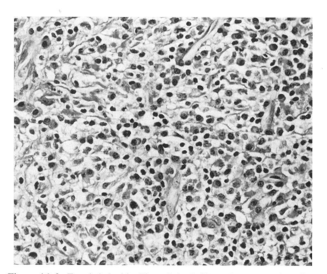

Figure 16–3. Zoon's balanitis. The cellular infiltrate is composed predominantly of plasma cells admixed with lymphocytes.

Balanitis Xerotica Obliterans (BXO) (Synonym: Lichen Sclerosus et Atrophicus, LSA)

CLINICAL

- LSA is an atrophic condition of epidermis and dermal connective tissue that involves genital and perianal skin of males and females. Extragenital skin involvement may or may not be present.
- *Balanitis xerotica obliterans* is the term applied to LSA of the glans penis and prepuce; usually involves older men (<4% prepubertal)
- Two forms of presentation:
  - Idiopathic or classic form:
    - Pathogenically, an autoimmune mechanism is favored; patients have increased organ-specific antibodies, for example, smooth muscle and parietal cell antibodies in males.
    - May be associated with vitiligo and alopecia areata.
    - Associated with characteristic clinical and pathologic features (see below).
  - Secondary BXO
    - Associated with phimosis
- Complications
  - Phimosis and urethral stricture.
  - Carcinoma—controversial; BXO may precede, coexist, or arise subsequent to carcinoma. Rare reports have documented the association of BXO with carcinoma.
- Treatment
  - Circumcision is mainstay.
  - Other forms: laser therapy, topical steroids, antifungal agents, retinoids.

GROSS/CLINICAL APPEARANCE

- Well-defined and marginated white patch on the glans or prepuce which may involve the urethral meatus.
- Lichen-type scale with rough surface may be a presenting sign.
- Longstanding cases: firm lesions due to prominent underlying fibrosis.

MICROSCOPIC

- Active disease
  - Epidermis
    - Orthokeratotic hyperkeratosis accompanied by striking atrophy of the epidermis (distinctive combination)
    - Basal cell layer vacuolation, secondary clefting of dermal-epidermal junction, and bulla (rare)
  - Dermis
    - Marked edema and homogenization of collagen in upper dermis
    - Perivascular or sheetlike lymphoplasmacytic infiltrate below edematous, homogenized zone
- Late and inactive disease
  - Four principal events occur over time:
    - The epidermis loses the basal cell layer, which becomes squamatized.
    - Homogenized upper dermis gradually becomes replaced by sclerotic collagen.
    - Inflammation in the mid-dermis is patchy or absent and now seen in superficial dermis.
    - Areas of epithelial hyperplasia may alternate with atrophy and in rare cases frank squamous atypia may be evident

DIFFERENTIAL DIAGNOSIS

- Lupus erythematosus
- Morphea
- Lichen planus

References

Campus GV, Alia F, Bosincu L. Squamous cell carcinoma and lichen sclerosus et atrophicus of the prepuce. Plast Reconstr Surg 89:692–694, 1992.

Datta C, Dutta SK, Chaudhuri A. Histopathological and immunological studies in a cohort of balanitis xerotica obliterans. J Indian Med Assoc 91:146–148, 1993.

Pride HB, Miller OF, Tyler WB. Penile squamous cell carcinoma arising from balanitis xerotica obliterans. J Am Acad Dermatol 29:469–473, 1993.

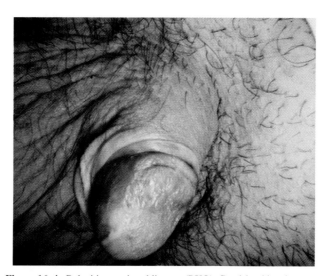

Figure 16–4. Balanitis xerotica obliterans (BXO). Grayish-white plaque on glans penis.

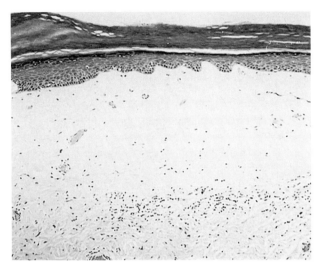

Figure 16–5. BXO, active phase. Edema and homogenization of upper dermis with scant perivascular inflammation below.

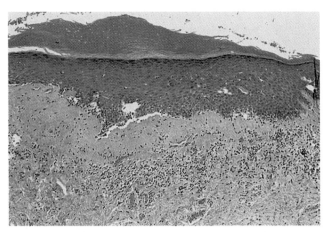

Figure 16–6. BXO, inactive phase. Sclerotic collagen and inflammation in the superficial dermis.

■ Infection

Syphilis

Clinical

- Syphilis is one of the most extensively studied diseases afflicting humans; its incidence was thought to be declining because of efficacious antibiotic therapy, but it has made a comeback with the acquired immunodeficiency syndrome (AIDS) epidemic
- The disease is produced by a microaerophilic gram-negative, *Treponema pallidum,* after a 9- to 90-day incubation period.
- Untreated disease in its classic form occurs in three stages: primary, secondary, and tertiary.
- Penis is involved in all three stages of disease:
  - Primary syphilis: early papule evolves into ulcer—syphilitic chancre at site of genital trauma during sexual contact accompanied by painless, nontender, rubbery, nonsuppurative lymphadenopathy.
  - Secondary syphilis: systemic symmetric mucocutaneous lesions accompanied by generalized lymphadenopathy; condyloma lata and mucous patches involving penis are part of the systemic disease.
  - Tertiary syphilis: gummatous inflammation.
- Treatment
  - Stage-dependent.
  - Predominantly antimicrobial, and successful if timely.
  - Centers for Disease Control (CDC) recommends all patients at risk for testing of human immunodeficiency (HIV) infection, which is also responsible for reactivation of the disease.

Gross/Clinical Appearance

- Primary syphilitic chancre: begins as a tiny papule, enlarges to ulcerate; single rounded painless ulcer with clear-cut margins and clean indurated base
- Secondary syphilis: condyloma lata lesions (may be large), maculopapular, annular, usually hyperpigmented skin lesion
- Tertiary syphilis: nodular gummas with central necrosis

Microscopic

- Histologic hallmarks—perivascular plasma cell infiltrate with endarteritis and endothelial proliferation.
- Syphilitic chancre:
  - Epidermal ulceration with acanthosis at margins, submucosa, or dermis shows inflammatory infiltrate of lymphocytes and plasma cells in sheets and perivascularly with proliferation of endothelial cells.
  - Lymph nodes exhibit follicular hyperplasia with marked plasma cell proliferation and endothelial prominence.
- Secondary syphilis:
  - Cutaneous lesion: epidermis may show parakeratotic scales, acanthosis, ulceration, spongiosis, exocytosis, dyskeratosis, and basal vacuolation.
  - Condyloma lata: prominent epithelial hyperplasia (pseudoepitheliomatous hyperplasia), ulceration, and exocytosis with neutrophils.
  - Dermis:
    - Plasma cell infiltrate with endothelial proliferation.
    - In up to 25% the plasma cell infiltrate may be absent.
    - Pronounced lymphocytic response resembling mycosis fungoides may be present.

- Tertiary syphilis:
  - Hard granulomas: nodular aggregates of perivascular inflammation with plasma cells.
  - Gummatous phase: central caseous necrosis with intense inflammation.

DIFFERENTIAL DIAGNOSIS

- Zoon's balanitis
- Tuberculosis
- Nonspecific inflammation

SPECIAL STAINS

- Warthin-Starry or Levaditi's stain:
  - Spiral organisms in epidermis, dermal capillaries, or lymph nodes.

- Organisms have 8 to 12 convolutions; caution is warranted in interpretation of reticulum fibers in the dermis.

References

Abell E, Marks R, Wilson-Jones E. Secondary syphilis: A clinicopathological review. Br J Dermatol 93:53–61, 1975.

Cochran RIE, Thomson J, Fleming KA et al. Histology simulating reticulosis in secondary syphilis. Br J Dermatol 95:251–254, 1976.

Hutchinson CM, Hook EW III. Syphilis in adults. Med Clin North Am 74:1389–1416, 1990.

Jeerapaet P, Ackerman AB. Histologic patterns of seondary syphilis. Arch Dermatol 107:373–377, 1973.

Poulsen A, Kobayasi T, Secher L et al. *Treponema pallidum* in macular and papular secondary syphilis skin eruptions. Acta Dermatol Venereol (Stockh) 66:251–258, 1986.

Sparling PF. Natural history of syphilis. In Holmes KK, Mardh P, Sparling PF (eds). *Sexually Transmitted Diseases*. New York, McGraw-Hill, 1990, chapter 19.

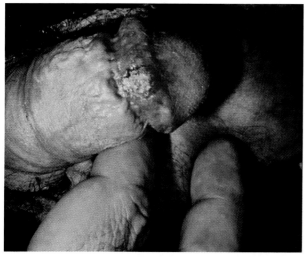

Figure 16–7. Primary syphilitic chancre. Single oval ulcer. Secondary infection in this case resulted in yellowish exudate at the base.

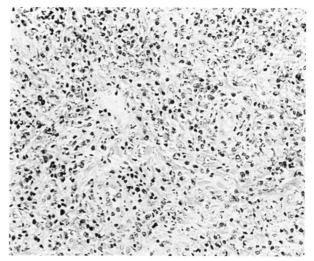

Figure 16–8. Syphilitic chancre. Perivascular chronic inflammation with endothelial proliferation. Plasma cells are a prominent component of the inflammatory infiltrate.

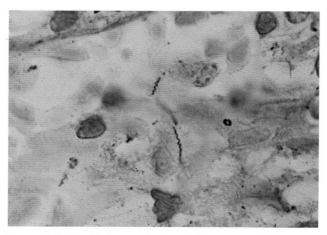

Figure 16–9. Warthin-Starry stain showing *Treponema pallidum* organisms.

Herpes Simplex

CLINICAL

- Herpes (from the Greek "to creep") is a double-stranded DNA virus which has two subtypes, herpes simplex virus types 1 (HSV-1) and 2 (HSV-2):
  - HSV-1 produces oral lesions.
  - HSV-2 produces predominantly genital lesions and 10% to 25% of oral lesions.
- Clinical manifestations are more severe and fulminant in the first episode than in recurrent disease.
- Incubation period is 2 to 12 days.
- Systemic symptoms: fever, malaise, headache.
- Local symptoms: pain, itching, urethral discharge, dysuria, tender lymphadenopathy.
- Complications: also affects sexual partners (women) and neonates.
  - Women: cervical dysplasia and carcinoma (putative role).
  - Neonates: aseptic meningitis, encephalitis, radiculopathy.
  - Disseminated disease: arthritis, hepatitis, hematologic disorders.
- Treatment
  - Options limited
  - Antiviral agents (acyclovir and foscarnet sodium) decrease intensity and duration but not curative

GROSS/CLINICAL APPEARANCE

- Multiple grouped discrete vesicles.
- Vesicles evolve into pustules.
- Pustules coalesce, erode, and form an ulcer with overlying crust.

MICROSCOPIC

- Unilocular or multilocular intraepithelial vesicles with profound acantholysis.
- Vesicle contains proteinaceous material and is surrounded by epidermal cells demonstrating marked reticular and ballooning degeneration.
- Cytopathic effect (CPE): intranuclear inclusions in multinucleated syncytial giant cells; seen chiefly in epidermal cells, but may be seen in adnexal structures, endothelial cells, and fibroblasts.
- Inclusions (Cowdry type A bodies) may be small, demarcated acidophilic bodies to large homogeneous ground-glass bodies surrounded by halos.

SPECIAL STAINS

- Fresh preparation ("Tzank smear")—Wright's, Giemsa, toluidine blue, or Papanicolau's stain
- Immunohistochemical stains for HSV-1 and -2

References

Ashley RL. Laboratory techniques in the diagnosis of herpes simplex infection. Genitourin Med 69:174–183, 1993.
McSorley J, Shapiro L, Brownstein MH, et al. Simplex and varicellazoster: Comparative cases. Int J Dermatol 13:69–75, 1974.
Nahmias AJ, Roizman D. Infection with herpes simplex virus 1 and 2. N Engl J Med 29:667–719, 1973.
Rudlinger R, Norval M. Herpes simplex virus infections: New concepts in an old disease. Dermatologica 178:1–5, 1989.

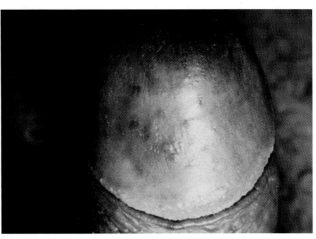

Figure 16–10. Herpes simplex. Grouped discrete vesicles of herpes are present on glans.

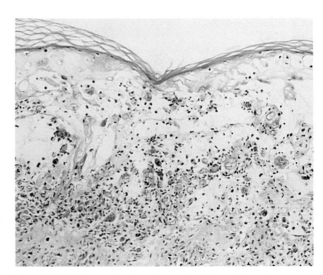

Figure 16–11. Herpes simplex. Intraepithelial vesicle with numerous multinucleated cells.

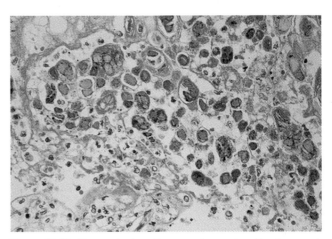

Figure 16–12. Herpes simplex. Numerous intranuclear Cowdry type A inclusion bodies forming homogeneous ground-glass bodies within multinucleated cells.

Lymphogranuloma Venereum (LGV)

CLINICAL

- Sexually transmitted disease caused by *Chlamydia trachomatis* subtypes L_1, L_2, L_3
- Occurrence sporadic in United States, and most Western countries; highly prevalent in Africa, Asia, South America
- Three- to 6-week incubation period; three stages of disease analogous to syphilis:
  - Primary genital stage: papule
  - Secondary inguinal stage: acute lymphadenitis with bubo formation
  - Chronic tertiary stage: genital ulcers, fistulas, elephantiasis, rectal strictures
- Treatment
  - Antibiotics: effective if administered in timely fashion

GROSS/CLINICAL APPEARANCE

- Lesion begins as a papule which transforms into a pustule and heals without treatment; therefore in 50% of patients the lesion may not be clinically examined.
- Inguinal bubo: pathognomonic—painful, unilateral enlargement (66%), which progresses to abscess and rupture (33%).

MICROSCOPIC

- Nonspecific and nondiagnostic
- Penile lesions: ulcer with exudate and polymorphs
- Base with granulation tissue, chronic inflammation, occasional granulomas
- Lymph nodes: follicular hyperplasia with elongated stellate abscess

SPECIAL STAINS

- Giemsa stain on smear from ulcer may demonstrate chlamydial inclusions in macrophages, evident as purple inclusions of elementary bodies; stain lacks specificity and sensitivity.

DIFFERENTIAL DIAGNOSIS

- Ulcerative sexually transmitted diseases:
  - Syphilis
  - Chancroid
  - Granuloma inguinale
  - Herpes

References

Faro S: Lymphogranuloma venereum, chancroid, and granuloma inguinale. Obstet Gynecol Clin North Am 16:517–530, 1989.
Sheldon WH, Heyman A. Lymphogranuloma venereum. Am J Pathol 23:653–664, 1947.

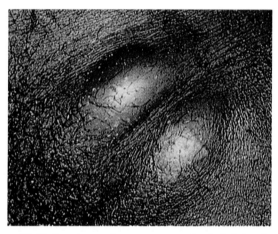

Figure 16–13. Lymphogranuloma venereum. Inguinal bubo due to enlarged lymph node. (From Morse SA, Moreland AA, Thompson SE (eds). *Atlas of Sexually Transmitted Diseases.* Philadelphia, JB Lippincott, p 6.9.)

Granuloma Inguinale (Synonyms: Donovanosis, Granuloma Venereum)

CLINICAL

- Chronic progressive sexually transmitted disease.
- Causative organism is a nonmotile, gram-negative, pleomorphic encapsulated intracellular organism of uncertain affiliation—*Calymmatobacterium donovani.*
- Rare in United States; common in central deserts of Australia, India, Carribean countries, and Africa.
- Incubation period: 8 to 80 days.

- Treatment
  - Antibiotics

GROSS/CLINICAL APPEARANCE

- Single or multiple papules which subsequently form ulcers that bleed readily and have granulation tissue at the base.
- Ulcers (hallmark of the disease) are nontender, indurated, and firm.
- Verrucous form of disease may mimic carcinoma (rare).

MICROSCOPIC

- Central ulceration bordered by acanthotic epidermis displaying features of pseudoepitheliomatous hyperplasia.
- The dermis shows:
  - Granulation tissue.
  - Microabscesses with neutrophils.
  - Large histiocytic cells (25–90 μm) with cytoplasmic vacuolation containing dark particulate inclusions (Donovan bodies).

SPECIAL STAINS

- Smear: Giemsa stain
- Tissue: Warthin-Starry

References

Beerman H, Sonck CE. The epithelial changes in granuloma inguinale. Am J Syphilis 36:501–510, 1952.

Fritz GS, Hubler WR, Dodson RF, et al. Mutilating granuloma inguinale. Arch Dermatol 111:1464–1465, 1975.

Richens J. The diagnosis and treatment of donovanosis (granuloma inguinale). Genitourin Med 67:441–452, 1991.

Sayal SK, Kar PK, Anand LC. A study of 255 cases of granuloma inguinale. Indian J Dermatol 32:91–97, 1987.

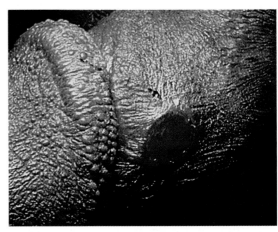

Figure 16–14. Granuloma inguinale. Discrete single penile ulcer at the shaft near the corona. (From Morse SA, Moreland AA, Thompson SE (eds). *Atlas of Sexually Transmitted Diseases.* Philadelphia, JB Lippincott, p 4.2.)

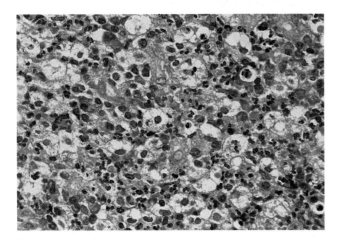

A

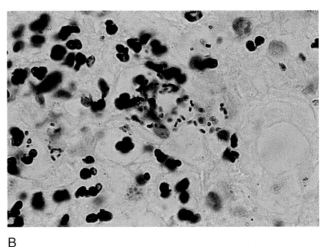

B

Figure 16–15. Granuloma inguinale. *A,* Large histiocytic cells with particulate bodies which are better appreciated by special stains. *B,* Warthin-Starry stain showing numerous Donovan bodies.

Chancroid (Synonym: Soft Chancre)

CLINICAL

- Acute ulcerative disease accompanied by lymphadenopathy in 50% of cases
- Caused by *Haemophilus ducreyi,* gram-negative, facultatively anaerobic, biochemically inert bacteria
- Recent increase in incidence in the United States, more prevalent in underdeveloped countries
- Incubation period: 4 to 10 days
- Treatment
  - Antibiotic therapy; difficult treatment in AIDS patients

GROSS/CLINICAL APPEARANCE

- Erythematous red, tender papule which erodes, becomes a pustule, and forms a shallow ulcer.
- Ulcer is nonindurated, has undermined edges, irregular red margins, and is usually covered by grayish-yellow purulent material.
- Lymphadenitis may spontaneously rupture with fistulas or secondary ulcers.

MICROSCOPIC

- Three distinctive zones are pathognomonic:
  - Surface zone at base of ulcer with fibrin, neutrophils, and debris
  - Intermediate wide zone of prominent neovascularization with endothelial proliferation and focal thrombi
  - Deep zone of cellular lymphoplasmacytic infiltration

SPECIAL STAINS

- Giemsa, Gram, or methylene blue stains: short rods.
- Smears preferable over tissue preparation.
- In smears organisms appear as a "railroad track" or "school of fish" pattern of alignment of short rods.

DIFFERENTIAL DIAGNOSIS

- Ulcerative sexually transmitted diseases:
  - Syphilis
  - Lymphogranuloma venereum
  - Granuloma inguinale
  - Herpes

References

Ducrey A. Experimentelle Untersuchungen über den Anteckungsstoff des weichen Schankers und über die Bubonen. Monatsheft Prakt Dermatol Hamburg 9:387–405, 1989.

Gaisin A, Heaton CL. Chancroid: Alias the soft chancre. Int J Dermatol 14:188–197, 1975.

Margolis RJ, Hood AF. Chancroid: Diagnosis and treatment. J Am Acad Dermatol 6:493–499, 1987.

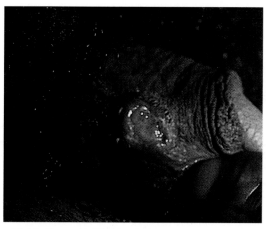

Figure 16–16. Chancroid. Discrete single ulcer with undermined edges. (From Morse SA, Moreland AA, Thompson SE (eds). *Atlas of Sexually Transmitted Diseases.* Philadelphia, JB Lippincott, p 3.5.)

Molluscum Contagiosum

CLINICAL

- Common viral mucocutaneous disorder caused by the molluscum contagiosum virus, a large brick-shaped DNA virus
- Incubation of 2 to 7 weeks
- Treatment
  - Curettage with application of podophyllin or silver nitrate or laser vaporization.
  - Most lesions regress spontaneously within 6 months to 1 year.
  - Treatment is to prevent transmission and autoinoculation.

GROSS/CLINICAL APPEARANCE

- Multiple spherical dome-shaped, discrete 3 to 6-mm papules with central umbilication through which milky-white contents can be extruded under pressure

MICROSCOPIC

- Cup-shaped invagination of acanthotic epidermis into the dermis.
- Cytoplasmic inclusions in cells of stratum malpighii; the basal layer is uninvolved. Inclusions progressively enlarge and reach surface and extrude through a craterlike lesion.
- Inclusions called Henderson-Patterson bodies contain viral particles which are eosinophilic but gradually acquire basophilia and granularity as they enlarge to replace the nucleus.
- Dermis usually lacks significant inflammation unless epidermal contents rupture into dermis.

References

Epstein WL. Molluscum contagiosum. Semin Dermatol 11:184–189, 1992.

Henao J, Freeman RG. Inflammatory molluscum contagiosum. Arch Dermatol 90:479–482, 1964.

Lutzner MA. Molluscum contagiosum, verruca and zoster viruses. Arch Dermatol 23:436–444, 1963.

Porter CD, Blake NW, Cream JJ, et al. Molluscum contagiosum virus. Mol Cell Biol Hum Dis Ser 1:233–257, 1992.

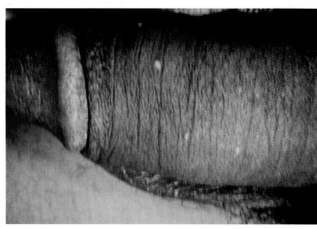

Figure 16–17. Molluscum contagiosum. Multiple grayish-white papules.

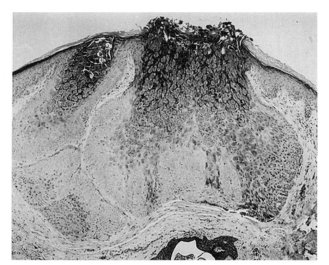

Figure 16–18. Molluscum contagiosum. Cup-shaped invagination of acanthotic epidermis with numerous inclusions.

CHAPTER 17

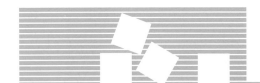

Neoplastic and Tumorous Lesions of the Penis

■ Condyloma

CLINICAL

- Most common tumorous lesion of the penis; caused by human papillomavirus (HPV) infection.
- Usually seen in young adults; the incidence has reached epidemic proportions in the last decade.
- The great majority of lesions are sexually transmitted; 60% to 90% of men are partners of women with HPV infection, and have warts or aceto-white lesions (clinically inapparent lesions enhanced by 3%–5% acetic acid).
- Genital condyloma in children should arouse suspicion of sexual abuse.
- Incubation period is from several weeks to months or even years (most often 3 months)
- Nondysplastic lesions are produced by HPV types 6 and 11, whereas HPV types 16, 18, 31, 33, and 35 are associated with dysplastic lesions.
- Treatment
  - Laser or topical podophyllin.
  - Therapy by both modes may induce marked bizzare cytologic changes. Frequent mitoses, absence of marked nuclear chromatin abnormalities, and intercellular edema are features of therapy-induced atypia.

GROSS/CLINICAL APPEARANCE

- Condyloma acuminatum:
  - Papillomatous pedunculated or sessile growths with roughened keratotic surface
  - Single lesions 1 to 4 mm in diameter × 1 to 15 mm in height; multiple lesions form plaquelike masses of several centimeters size (giant condyloma of Buschke-Löwenstein)
- Condyloma plana (flat warts): flesh-colored or hypopigmented flat or minimally elevated papules
- Bowenoid papulosis: discussed later
- Location on penis: corona of glans, fossa navicularis, urethra, penile meatus
- May also involve scrotum or perineal areas

MICROSCOPIC

- Acanthosis
- Papillomatosis
- Hyperkeratosis with parakeratosis
- Cytoplasmic clearing with atypia—koilocytic atypia (pleomorphism, mitoses, raisinoid nuclei, binucleation)
- Basal cell layer proliferation
- Severe degrees of atypia due to complication by dysplasia or therapy (e.g., podophyllin application)

SPECIAL STUDIES

- Immunohistochemical stains for HPV capsid antigen.
  - Likelihood of positive staining decreases with increasing grades of dysplasia and is usually negative in cancer.
- DNA hybridization for HPV subtyping.

DIFFERENTIAL DIAGNOSIS

- Verruca vulgaris caused by HPV types 2, 3, 4 on or near genital skin
- Molluscum contagiosum
- Seborrheic keratosis
- Fibroepithelial polyp
- Condyloma lata of secondary syphilis
- Pearly penile papule

References

Margolis S. Genital warts and molluscum contagiosum. Urol Clin North Am 11:163–170, 1984.

Nuovo GJ, Hochman HA, Eliezri HA, et al. Detection of human papillomavirus DNA in penile lesions histologically negative for condylomata. Analysis by in-situ hybridization and the polymerase chain reaction. Am J Surg Pathol 14:829–836, 1990.

Oriel JD. Natural History of genital warts. Br J Venereal Dis 47:1–13, 1971.

Rosenberg SK, Reid R. Sexually transmitted papilloma viral infections in the male—I. Anatomic distribution and clinical features. Urology 29:488–492, 1987.

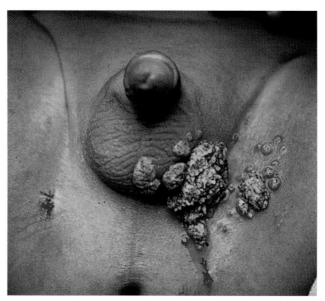

Figure 17–1. Genital condylomata in a child. (Courtesy of Julian Wan, M.D., Department of Urology, State University of New York at Buffalo.)

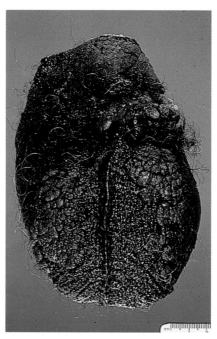

Figure 17–2. Scrotal condyloma. Numerous, often confluent lesions with massive edema resulted in radical surgery requiring excision of entire scrotal skin.

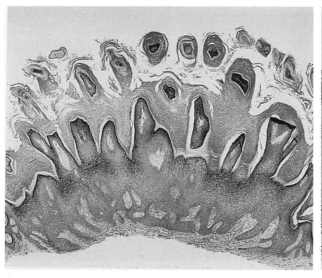

A

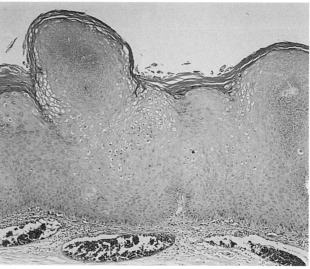

B

Figure 17–3. Condyloma. *A*, Acanthosis, hyperkeratosis, and papillomatosis form the distinctive architecture of this lesion. *B*, Acanthosis, papillomatosis, and koilocytic atypia with occasional dyskeratosis.

■ Hirsutoid Papillomas (Synonym: Pearly Penile Papules)

CLINICAL

- Occur in 10% to 20% of normal males
- No clinical significance
- Most likely represent embryologic remnants of a copulative organ that is well developed in other mammals
- No association with infectious agents and no malignant transformation
- Treatment: none

GROSS/CLINICAL APPEARANCE

- One- to 3-mm yellow-white papules located on corona or frenulum; may resemble hair.
- Individual lesions are domelike, and arranged in a row.

MICROSCOPIC

- Acanthosis with central fibrovascular core (angiofibroma).
- Glands are absent, may resemble fibroepithelial polyp.

DIFFERENTIAL DIAGNOSIS

- Condyloma

References

Glicksman JM, Freeman RG. Pearly penile papules. A statistical study of incidence. Arch Dermatol 93:56–59, 1966.

Johnson BL, Baxter DL. Pearly penile papules. Arch Dermatol 90:166–167, 1964.

Tannenbaum MH, Becker SW. Papillae of the corona of the glans penis. J Urol 93:391–395, 1965.

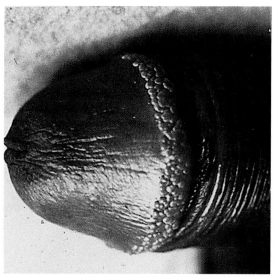

Figure 17–4. Hirsutoid papulosis. Numerous, small, yellow-white papules located on the corona. (From Hasmat AI, Das S. *The Penis.* Baltimore, Waverly Press, p 94.)

■ Verruciform Xanthoma

CLINICAL

- Warty mucocutaneous lesion that most often involves the oral cavity but which may, very rarely, involve genital skin (penile or scrotal)
- Treatment: Excision

GROSS/CLINICAL APPEARANCE

- Well-circumscribed exophytic, papillary, or ulcerated lesion 0.2 to 3.0 cm.
- Lesion may be white, gray, pink, or yellow.

MICROSCOPIC

- Irregular acanthosis
- Hyperkeratosis
- Focal parakeratosis
- Neutrophilic infiltrate in epidermis
- Papillomatosis with elongated and deep rete ridges
- Characteristic xanthomatous cell infiltrate between the rete ridges and superficial dermis

SPECIAL STAINS

- Immunohistochemistry: KP-1 (macrophage marker): positive in histiocytes
- Histochemistry:
  - Oil red O: occasionally lipid-positive
  - PAS: occasionally positive

DIFFERENTIAL DIAGNOSIS

- Xanthomatous lesions:
  - Dystrophic xanthoma
  - Histiocytosis X
  - Cutaneous lipidoses
- Verrucous lesions:
  - Condyloma acuminatum
  - Condyloma lata
  - Verrucous carcinoma

References

Barr RJ, Plank CJ. Verruciform xanthoma of the skin. J Cutan Pathol 7:422–428, 1980.

Kraemer BB, Schmidt WA, Foucar E, et al. Verruciform xanthoma of the penis. Arch Dermatol 117:224–228, 1981.

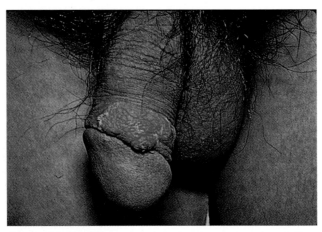

Figure 17–5. Verruciform xanthoma, gross. Exophytic and cerebriform lesion involving the foreskin. (From Kraemer BB, Schmidt WA, Fovear E, et al. Verruciform xanthoma of penis. *Arch Dermatol* 117:516–518, 1981.)

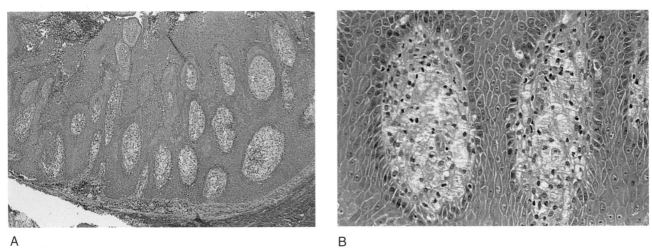

A   B

Figure 17–6. Verricuform xanthoma. *A*, Exophytic papillary lesion that resembles condyloma. *B*, Acanthotic epidermis with elongated and deep rete ridges separated by xanthomatous and chronic inflammation.

■ Penile Cysts

- Epidermal inclusion cyst
  - Commonest location: shaft
  - Size: 0.1 to 1.0 cm
- Mucoid cysts:
  - Ectopic urethral mucosa
  - Lining of stratified columnar epithelium with mucous cells
  - Mucoid contents, unilocular
  - From 0.2 to 2.0 cm
- Median raphe cysts: developmental—incomplete closure of the genital fold

- Lined by pseudostratified columnar epithelium
- Uni- or multilocular

References

Asarch RG, Golitz LE, Sausker WF, et al. Median raphe cysts of the penis. Arch Dermatol 115:1084–1086, 1979.

Cole LA, Helwig EB. Mucoid cysts of the penile skin. J Urol 115:397–400, 1976.

Golitz LE, Robin M. Median raphe canals of the penis. Cutis 27:170–172, 1981.

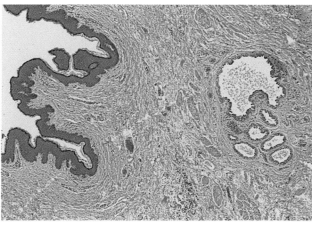

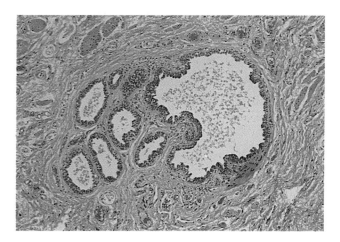

A   B

Figure 17–7. Median raphe cyst lined by low cuboidal-to-columnar pseudostratified epithelium. (*A*, low power. *B*, high power.)

■ Peyronie's Disease (Synonyms: Plastic Induration of the Penis, Fibrous Sclerosis of the Penis, Fibrous Cavernitis)

CLINICAL

- Disease presenting with a painful erection accompanied by distortion, bending, or constriction of the erect penis.
- Affects men between ages of 20 and 80 years (median 53 years); uncommon in men less than 40 years old.
- Painful erection most common presenting symptom (two thirds of patients).
- "Tumorous" presentation: palpated as a firm nodule or plaque on dorsal surface; multiple plaques may be present.
- Examination of the flaccid penis may be unremarkable.
- Ten percent to 20% of patients have Dupuytren's contracture, (palmar or plantar fibromatosis).

- Pathogenetic theories postulate a relationship to fibromatosis, postinflammatory fibrosing reaction (e.g., after urethritis), or posttraumatic (postcoital or postinstrumentation trauma).
- Treatment
  - Surgical excision of plaque
  - Others: radiotherapy or steroid injections
  - Prosthesis

GROSS/CLINICAL APPEARANCE

- Distortion or bending of erect penis
- Firm nodules or plaques on dorsum of penis

MICROSCOPIC

- Fibrosis of the tunica albuginea and Buck's fascia; it does not involve corpus cavernosum.

- Histologic features not as dramatic as clinical presentation.
  - Early stage: fibrous connective tissue with or without perivascular inflammation resembling fibromatosis.
  - Late stage: fibrous or collagenized tissue.
- Ossification or calcification may occur.

DIFFERENTIAL DIAGNOSIS

- Leiomyoma
- Leiomyosarcoma

References

Enzinger FM, Weiss SW. Fibromatoses. In Enzinger FM, Weiss SW (eds). *Soft Tissue Tumors*, ed 3. St Louis, Mosby–Year Book, 1995, pp 207–208.

Smith BH. Subclinical Peyronie's disease. Am J Clin Pathol 52:385–390, 1969.

Wilson SK, Delk JR. A new treatment for Peyronie's disease: Modeling the penis over an inflatable penile prosthesis. J Urol 152:1121–1123, 1994.

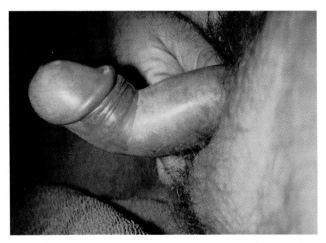

Figure 17–8. Peyronie's disease. Bending of erect penis. (Courtesy of Dr. Hans Stricker, Department of Urology, Henry Ford Hospital, Detroit.)

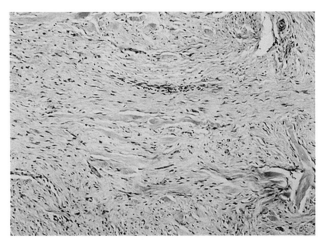

Figure 17–9. Peyronie's disease. Histology of fibrous plaque composed of mature fibrocollagenous tissue.

■ Lipogranulomas (Synonyms: Paraffinomas, Sclerosing Lipogranulomas, Tancho's Nodules)

CLINICAL

- Involve penile or scrotal skin and paratesticular soft tissue.
- Etiology: penile injection of extraneous substances such as paraffin, silicone, oil, or wax for penile enlargement or sexual gratification. In the scrotum, trauma, cold weather, injection of foreign material, and application of topical ointments have been linked.
- Occurs in younger men (usually <40 years).
- Biopsy is necessitated in the absence of clinical history of injection.
- Treatment: Excision

GROSS/CLINICAL APPEARANCE

- Localized plaque or mass of several centimeters in greatest dimension.
- Mass is tender, indurated.

MICROSCOPIC

- Lipid vacuoles of variable sizes in a sclerotic stroma
- Histiocytic or foreign body granulomatous inflammation with lymphocytes, plasma cells, and eosinophils

SPECIAL STAINS

- Lipid stain: positive (does not rule out lipomatous tumors)

- Cytokeratin: negative (helpful to rule out signet ring cell carcinoma and adenomatoid tumor)

DIFFERENTIAL DIAGNOSIS

- Signet ring carcinoma
- Adenomatoid tumor
- Atypical lipoma (sclerosing liposarcoma)
- Malacoplakia

References

Oertel YC, Johnson FB. Sclerosing lipogranuloma of male genitalia. Review of 23 cases. Arch Pathol 101:321–326, 1977.

Smetana HF, Bernhard W. Sclerosing lipogranuloma. Arch Pathol 50:296–325, 1950.

Steward RC, Beason ES, Hayes CW. Granulomas of the penis from self-injection with oils. Plast Reconstr Surg 64:108–111, 1979.

Takihara H, Takahashi M, Ueno T, et al. Sclerosing lipogranuloma of the male genitalia: Analysis of the lipid constituents and histological study. Br J Urol 71:58–62, 1993.

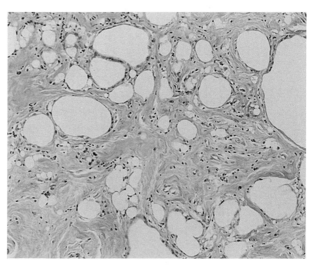

Figure 17–10. Lipogranuloma. Lipid granulomata of variable sizes, interspersed amidst a sclerotic stroma.

■ Premalignant Lesions: Penile Intraepithelial Neoplasia and Carcinoma in Situ

- Nomenclature controversial.
- Three eponyms used for histologically similar but clinically and biologically different lesions:
  - Erythroplasia of Queyrat (EQ).
  - Bowen's disease (BD).
  - Bowenoid papulosis.
- EQ and BD may be related except that they have different sites of predilection and the latter is associated with visceral malignancies.
- Distinguishing features are summarized in Table 17–1.
- Treatment of penile intraepithelial neoplasia and carcinoma in situ
  - Multiple deep biopsies that exclude invasion are a prerequisite.
  - Local excision.
  - Topical 5-fluorouracil (if hair follicles not involved).
  - Laser therapy in BP cases.

Erythroplasia of Queyrat (EQ)

CLINICAL

- Bright-red, well-defined, minimally raised, glistening, velvety plaques.
- Wide age range, most patients in fifth to sixth decade of life.
- Ten percent of patients develop invasive carcinoma and 2% will have distant metastases.

GROSS/CLINICAL APPEARANCE

- Most commonly presents as a single lesion
- Shiny, elevated, reddish, velvety erythematous plaque
- Most frequent sites: glans and prepuce
- Less common: urethral meatus, frenulum, neck of penis

HISTOLOGY

- Full-thickness alteration of squamous epithelium with loss of polarity, proliferation of pleomorphic hyperchromatic cells, dyskeratosis, multinucleation, and numerous typical and atypical mitoses
- Chronic inflammation in underlying stroma with vascular proliferation

DIFFERENTIAL DIAGNOSIS

- Plasma cell (Zoon's) balanitis
- Candidiasis
- Drug eruptions
- Benign dermatoses
- Lichen planus
- Psoriasis

Bowen's Disease

CLINICAL

- Eponym used to designate squamous carcinoma in situ of both sun-exposed and unexposed skin.

Table 17–1

DISTINGUISHING FEATURES OF ERYTHROPLASIA OF QUEYRAT, BOWEN'S DISEASE, AND BOWENOID PAPULOSIS

Features	Erythroplasia of Queyrat	Bowen's Disease	Bowenoid Papulosis
Site	Glans, prepuce	Penile shaft	Penile shaft
Age	5th and 6th decades	4th and 5th decades	3rd and 4th decades
Lesion	Erythematous plaque	Scaly plaque	Papules
Hyperkeratosis	–	+	+
Maturation	–	–	+
Sweat gland involvement	–	–	+
Pilosebaceous involvement	–	+	–
Progress to carcinoma	10%	5%–10%	–
Association with internal cancer	–	+	–
Spontaneous regression	–	–	+

- Lesion involves skin of the shaft and does not have the erythematous appearance of EQ.
- Age: fourth and fifth decades (one decade earlier than EQ).
- Five percent to 10% of patients progress to invasive cancer.
- Associated with internal (visceral) malignancies, for example, lung, gastrointestinal, and urothelial carcinoma

GROSS/CLINICAL APPEARANCE

- Solitary, dull, painless plaquelike lesion
- Location:
  - Shaft and hair-bearing penile skin, rarely glans
  - Inguinal and suprapubic areas

MICROSCOPIC

- Histologically identical to EQ.
- Some subtle differences are due to differences in location. Bowen's disease shows hyperkeratosis, and involves pilosebaceous structures.

Bowenoid Papulosis (BP)

CLINICAL

- Multicentric lesion occurring in young adults, with a predilection for penile shaft or perineum.
- Age: third and fourth decades (mean age 29.5 years).
- Associated with HPV types 6, 16, and 39.
- Spontaneous regression or recurrence characterizes biologic course.
- Squamous carcinoma has been reported as arising from bowenoid papulosis but it is uncertain whether the reported cases were truly BP lesions or if they were BD or EQ lesions. Most experts doubt the malignant potential of bowenoid papulosis.

GROSS/CLINICAL APPEARANCE

- Multiple, erythematous, hyperpigmented papular, 2 to 3-mm (up to 1 cm) lesions which may resemble condyloma acuminatum or condyloma latum

MICROSCOPIC

- Most cases histologically indistinguishable from BD or EQ; the diagnosis should be made only after clinicopathologic correlation.
- BP lesions may show full-thickness atypical keratinocytes and mitoses, but usually more maturation of keratinocytes is seen in these lesions compared with BD or EQ.
- The atypia of keratinocytes is usually observed in upper sweat glands, whereas pilosebaceous units are usually spared—a pattern that is reversed in BD.

References

Aynaud O, Ionesco M, Barrasso R. Penile intraepithelial neoplasia: Specific clinical features correlate with histologic and virologic findings. Cancer 74:1762–1767, 1994.

Callen JP, Headington JT. Bowen's and non-Bowen's squamous intraepithelial neoplasia of the skin: Relationship to internal malignancy. Arch Dermatol 116:422–426, 1980.

Eisen RF, Bhawan J, Cahn TH. Spontaneous regression of bowenoid papulosis of the penis. Cutis 32:269–272, 1983.

Gerber GS. Carcinoma in situ of the penis. J Urol 151:829–833, 1994.

Graham JH, Helwig EB. Erythroplasia of Queyrat: A clinicopathologic and histochemical study. Cancer 32:1396–1414, 1973.

Kaye V, Zhang G, Dehner LP, et al. Carcinoma in situ of penis: Is distinction between erythroplasia of Queyrat and Bowen's disease relevant? Urology 36:479–482, 1990.

Patterson JW, Kao GF, Graham JH, et al. Bowenoid papulosis: A clinicopathologic study with ultrastructural observations. Cancer 57:823–836, 1986.

Wade TR, Kopf AW, Ackerman AB. Bowenoid papulosis of the penis. Cancer 42:1890–1903, 1978.

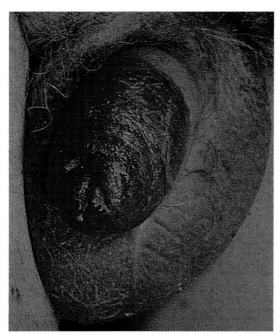

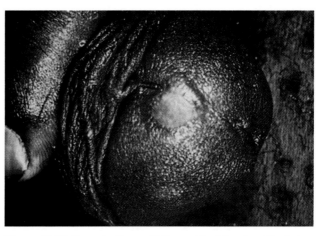

Figure 17–12. Bowen's disease. Dull, grayish-white plaquelike lesion. Histologically, this lesion shows features of squamous carcinoma in situ.

Figure 17–11. Erythroplasia of Queyrat. Extensive involvement by reddish velvety erythematous plaque. (From Aurach WW, Christensen HE. Metastasizing erythroplasia of Queyrat. Acta Derm (Stockh) 56:409–412, 1976.)

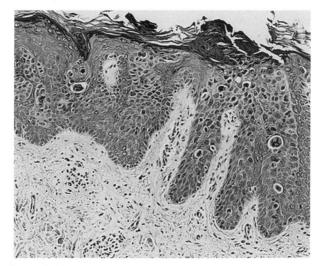

Figure 17–13. Histology of erythroplasia of Queyrat and Bowen's disease is a squamous carcinoma in situ with loss of polarity and frequent mitoses.

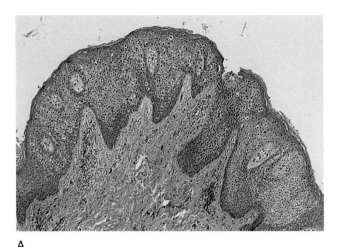

A

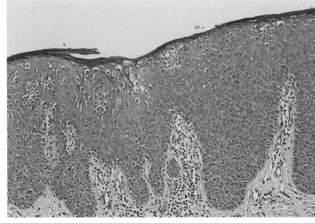

B

Figure 17–14. Bowenoid papulosis (BP). Dysplasia is present at all levels, although maturation of keratinocytes is apparent. Some BP lesions may be histologically indistinguishable from erythroplasia of Queyrat or Bowen's disease. (*A*, low power. *B*, high power.)

◾ Squamous Cell Carcinoma

CLINICAL

- Affects less than 0.5% of male population in Western countries; higher incidence in Uganda, Brazil, Jamaica, Mexico, and Haiti; African-American-to-white ratio in United States: 2:1.
- Risk factors:
  - Lack of circumcision
  - Poor hygiene and accumulation of smegma
  - Phimosis
  - HPV infection
  - Ultraviolet radiation
- Disease of older men: age range 20 to 90 years; rare in men less than 40 years old
- Presenting symptoms: mass, pain, discharge, difficulty in voiding, lymphadenopathy
- Mode of spread: lymphatic—inguinal lymph nodes; hematogenous—rare, distant metastatic sites include liver, lung, and bone
- Treatment
  - Surgical:

- Depends on location and tumor size:
  - Local excision including circumcision
  - Partial or total penectomy
  - Lymph node dissection
- Radiation: phallus preservation in small lesions and younger men
- Chemotherapy: high-volume nodal and distant metastasis

GROSS/CLINICAL APPEARANCE

- Mass, ulceration, or nodular growth are chief presenting forms; average size 2 to 5 cm.
- Grayish-white appearance with necrosis and hemorrhage.
- Lesions may be classified as:
  - Superficial spreading: extensive dysplasia, in situ component with areas of invasion; margins important.
  - Ulcerative or infiltrative: deep invasion characteristic.
  - Fungating and exophytic.
  - Multicentric: multiple gross lesions.
- Location: glans (48%); prepuce (21%); glans, prepuce, and shaft (14%); glans and prepuce (9%); coronal sulcus (6%); shaft (2%)

Staging Systems

JACKSON'S STAGING SYSTEM

Stage	Description
Stage I	Confined to glans, prepuce, or both
Stage II	Extending onto penile shaft
Stage III	Operable inguinal lymph node metastases
Stage IV	Inoperable inguinal lymph node, adjacent structure, or distant metastasis

AMERICAN JOINT COMMITTEE ON CANCER (TNM)

Primary Tumor (T)

TX	Primary tumor cannot be assessed
T0	No evidence of primary tumor
Tis	Carcinoma in situ
Ta	Noninvasive verrucous carcinoma
T1	Tumor invades subepithelial connective tissue
T2	Tumor invades the corpus spongiosum or cavernosum
T3	Tumor invades the urethra or prostate
T4	Tumor invades other adjacent structures

Regional Lymph Nodes (N)

NX	Regional lymph node cannot be assessed
N0	No regional lymph node metastasis
N1	Metastasis in a single superficial inguinal lymph node
N2	Metastases in multiple or bilateral superficial inguinal lymph nodes
N3	Metastasis in deep inguinal or pelvic lymph nodes, unilateral or bilateral

Distant Metastasis (M)

MX	Presence of distant metastasis cannot be assessed
M0	No distant metastasis
M1	Distant metastasis

MICROSCOPIC

- Features of invasive squamous carcinoma
  - Desmoplasia.
  - Nests, cords, trabeculae, and sheets.
  - Intercellular bridges, intracellular keratin, and keratin pearls define squamous differentiation.
- Grading based on degree of differentiation after Broders' system. Maiche et al. have proposed a system based on degree of keratinization, mitotic activity, cellular atypia, and intensity of inflammation.

Grading of Squamous Carcinoma

MODIFIED BRODERS' SYSTEM

Grade		Histologic Features
1	Well	Prominent intercellular bridges Prominent keratin pearl formation Minimal cytologic atypia Rare mitoses
2/3	Moderate	Occasional intercellular bridges Fewer keratin pearls Increased mitotic activity Moderate nuclear atypia
4	Poorly	Marked nuclear pleomorphism Numerous mitoses Necrosis No keratin pearls

SCORING SYSTEM ACCORDING TO MAICHE ET AL

Degree of Keratinization

0 points:	No keratin pearls; keratin in less than 25% of cells
1 point:	No keratin pearls, keratin in 25% to 50% of cells
2 points:	Keratin pearls incomplete or keratin in 50% to 75% of cells
3 points:	Keratin pearls complete or keratin in more than 75% of cells

Mitotic Activity

0 points:	10 or more mitotic cells per field
1 point:	6–9 mitotic cells per field
2 points:	3–5 mitotic cells per field
3 points:	0–2 mitotic cells per field

Cellular Atypia

0 points:	All cells atypical
1 point:	Many atypical cells per field
2 points:	Moderate number of atypical cells per field
3 points:	Few atypical cells per field

Inflammatory Cells

0 points:	No inflammatory cells present
1 point:	Inflammatory cells (lymphocytes) present

Grade 1:	8–10 points
Grade 2:	5–7 points
Grade 3:	3–4 points
Grade 4:	0–2 points

References

Cubilla AL, Barreto J, Caballero C, et al. Pathologic features of epidermoid carcinoma of the penis: A prospective study of 66 cases. Am J Surg Pathol 17:753–763, 1993.

Johnson DE, Fuerst DE, Ayala AG. Cancer of the penis: Experience with 153 cases. Urology 1:404–408, 1973.

Jones WG, Hamers H, Van Den Bogaert W. Penis cancer. A review by the joint radiotherapy committee of the European Organization for Research and Treatment of Cancer (EORTC) genitourinary and radiotherapy groups. J Surg Oncol 40:227–231, 1989.

Lucia MS, Miller GJ: Histopathology of malignant lesions of the penis. Urol Clin North Am 19:227–246, 1992.

Maiche AG, Pyrhonen S, Karkinen M. Histological grading of squamous cell carcinoma of the penis. A new grading system. Br J Urol 67:522–526, 1991.

Narayana AS, Olney LE, Loening SA, et al. Carcinoma of the penis. Cancer 49:2185–2191, 1982.

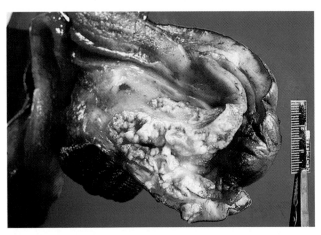
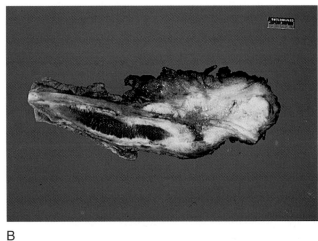

A

B

Figure 17–15. Squamous cell carcinoma. *A,* Cut section of a fungating and infiltrative mass involving the distal penis. *B,* Cut section of another case showing extensive deep infiltration by carcinoma.

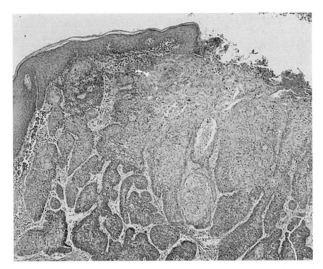
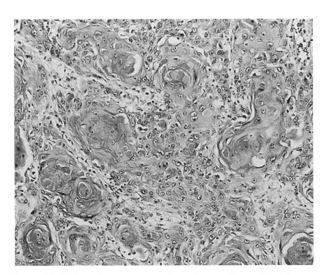

Figure 17–16. Squamous cell carcinoma. Area of ulceration beneath which is invasive squamous carcinoma. Note transition from the non-neoplastic mucosa.

Figure 17–17. Invasive squamous cell carcinoma. Nests of invasive neoplastic cells with intracytoplasmic keratin.

▪ Histologic Variants of Squamous Cell Carcinoma

Verrucous Carcinoma

- Verrucous carcinoma is a well-differentiated squamous cell carcinoma described in oral cavity, larynx, vulva, vagina, anus, and penis.
- It accounts for 5% to 16% of penile malignancies.
- Tumors grow locally and do not metastasize; multiple recurrences occur if inadequately treated.
- Hybrid squamous verrucous carcinoma: cellular anaplasia, increased mitoses, rupture of basement membrane in an otherwise typical verrucous carcinoma. These tumors are biologically similar to verrucous carcinoma (caution: few cases evaluated). Up to 25% of verrucous carcinoma may have a hybrid component.
- Treatment
  - Local excision (high recurrence rate).
  - Partial or radical penectomy.
  - Radiation therapy should be avoided because of reported dedifferentiation (controversial).

GROSS/CLINICAL APPEARANCE

- Large, fungating, frequently ulcerated warty lesion that on cut section burrows through normal tissues.
- Most lesions start on coronal sulcus and spread to the glans or prepuce.

MICROSCOPIC

- Exophytic and endophytic growth component
- Acanthosis, papillomatosis, hyperkeratosis
- Broad-based bulbous pattern of invasion
- Cytologic atypia minimal and confined to deeper portions of tumor
- Inflammatory zone at tumor-host interface

DIFFERENTIAL DIAGNOSIS

- Giant condyloma of Buschke-Löwenstein (controversial: some of the reported cases are verrucous carcinoma; terminology is often used interchangeably)
- Well-differentiated squamous carcinoma (conventional type)

References

Cubilla AL, Barreto J, Caballero C, et al. Pathologic features of epidermoid carcinoma of the penis: A prospective study of 66 cases. Am J Surg Pathol 17:753–763, 1993.

Fukunaga M, Yokoi K, Miyazawa Y, et al. Penile verrucous carcinoma with anaplastic transformation following radiotherapy. Am J Surg Pathol 18:501–505, 1994.

Johnson DE, Lo RK, Srigley J, et al. Verrucous carcinoma of the penis. J Urol 133:216–218, 1985.

McKee PH, Lowe D, Haigh RJ. Penile verrucous carcinoma. Histopathology 7:897–906, 1983.

Yeager JK, Findlay RF, McAleer IM. Penile verrucous carcinoma. Arch Dermatol 126:1208–1210, 1990.

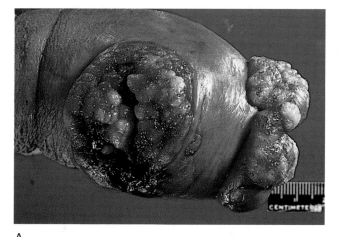

A

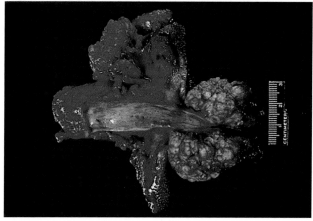

B

Figure 17–18. Verrucous carcinoma. This is a large exophytic and papillary lesion involving the prepuce which has burrowed through the glans and exited on the side of the penile shaft (*A*). This specimen open through the urethra shows a large mass destroying most of the penis (*B*). (From Fletcher CDM (ed). Male genital tumors. In *Diagnostic Histopathology of Tumors*. Edinburgh, Churchill Livingstone, 1995, p 605.)

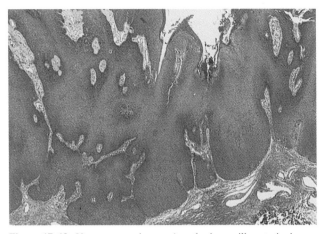

Figure 17–19. Verrucous carcinoma. Acanthosis, papillomatosis, hyperkeratosis (exophytic component).

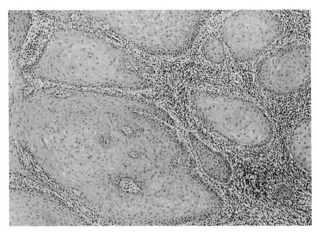

Figure 17–20. Verrucous carcinoma. Close view of advancing edge showing bulbous projections invading superficial dermis by pushing-border type of invasion (endophytic component).

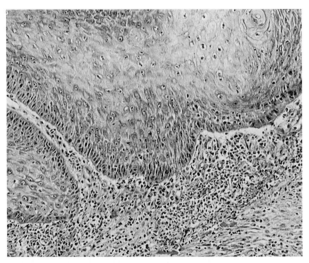

Figure 17–21. Verrucous carcinoma. Blunt bulbous nests of squamous cells with bland cytologic features. Note the presence of inflammation at the tumor-host interface.

Spindle Cell (Sarcomatoid) Squamous Cell Carcinoma

CLINICAL

- Rare variant of dedifferentiated squamous cell carcinoma.
- In purely spindle cell variants immunohistochemistry or ultrastructural examination may be necessary to prove epithelial differentiation.
- Large, bulky, polypoid, grayish-white, fleshy lesions, appearing different from the conventional exophytic or ulcerative squamous cell carcinoma.
- Location: glans penis.

- Prognostic significance unclear as very few tumors reported, but tumors may behave aggressively as they present at an advanced stage.
- Treatment
  - Radical penectomy with or without adjuvant therapy

GROSS/CLINICAL APPEARANCE

- Polypoid, grayish-white, fleshy, with or without surface ulceration.
- Necrosis may be variable.

MICROSCOPIC

- Predominantly anaplastic spindle cell tumor admixed focally with a variable amount of obvious squamous differentiation.
- Squamous component may be very small and may be found only after careful search and examination of multiple sections.
- Spindle cell component demonstrates considerable pleomorphism and mitotic activity.
- The surface may be ulcerated, but finding of squamous dysplasia at the surface is helpful to prove squamous lineage of the neoplasm.
- Heterologous differentiation: neoplastic cartilage or osseous production by the tumor is rare in penile carcinoma (some authors refer to these tumors as carcinosarcoma).

IMMUNOHISTOCHEMISTRY

- Cytokeratin: positive (usually focal)
- Vimentin: positive

DIFFERENTIAL DIAGNOSIS

- Leiomyosarcoma
- Malignant fibrous histiocytoma

References

Cubilla AL, Barreto J, Caballero C, et al. Pathologic features of epidermoid carcinoma of the penis: A prospective study of 66 cases. Am J Surg Pathol 17:753–763, 1993.

Manglani KS, Manaligod JR, Biswamay R. Spindle cell carcinoma of the glans penis: A light and electron microscopic study. Cancer 46:2266–2272, 1980.

Wood EW, Gardner WA Jr, Brown FM. Spindle cell squamous carcinoma of the penis. J Urol 107:990–991, 1972.

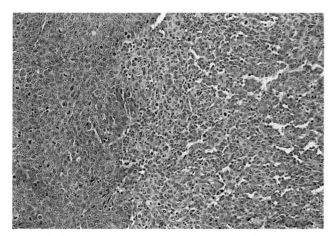

Figure 17–22. Sarcomatoid squamous carcinoma. Transition of poorly differentiated squamous carcinoma (*left*) into undifferentiated oval-to-spindled cells.

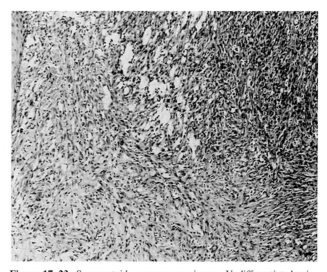

Figure 17–23. Sarcomatoid squamous carcinoma. Undifferentiated spindle-shaped cells focally with myxoid stroma and vague fascicular arrangement.

■ Other Tumors

Basal Cell Carcinoma

CLINICAL

- Although basal cell carcinoma is the most common malignant skin tumor in other regions of the body, it is very uncommon on penile or scrotal skin.

- Age range: 37 to 79 years.
- Clinically indolent neoplasm after adequate excision.
- Treatment: Local excision

GROSS/CLINICAL APPEARANCE

- Papular, nodular, or ulcerated lesion of variable size.

Microscopic

- Nests or fingerlike buds extending from the epidermis.
- Uniform basaloid cells with peripheral palisading.
- Focal squamous differentiation may be present.
- Retraction artifact at the periphery: peritumoral lacunae or cleftlike spaces.
- Adjacent stroma is fibrotic, desmoplastic, or may appear mucinous or myxoid.

References

Goldminz D, Scott G, Klaus S. Penile basal cell carcinoma. Report of a case and review of the literature. J Am Acad Dermatol 20:1094–1097, 1989.

Hall TC, Britt DB, Woodhead DM. Basal cell carcinoma of the penis. J Urol 99:314–315, 1968.

McGregor DH, Tanimura A, Weigel JW. Basal cell carcinoma of penis. Urology 20:320–323, 1982.

Rahbari H, Mehregan AH: Basal cell epitheliomas in usual and unusual sites. J Cutan Pathol 6:425–431, 1979.

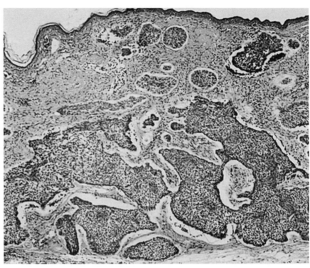

Figure 17–24. Basal cell carcinoma. Characteristic invasive basaloid cell nests with typical peripheral palisading.

Malignant Melanoma

Clinical

- Involvement of penis by malignant melanoma is rare, and accounts for approximately 1% of all penile cancers.
- Age: Fifth to sixth decade, which is an older age group than that of other cutaneous melanomas.
- The tumor is more common in white men and rare in African-American men, in whom squamous carcinoma is more common.
- Staging system:
  - Stage I: tumor confined to the penis.
  - Stage II: metastatic neoplasm to lymph nodes.
  - Stage III: distant metastases.
- Prognosis depends on depth of invasion (Clark level and Breslow thickness) and stage; more than half of patients are stage II at presentation.
- Malignant melanoma of soft parts (clear cell sarcoma) has also been reported to involve the penis.
- Treatment
  - Stage I: wide local excision or partial penectomy with or without superficial inguinal lymph node dissection
  - Stage II: wide local excision or partial penectomy with bilateral inguinal lymph node dissection
  - Stage III: palliative therapy

Gross/Clinical Appearance

- Black, brown, or blue variegated papule or ulcerated plaque.
- Majority of cases involve glans and prepuce, but shaft may be involved.

Microscopic

- Identical to mucocutaneous counterparts.
- Nodular, superficial spreading and acral lentiginous types have been reported.

Special Stains

- S-100 protein: positive
- HMB-45: positive

Differential Diagnosis

- Paget's disease must be considered in differential diagnosis of in situ melanoma.

References

Begun FT, Grossman HB, Diokno AC, et al. Malignant melanoma of the penis and male urethra. J Urol 132:123–125, 1984.

Jaeger N, Wirtler H, Tschubel K. Acral lentiginous melanoma of penis. Eur Urol 8:182–184, 1982.

Johnson DE, Ayala AG. Primary melanoma of the penis. Urology 2:174–177, 1973.

Manivel JC, Fraley EE. Malignant melanoma of the penis and male urethra: 4 case reports and literature review. J Urol 1988; 139:813–816.

Oldbring J, Mikulowski P. Malignant melanoma of the penis and male urethra. Report of nine cases and review of the literature. Cancer 59:581–587, 1987.

Stillwell TJ, Zincke H, Gaffey TA, et al. Malignant melanoma of the penis. J Urol 140:72–75, 1988.

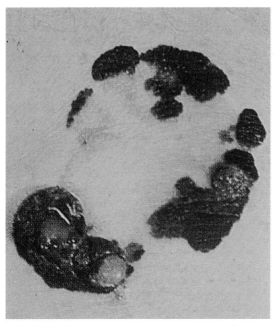

Figure 17–25. Malignant melanoma. Clinically unevenly pigmented lesion with variegated appearance and ill-defined edges.

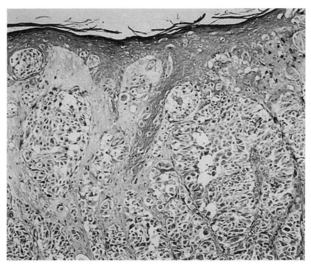

Figure 17–26. Malignant melanoma. Nests of malignant cells in dermis along with junctional component.

Metastatic Tumors

CLINICAL

- Although the penis has a rich and complex vascular circulation interconnected to the pelvic organs, metastasis to the penis is rare and usually a late manifestation of systemic disease.
- Tumors metastatic to penis:
  - Common: prostate (most frequent), bladder, rectosigmoid colon, kidney.
  - Rare: testis, ureter, lung, pancreas, nasopharynx, bone.
- Priapism, hematuria, dysuria, or palpable mass is presenting symptom.
- Modes of spread to penis:
  - Retrograde venous dissemination (commonest).
  - Retrograde lymphatic dissemination, with or without prior lymph node involvement.
  - Arterial dissemination.
  - Direct extension.
  - Perineural tumor infiltration.
- Prognosis: poor.
- Treatment
  - Total penectomy: relief of pain and symptoms
  - Palliative

GROSS/CLINICAL APPEARANCE

- Single or usually multiple palpable nodules which may ulcerate

MICROSCOPIC

- Corpus cavernosum is most frequent site of metastatic spread with diffuse involvement including tumor in vascular spaces.
- Tumor histologically resembles primary neoplasm.

References

Haddad FS. Penile metastases secondary to bladder cancer. Review of the literature. Urol Int 39:125–142, 1984.

Ordonez NG, Ayala AG, Bracken RB. Renal cell carcinoma metastatis to penis. Urology 19:417–419, 1982.

Perez-Mesa C, Oxenhandler R. Metastatic tumors of the penis. J Surg Oncol 42:11–15, 1989.

Powell BL, Craig JB, Muss HB. Secondary malignancies of the penis and epididymis: A case report and review of the literature. J Clin Oncol 3:110–116, 1985.

Powell FC, Venencie PY, Winkelmann RK. Metastatic prostate carcinoma manifesting as penile nodules. Arch Dermatol 20:1604–1606, 1984.

Robey EL, Schellhammer PF. Four cases of metastases to the penis and review of the literature. J Urol 132:992–994, 1984.

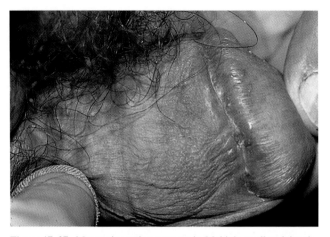

Figure 17–27. Metastatic carcinoma to penis. Multiple small nodular elevations involving the coronal sulcus area.

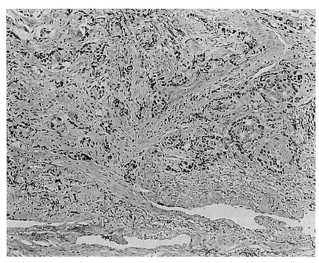

Figure 17–28. Metastatic adenocarcinoma to penis. The corpus cavernosum shows extensive neoplasm within vascular spaces.

■ Soft Tissue Tumors of the Penis

- Soft tissue tumors involving the penis are summarized in Table 17–2.
- Sarcomas are the most common nonsquamous malignancies of the penis—5% of all penile cancers.
- Age: Fifth to sixth decade, except rhabdomyosarcoma, which occurs in children.
- Spindle cell carcinoma must be excluded by ultrastructural studies or immunohistochemistry.
- Most sarcomas involve the shaft, except Kaposi's sarcoma, which has a predilection for the glans.

Table 17–2
SOFT TISSUE TUMORS OF THE PENIS

	Benign	**Malignant**
Vascular	Hemangioma	Kaposi's sarcoma
	Glomus tumor	Angiosarcoma
		Epithelioid hemangioendothelioma
Neurogenic	Neurofibroma	Malignant peripheral nerve sheath tumor
	Schwannoma	
Myogenic	Leiomyoma	Leiomyosarcoma
		Rhabdomyosarcoma
Fibrous	Dermatofibroma	Fibrosarcoma
		Malignant fibrous histiocytoma

- The most common soft tissue sarcomas involving the penis—Kaposi's sarcoma and leiomyosarcoma—are discussed here.

Kaposi's Sarcoma

- With the AIDS epidemic increased numbers of cases are reported.
- Twenty percent of AIDS patients have penile tumors, and in 3% of AIDS patients penile sarcoma is the presenting symptom.
- Glans penis or shaft, or both, are commonly involved.
- Local excision or radiation therapy is helpful.

Leiomyosarcoma

- Superficial type:
  - Arises from smooth muscle of the glans penis or the dermis of the shaft.
  - Forms a subcutaneous nodule.
  - Local excision may be adequate, but recurrences may occur.
- Deep type:
  - Arises from smooth muscle of the corpora cavernosa.
  - Tumors invade deeply, involve urethra, and metastasize early.
  - Radical surgery is required.
  - Poor prognosis.

References

Bayne P, Wise G. Kaposi's sarcoma of penis and genitalia. Urology 31:22–25, 1988.

Dalkin B, Zaontz MR. Rhabdomyosarcoma of the penis in children. J Urol 141:908–909, 1989.

Dehner LP, Smith BH. Soft tissue tumors of the penis. A clinicopathologic study of 46 cases. Cancer 25:1431–1447, 1970.

Deutch M, Lee RLS, Mercado R. Hemangioendothelioma of the penis with late appearing metastases: Report of a case with review of the literature. J Surg Oncol 5:27–34, 1973.

Isa SS, Almaraz R, Magovern J. Leiomyosarcoma of the penis: Case report and review of the literature. Cancer 54:939–942, 1984.

Lowe FC, Lattimer G, Metroka CE. Kaposi's sarcoma of the penis in patients with acquired immunodeficiency syndrome. J Urol 142: 1475–1477, 1989.

Pow-sang MR, Orihuela E. Leiomyosarcoma of the penis. J Urol 151: 1643–1645, 1994.

Valadez RA, Waters WB. Leiomyosarcoma of penis. Urology 27:265–267, 1986.

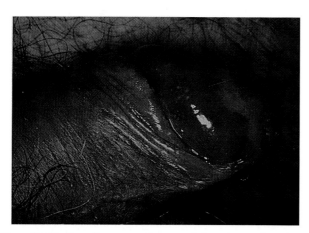

Figure 17–29. Kaposi's sarcoma. Corona and glans show moist red neoplasm. (From Andriole GL, Macher AM, Reichert CM, et al: AIDS case for diagnosis. *Milit Med* 515:m51, 1986.)

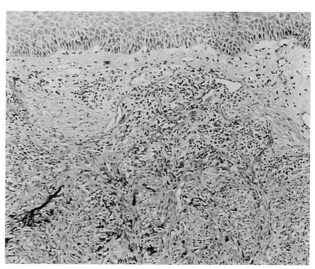

Figure 17–30. Kaposi's sarcoma. Spindle cell proliferation of relatively uniform cells with increased and dilated capillary spaces and extravasated red blood cells.

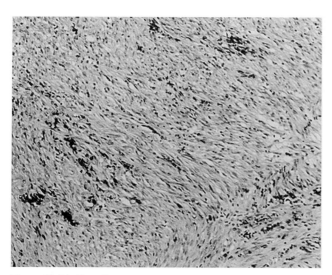

Figure 17–31. Kaposi's sarcoma. Spindle cell proliferation of relatively uniform cells, associated with extravasated red blood cells.

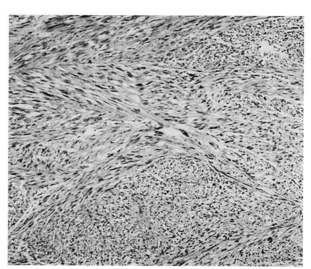

Figure 17–32. Leiomyosarcoma. Interlacing fascicles of neoplastic smooth muscle cells with nuclear pleomorphism and fibrillar eosinophilic cytoplasm.

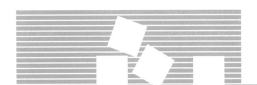

CHAPTER 18

Diseases of the Scrotum

■ Normal Anatomy and Histology

- Contains the testis and lower part of the spermatic cord.
- Divided into two halves by a cutaneous raphe which continues ventrally to the inferior penile surface and dorsally along the midline of the perineum to the anus.
- The left scrotum is usually lower because of longer spermatic cord.
- The scrotum is composed of the skin, dartos muscle, and external cremasteric and internal spermatic fasciae. The dermis contains hair follicles and adnexal structures; although scattered fat cells are present there is no distinct subcutaneous adipose tissue layer.
- Blood supply: external and internal pudendal arteries, cremasteric and testicular arteries.
- Lymphatic drainage: superficial inguinal lymph nodes.
- Embryology: the scrotum develops from the genital swellings that meet each other ventral to the anus and unite, forming two sacs.

■ Hidradenitis Suppurativa

CLINICAL

- Chronic, suppurative inflammatory disease seen in diseases of the follicular occlusion
- Triad—hidradenitis suppurativa, acne conglobata, and perifollicular capitis.
- The term is a slight misnomer as the disease is, by definition, an inflammatory process of apocrine and eccrine glands and ducts which are secondarily involved by the initiating event, follicular hyperkeratosis.
- Sequence of events: follicular hyperkeratosis—damming effect and retention of follicular and sweat gland products; rupture of pilosebaceous structures; extrusion of keratin with apocrine and eccrine products and commensal bacte-

ria into dermis; necrotizing granulomatous reaction with abscess; finally, extension to surface as sinus tract.
- Hormonal, genetic, mechanical (obesity, friction), and environmental factors predispose to hidradenitis suppurativa.
- Microbiologic cultures often negative; superinfection is usually due to staphylococcal, streptococcal, or mixed microbial agents, including anaerobic organisms and actinomycotic species.
- Treatment
  - Incision and drainage or localized excision with or without antibiotic therapy

GROSS/CLINICAL APPEARANCE

- Erythematous papules that progress to fluctuant nodules with draining sinuses; conglomeration of numerous involved follicles forms large plaques
- Location: periscrotal and scrotal skin; axillae; perianal, areolar, and periumbilical regions

MICROSCOPIC

- Epidermal ulceration with sinus tract
- Deep dermal necrotizing acute inflammation with foreign body granulomatous inflammation surrounded by granulation tissue and peripheral fibrosis

References

Brunsting HA. Hidradenitis and other variants of acne. Arch Dermatol Syphilol 65:303–315, 1952.
Shelly WB, Cahn MM. The pathogenesis of hidradenitis suppurativa in man. Arch Dermatol 72:562–565, 1955.

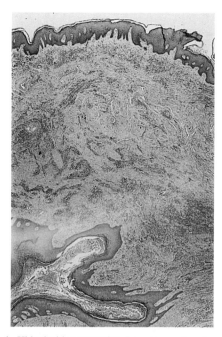

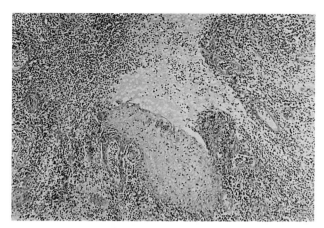

Figure 18–2. Hidradenitis suppurativa. Portion of sinus tract wall with surrounding acute inflammation and granulation tissue.

Figure 18–1. Hidradenitis suppurativa. Low-power view shows deep dermal epithelial sinus with surrounding inflammation and fibrosis.

■ Scrotal Calcinosis

CLINICAL

- Occurs in two settings: (1) calcification of preexisting epidermoid or pilar cysts; (2) involvement of dermal connective tissue in the absence of demonstrable cysts—idiopathic scrotal calcinosis.
- It is plausible that idiopathic scrotal calcinosis represents an end-stage phenomenon of numerous "old" epidermoid cysts which over time have lost their cyst wall.
- Treatment
  - Unnecessary for asymptomatic and uninflamed lesions
  - Surgical incision for recurrent, infected, or extensive cysts

GROSS/CLINICAL APPEARANCE

- Multiple (up to 50), firm-to-hard nodules, ranging in size from a few millimeters up to 2 to 3 cm; occasionally a single hard nodule may be present.
- Overlying skin may be intact but may ulcerate, exuding cheesy material.

MICROSCOPIC

- Epidermis may be ulcerated or thinned out.
- Granules and globules of hematoxylinophilic calcific material within dermis.
- Giant cell granulomatous inflammation or recognizable cyst wall may be identified.

DIFFERENTIAL DIAGNOSIS

- Calcified parasites.

References

Akosa AB, Gilliland EA, Ali MH, et al. Idiopathic scrotal calcinosis: A possible aetiology reaffirmed. Br J Plast Surg 42:324–327, 1989.

Fetsch JF, Montgomery EA, Meis JM. Calcifying fibrous pseudotumor. Am J Surg Pathol 17:502–508, 1993.

Malcolm A. Idiopathic calcinosis of the scrotum. Br J Urol 54:190, 1982.

Shapiro L, Platt N, Torres-Rodriguez VM. Idiopathic calcinosis of the scrotum. Arch Dermatol 102:199–204, 1970.

Song DH, Lee KH, Kang WH. Idiopathic calcinosis of the scrotum: Histopathologic observations of fifty-one nodules. J Am Acad Dermatol 19:1095–1101, 1988.

Swinehart JM, Golitz LE. Scrotal calcinosis. Dystrophic calcification of epidermoid cysts. Arch Dermatol 118:985–988, 1982.

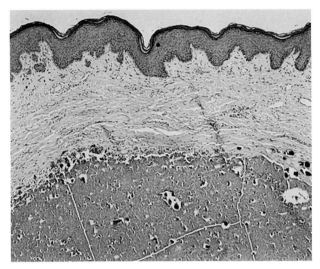

Figure 18–3. Scrotal calcinosis. Basophilic aggregates within dermis. Note the absence of a cyst wall lining.

■ Paget's Disease

CLINICAL

- Extramammary Paget's disease involving penile or scrotal skin is rare.
- Association with underlying carcinoma (adnexal or visceral) has been demonstrated in majority of cases.
- Urinary bladder, urethral, and prostate cancer are most commonly associated.
- Age: sixth to seventh decade.
- Presenting symptoms: itching, serosanguineous discharge
- Treatment
  - Local excision with close follow-up

GROSS/CLINICAL APPEARANCE

- Scaly, eczematous, erythematous, well-circumscribed lesion

MICROSCOPIC

- Atypical intraepidermal proliferation of large cells with abundant vacuolated cytoplasm; large vesicular nuclei with prominent nucleoli.
- Atypical cell clusters at the tips of the rete ridges.
- Hyperkeratosis, parakeratosis, and papillomatosis are commonly seen.

SPECIAL STAINS AND IMMUNOHISTOCHEMISTRY

- Stains for intracytoplasmic neutral and acid mucins:
  - PAS

- Alcian blue (pH 2.5)
  - Mucicarmine
- Immunohistochemistry:
  - CEA and EMA: positive
  - S-100 protein: negative (rules out melanoma)
  - HMB-45: negative (rules out melanoma)

DIFFERENTIAL DIAGNOSIS

- Squamous cell carcinoma in situ (Bowen's disease)
- Malignant melanoma in situ

References

Helwig EB, Graham JH. Anogenital extramammary Paget's disease primarily involving the scrotum. Cancer 63:970–975, 1989.

Hoch WH. Adenocarcinoma of the scrotum (extramammary Paget's disease). A case report and review of the literature. J Urol 132:137–139, 1984.

Mitsudo S, Nakanishi I, Koss L. Paget's disease of the penis and adjacent skin. Its association with fatal sweat gland carcinoma. Arch Pathol Lab Med 105:518–520, 1981.

Ordonez NG, Awalt H, Mackay B. Mammary and extramammary Paget's disease: An immunohistochemical and ultrastructural study. Cancer 59:1173–1183, 1987.

Perez MA, Larossa DD, Tomaszewski JE. Paget's disease primarily involving the scrotum. Cancer 63:970–975, 1989.

Takahashi Y, Komeda H, Horie M, et al. Paget's disease of the scrotum. Acta Urol Jpn 34:1069–1072, 1988.

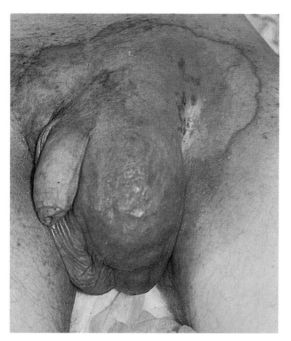

Figure 18–4. Paget's disease. Scaly eczematous and erythematous, apparently well-circumscribed, lesion.

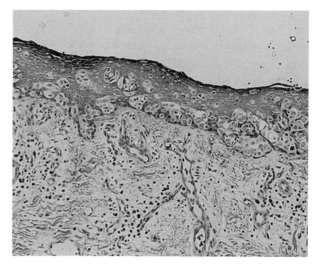

Figure 18–5. Paget's disease. Large atypical intraepidermal neoplastic cells with abundant vacuolated cytoplasm.

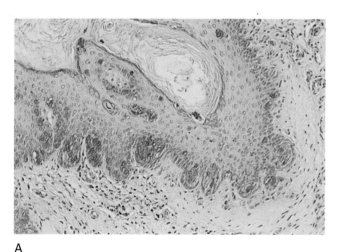

A

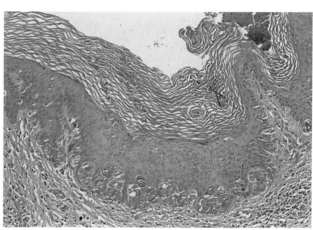

B

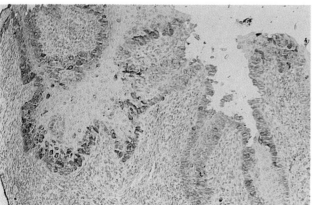

C

Figure 18–6. Paget's disease. *A,* Mucicarmine stain. *B,* Alcian blue stain. *C,* Immunohistochemistry showing positive reaction with epithelial membrane antigen.

■ Squamous Cell Carcinoma (Synonyms: Pott's Cancer, Chimney-Sweeps' Cancer)

CLINICAL

- First well-documented malignancy to be associated with occupational exposure. In the eighteenth century Pott noted that persons exposed to soot and dust (chimney sweeps and cotton factory workers) had a higher-than-average incidence of scrotal carcinoma.
- Other occupations known to be associated as risk factors include tar workers, paraffin and shale oil workers, machine operators in engineering industries, petroleum wax pressmen, workers in the screw-making industry, and automatic lathe operators.
- Carcinogen: 3′, 4′-benzpyrene.
- Other risk factors: psoriasis treated with coal tar and arsenic, condyloma acuminatum (HPV infection), multiple cutaneous epitheliomas.
- Incidence of scrotal squamous carcinoma is much lower than that of penile squamous carcinoma.
- Age: sixth to seventh decade; interestingly, right scrotum is more commonly involved than left and the tumor appears to be relatively less common in African-American men.
- Treatment

STAGING OF SQUAMOUS CELL CARCINOMA ACCORDING TO LOWE

Stage	Description
A1	Localized to scrotal wall
A2	Locally extensive tumor invading adjacent structure (testis, spermatic cord, penis, pubis, perineum)
B	Metastatic disease involving inguinal lymph nodes only
C	Metastatic disease involving pelvic lymph nodes without evidence of distant spread
D	Metastatic disease beyond pelvic lymph nodes or metastases to distant organs

- Radical surgery with bilateral superficial inguinal lymph node dissection
- Overall prognosis is poor, 5-year survival. Stage A, 70%; stage B, 44%; stages C and D, little chance of long-term survival

GROSS/CLINICAL APPEARANCE

- Early lesion is a slowly growing pimple, wart, or nodule usually on anterolateral aspect of scrotum.
- Ulcerative lesions (late): raised, rolled edges, with variable amounts of seropurulent discharge.
- Invasion of scrotal contents or penis may be present in advanced lesions.

MICROSCOPIC

- Well, moderate, or poorly differentiated invasive squamous cell carcinoma with variable amounts of keratin production

DIFFERENTIAL DIAGNOSIS

- Sebaceous cyst
- Eczema, folliculitis, psoriasis
- Syphilis
- Tuberculous epididymitis involving scrotum
- Basal cell carcinoma

References

Andrews PE, Farrow GM, Oesterling JE. Squamous cell carcinoma of the scrotum: Long-term followup of 14 patients. J Urol 146:1299–1304, 1991.

Lowe FC: Squamous cell carcinoma of the scrotum. J Urol 130:423–427, 1983.

Parys BT, Hutton JL. Fifteen-year experience of carcinoma of the scrotum. Br J Urol 68:414–417, 1991.

Pott P. Cancer scroti. In Hawes L, Clarke W, Collins R (eds). *Chirurgical Works*, vol 5. London, Longman, 1775, p 63.

Ray B, Whitmore WF. Experience with carcinoma of the scrotum. J Urol 117:741–745, 1977.

Waldron HA. On the history of scrotal cancer. Ann R Coll Surg 65:420–422, 1983.

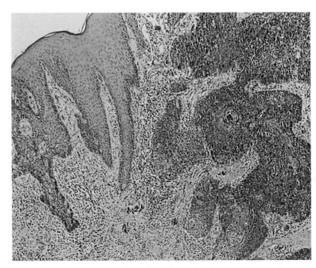

Figure 18–7. Invasive, moderately differentiated squamous carcinoma of scrotum.

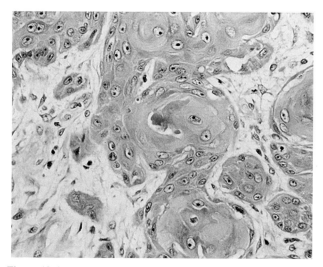

Figure 18–8. Invasive, well-differentiated squamous carcinoma of scrotum. High-power view, with characteristic cytologic features of squamous neoplasia.

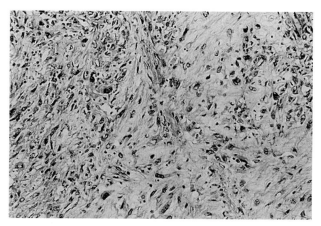

Figure 18–9. High-grade sarcoma of scrotum. Undifferentiated high-grade sarcoma with anaplastic oval-to-spindle–shaped cells.

■ Other Tumors

Basal Cell Carcinoma

- Five percent to 15% of all scrotal malignancies.
- Clinically present as plaques or ulcers.
- Age 42 to 82 years (mean 65 years).
- Predilection for left side of scrotum.
- Metastatic rate of 13% is reported, which is distinctly higher than basal cell carcinoma at other sites.

Sarcomas

- Sarcoma excluding extension from testis or paratesticular structures is very rare.
- Leiomyosarcoma is the most common sarcoma.
- Other sarcomas: liposarcoma, malignant fibrous histiocytoma, mixed liposarcoma with leiomyosarcoma.

References

Dalton DP, Rushovich AM, Victor TA, et al. Leiomyosarcoma of the scrotum in a man who had received scrotal irradiation as a child. J Urol 139:136–138, 1988.

Moon TD, Sarma DP, Rodriquez FH. Leiomyosarcoma of the scrotum. J Am Acad Dermatol 20:290–292, 1989.

Naito S, Kaji S, Kumazawa J. Leiomyosarcoma of the scrotum. Case report and review of literature. Urol Int 43:242–244, 1988.

Suster S, Wong TY, Moran CA. Sarcomas with combined features of liposarcoma and leiomyosarcoma. Study of two cases of an unusual soft-tissue tumor showing dual lineage differentiation. Am J Surg Pathol 17:905–911, 1993.

Washecka RM, Sidhu G, Surya B. Leiomyosarcoma of scrotum. Urology 34:144–146, 1989.

Watanabe K, Ogawa A, Komatsu H, et al. Malignant fibrous histiocytoma of the scrotal wall: A case report. J Urol 140:151–152, 1988

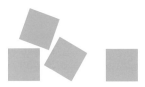

INDEX

Note: Page numbers in *italics* refer to illustrations; page numbers followed by t refer to tables.

L

Large cell calcifying Sertoli cell tumor, 152–153, *153*
Leiomyoma, of paratesticular region, 184, *185*
    of prostate gland, 83, 86–87, *87*
Leiomyosarcoma, of paratesticular region, 184, *185*
    of penis, 218, *219*
    of prostate gland, 87–88
    of scrotum, 225
Leukemia, of prostate gland, 90–91
    of testis, 165, *167*
Leydig cell(s), 101, *103*
    ectopic, *103*
Leydig cell tumor, 148–150, *149, 150*
Lichen sclerosus et atrophicus, of penis, 193, *193, 194*
Lipogranuloma, of penis, 206–207, *207*
Liposarcoma, of paratesticular region, 184, *185*
    of prostate gland, 89
    of scrotum, 225
Lymphogranuloma venereum, 197, *197*
Lymphoma, of prostate gland, 90, *90*
    of testis, 120t, 128t, 163–164, *164*
    vs. seminoma, 120t

M

Malacoplakia, of prostate gland, 23, *24*
    of testis, 170–171, *171*
Malignant fibrous histiocytoma, of paratesticular region, 184
    of prostate gland, 89
    of scrotum, 225
Median raphe cyst, of penis, 205
Melanoma, of penis, 216, *217*
Melanosis, of prostate gland, 41, *41*
Melanotic neuroectodermal tumor, 182, *182*
Mesenchymal tumor, of prostate gland, 82–89
Mesonephric hyperplasia, of prostate gland, 40, *40*
Mesothelioma, of tunica vaginalis, 176, *177,* 177t
Metastases, to penis, 217, *218*
    to prostate gland, 91–92, *92*
    to seminal vesicles, 97, *97*
    to testis, 128t, 166–167, *167*
Michaelis-Gutmann bodies, in malacoplakia, 23, *24*
Mixed germ cell tumor, of testis, *136,* 141–142, 141t, *142*
Mixed germ cell–sex cord tumor, unclassified, 160–161, 161t, *162*
Mixed gonadal-stromal tumor, of testis, 157–159, *159*
Molluscum contagiosum, of penis, 200, *200*
Monorchidism, 108
Mucinous adenocarcinoma, of prostate gland, 62, *62, 63*
Mucinous cystadenoma, of tunica, 178
Mucinous metaplasia, of prostate gland, 15, *15*
Mucinous tumor, 178, *179*
Mucoid cyst, of penis, 205
Müllerian tumor, 178, *178*
Multiple myeloma, of prostate gland, 91, *91*

Mumps orchitis, 110–111, *111*
Mycobacterium tuberculosis, of testis, 113, 113

N

Nephrogenic adenoma, 37, *37*
Nerves, prostate cancer infiltration of, 50, *56*
Neurofibrosarcoma, of prostate gland, 89
Nevus, blue, of prostate gland, 41, *41*
Nodular prostatic hyperplasia, 29, *30*
    vs. prostatic intraepithelial neoplasia, *46*
Nodule, spindle cell, of prostate gland, 84, *85*
    stromal, of prostate gland, 82, *82, 83*
Nonspecific (idiopathic) granulomatous orchitis, 111–112, *112*

O

Orchitis, acute, 109, *109*
    chronic, 110, *110*
    granulomatous, nonspecific (idiopathic), 111–112, *112*
    in fungal infection, 114
    in syphilis, 112–113
    in tuberculosis, 113, *113*
    mumps, 110–111, *111*
Osteosarcoma, of prostate gland, 89

P

Paget's disease, of scrotum, 222, *223*
Paneth cell–like metaplasia, of prostate gland, 16, *16*
Papillary cystadenofibroma, of tunica, 178
Papillary serous tumor, of tunica, 178
Papillary cystadenoma, of epididymis, 181, *181*
Papilloma, hirsutoid, of penis, 203, *203*
    inverted, of prostatic urethra, 39, *39*
Papulosis, bowenoid, 208, 208t, *210*
Paraffinoma, of penis, 206–207, *207*
Paraganglion tissue, of prostate gland, *9*
Paratesticular region, adenomatoid tumor of, 179, *180, 181*
    leiomyoma of, 184, *185*
    leiomyosarcoma of, 184, *185*
    liposarcoma of, 184, *185*
    mucinous cystadenoma of, 178
    papillary cystadenofibroma of, 178
    papillary cystadenoma of, 181, *181*
    retinal anlage tumor of, 182, *182*
    rhabdomyosarcoma of, 183, *183, 184*
    serous cystadenoma of, 178
Penile intraepithelial neoplasia, 207–208, 208t, *209, 210*
Penis, anatomy of, 189, *190*
    balanitis xerotica obliterans of, 193, *193, 194*
    balanoposthitis of, 191–192, *192*
    basal cell carcinoma of, 215–216, *216*
    bowenoid papulosis of, 208, 208t, *210*
    Bowen's disease of, 207–208, 208t, *209*